Contemporary Management of Temporomandibular Joint Disorders

Editors

DANIEL E. PEREZ
LARRY M. WOLFORD

ORAL AND MAXILLOFACIAL SURGERY CLINICS OF NORTH AMERICA

www.oralmaxsurgery.theclinics.com

Consulting Editor
RICHARD H. HAUG

February 2015 • Volume 27 • Number 1

ELSEVIER

1600 John F. Kennedy Boulevard • Suite 1800 • Philadelphia, Pennsylvania, 19103-2899

http://www.oralmaxsurgery.theclinics.com

ORAL AND MAXILLOFACIAL SURGERY CLINICS OF NORTH AMERICA Volume 27, Number 1
February 2015 ISSN 1042-3699, ISBN-13: 978-0-323-35447-9

Editor: John Vassallo; j.vassallo@elsevier.com
Developmental Editor: Colleen Viola

Oral and Maxillofacial Surgery Clinics of North America (ISSN 1042-3699) is published quarterly by Elsevier Inc., 360 Park Avenue South, New York, NY 10010-1710. Months of issue are February, May, August, and November. Business and Editorial Offices: 1600 John F. Kennedy Blvd., Suite 1800, Philadelphia, PA 19103-2899. Periodicals postage paid at New York, NY and additional mailing offices. Subscription prices are $385.00 per year for US individuals, $567.00 per year for US institutions, $175.00 per year for US students and residents, $455.00 per year for Canadian individuals, $680.00 per year for Canadian institutions, $520.00 per year for international individuals, $680.00 per year for international institutions and $235.00 per year for Canadian and foreign students/residents. To receive student/resident rate, orders must be accompanied by name or affiliated institution, date of term, and the *signature* of program/residency coordinator on institution letterhead. Orders will be billed at individual rate until proof of status is received. Foreign air speed delivery is included in all *Clinics* subscription prices. All prices are subject to change without notice. **POSTMASTER:** Send address changes to *Oral and Maxillofacial Surgery Clinics of North America*, Elsevier Periodicals Customer Service, 11830 Westline Industrial Drive, St. Louis, MO 63146. Tel: 1-800-654-2452 (U.S. and Canada); 314-447-8871 (outside U.S. and Canada). Fax: 314-447-8029. E-mail: journalscustomerservice-usa@elsevier.com (for print support); journalsonlinesupport-usa@elsevier.com (for online support).

Reprints. For copies of 100 or more, of articles in this publication, please contact the Commercial Reprints Department, Elsevier Inc., 360 Park Avenue South, New York, NY 10010-1710. Tel.: 212-633-3874; Fax: 212-633-3820; Email: reprints@elsevier.com.

Oral and Maxillofacial Surgery Clinics of North America is covered in *MEDLINE/PubMed (Index Medicus)*, *Science Citation Index Expanded (SciSearch®)*, *Journal Citation Reports/Science Edition*, and *Current Contents®/Clinical Medicine*.

Contributors

CONSULTING EDITOR

RICHARD H. HAUG, DDS
Carolinas Center for Oral Health, Charlotte,
North Carolina

EDITORS

DANIEL E. PEREZ, DDS
Clinical Assistant Professor, Department of
Oral and Maxillofacial Surgery, University of
Texas Health Science Center, San Antonio,
San Antonio, Texas

LARRY M. WOLFORD, DMD
Clinical Professor, Departments of Oral and
Maxillofacial Surgery and Orthodontics Texas,
A&M University Health Science Center Baylor
College of Dentistry, Baylor University Medical
Center, Dallas, Texas

AUTHORS

RUY CARRASCO, MD
Chair, Division of Rheumatology,
Rheumatology, Dell Children's Medical Center
of Central Texas, Austin, Texas

DANIEL SERRA CASSANO, DDS
Department of Pediatric Dentistry, Faculdade
de Odontologia de Araraquara, Universidade
Estadual Paulista - UNESP Araraquara School
of Dentistry; Private practice, Araraquara,
SP - Brazil

VANESSA CASTRO, DDS
Private Practice, Salvador-Bahia, Brazil;
Residency of Oral and Maxillofacial Surgery,
Federal Bahia University, Salvador, Bahia,
Brazil

JOÃO ROBERTO GONÇALVES, DDS, PhD
Department of Pediatric Dentistry, Faculdade
de Odontologia de Araraquara, Univ Estadual
Paulista - UNESP Araraquara School of
Dentistry, Araraquara, Brazil

**RAÚL GONZÁLEZ-GARCÍA, MD, PhD,
FEBOMFS**
Consultant Surgeon, Department of Oral
and Maxillofacial-Head and Neck Surgery,
University Hospital Infanta Cristina;

International Member of the American
Society of Temporomandibular Surgeons
(ASTMJS), Active Member of the European
Society of Temporomandibular Surgeons
(ESTMJS), Honorary Professor, University
of Extremadura (UEx) School of Medicine,
Badajoz, Spain

DAVID HOFFMAN, DDS
Director, Oral & Maxillofacial Surgery,
Staten Island University Hospital, Staten
Island, New York

AARON LIDDELL, DMD, MD, FACS
Former Chief Resident, Oral & Maxillofacial
Surgery, University of Texas HSC San Antonio,
San Antonio, Texas

PUSHKAR MEHRA, BDS, DMD
Associate Professor and Chairman,
Department of Oral and Maxillofacial Surgery,
Boston University Henry M. Goldman School of
Dental Medicine, Boston, Massachusetts

LOUIS G. MERCURI, DDS, MS
Visiting Professor, Department of Orthopedic
Surgery, Rush University Medical Center,
Chicago, Illinois; Clinical Consultant, TMJ
Concepts, Ventura, California

REZA MOVAHED, DMD
Private Practice, Clinical Assistant Professor, Orthodontics, Saint Louis University, St Louis, Missouri

MOHAMMED NADERSHAH, BDS, MSc
Assistant Professor, Department of Oral and Maxillofacial Surgery, Faculty of Dentistry, King Abdul Aziz University, Jeddah, Saudi Arabia; Formerly, Resident, Department of Oral and Maxillofacial Surgery, Boston Medical Center, Boston University Henry M. Goldman School of Dental Medicine, Boston, Massachusetts

DANIEL E. PEREZ, DDS
Clinical Assistant Professor, Department of Oral & Maxillofacial Surgery, University of Texas Health Science Center, San Antonio, San Antonio, Texas

LEANN PUIG, DMD
OMFS Resident, Kings County Hospital, Brooklyn, New York

LUCIANO REZENDE, DDS, MSc
Department of Pediatric Dentistry, Faculdade de Odontologia de Araraquara, Universidade Estadual Paulista - UNESP Araraquara School of Dentistry; Private Practice, Araraquara, SP - Brazil

DANIEL B. RODRIGUES, DDS
Clinical Professor, Residency of Oral and Maxillofacial Surgery, Federal Bahia University; Private Practice, Salvador, Bahia, Brazil

LARRY M. WOLFORD, DMD
Clinical Professor, Departments of Oral and Maxillofacial Surgery and Orthodontics Texas, A&M University Health Science Center Baylor College of Dentistry, Baylor University Medical Center, Dallas, Texas

Contents

The temporomandibular joint (TMJ) is one of the many joints involved in the inflammatory arthritides. As imaging of joints has developed, so have the data regarding extent and prevalence of TMJ involvement in these diseases. TMJ disease is especially prevalent in juvenile arthritis. The adult and pediatric inflammatory arthritides share common pathophysiology but are still markedly different. The preponderance of TMJ arthritis research exists in juvenile arthritis. This article discusses classification, treatment, and TMJ involvement in juvenile idiopathic arthritis.

One of the most well-known yet perhaps controversial conditions affecting temporomandibular dysfunction (TMD) and the signs and symptoms of facial pain and clinical outcomes after orthognathic surgery procedures is temporomandibular joint internal derangement. This article provides an overview of the mutual relationship between orthognathic surgery and TMD, with especial consideration to internal derangement. The existing literature is reviewed and analyzed and the pertinent findings are summarized. The objective is to guide oral and maxillofacial surgeons in their clinical decision making when contemplating orthognathic surgery in patients with preexisting TMD.

Temporomandibular joint (TMJ) ankylosis is a pathologic condition where the mandible is fused to the fossa by bony or fibrotic tissues. This interferes with mastication, speech, oral hygiene, and normal life activities, and can be potentially life threatening when struggling to acquire an airway in an emergency. Trauma is the most common cause of TMJ ankylosis, followed by infection. Diagnosis of TMJ ankylosis is usually made by clinical examination and imaging studies. The management goal in TMJ ankylosis is to increase the patient's mandibular function, correct associated facial deformity, decrease pain, and prevent reankylosis.

Combined orthognathic and total joint reconstruction cases can be predictably performed in 1 stage. Use of virtual surgical planning can eliminate a significant time requirement in preparation of concomitant orthognathic and temporomandibular joint (TMJ) prostheses cases. The concomitant TMJ and orthognathic surgery–computer-assisted surgical simulation technique increases the accuracy of combined cases. In order to have flexibility in positioning of the total joint prosthesis, recontouring of the lateral aspect of the rami is advantageous.

Condylar resorption (CR) is a common sequela of some temporomandibular joint (TMJ) abnormalities. CR can result in jaw deformities and dysfunction, malocclusion, pain, headaches, and airway obstruction. Most cases can be classified into 1 of 4 categories based on cause: (1) adolescent internal CR; (2) reactive (inflammatory) arthritis; (3) autoimmune and connective tissue diseases; and (4) other end-stage TMJ pathologic abnormality. MRI is helpful in differentiating the cause and defining treatment options. This article presents the nature and progression of the different TMJ CR pathologic abnormalities, clinical and imaging characteristics, and treatment options to produce predictable and stable outcomes.

Several open surgeries have been proposed for the treatment of internal derangement (ID) of the temporomandibular joint (TMJ), although minimally invasive temporomandibular joint surgery (MITMJS) plays a major role in the treatment of ID and has been widely used for the treatment of ID of the TMJ. Arthrocentesis, arthroscopic lysis and lavage, and operative or advanced arthroscopy are the 3 most relevant techniques for MITMJS; clear indications for their application and a detailed description of each technique are presented. Also, clinical outcomes for each technique from the most relevant studies in the literature are reported.

Although limited, there is evidence to support the assumption that temporomandibular joint (TMJ) articular disc repositioning indeed works; to date, there is no evidence that TMJ articular disc repositioning does not work. Despite the controversy among professionals in private practice and academia, TMJ articular disc repositioning is a procedure based on (still limited) evidence; the opposition is based solely on clinical preference and influenced by the ability to perform it or not.

Temporomandibular joint (TMJ) surgery can be divided into 3 types of surgery: Arthroscopy, arthroplasty, and total joint replacement. The complications associated with these procedures increase with complexity. They all include injury to adjacent structures, infections, and bleeding problems.

Dislocation of the temporomandibular joint is one of many pathophysiologic joint conditions that the oral and maxillofacial surgeon is challenged with managing.

Managing a dislocated joint will inevitably be the challenge of most surgeons or physicians, whether in private or academic practice. Accordingly, this article addresses the pathophysiology associated with dislocation, in addition to treatment strategies aimed at managing acute, chronic, and recurrent dislocation.

This article discusses hemifacial microsomia and Treacher Collins syndrome relative to the nature of these congenital deformities as well as the clinical, radiographic, and diagnostic characteristics. These patients often have severe facial deformities with hypoplasia or aplasia of the temporomandibular joints (TMJs) and mandible. The surgical treatment options are presented, including the advantages and disadvantages of autogenous tissues versus patient-fitted total joint prostheses to reconstruct the TMJs and mandible as well as counterclockwise rotation of the maxillomandibular complex.

Condylar hyperplasia (CH) is a progressive and pathologic overgrowth of either or both mandibular condyles, which can affect the neck, ramus, or body of the mandible. It may lead to facial asymmetry, malocclusion, speech, and masticatory problems. Identifying the specific type of condylar hyperplasia is crucial. Serial radiographs, dental models, clinical evaluations, and bone scan techniques are usually the best diagnostic methods to determine the type of CH and if the growth process is still active. The protocol of surgical procedures recommended in this article for CH has been proven to treat the condylar pathology and correct the jaw deformity.

ORAL AND MAXILLOFACIAL SURGERY CLINICS OF NORTH AMERICA

THE CLINICS ARE NOW AVAILABLE ONLINE!
Access your subscription at:
www.theclinics.com

Preface

Contemporary Management of Temporomandibular Joint Disorders

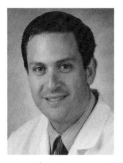 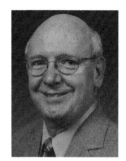

Daniel E. Perez, DDS   Larry M. Wolford, DMD

Editors

Over the last 30 years, TMJ surgery has endured major difficulties and undergone enormous changes. In the 1980s, TMJ surgery was in its relative infancy when Proplast/Teflon was introduced as the "wonder product" and was used extensively for TMJ surgery patients as a disc replacement and for total joint prostheses; for a time, it was the material of choice for TMJ reconstruction until it disintegrated and was ultimately recalled by the FDA in 1991. Thousands of patients were injured by these products and lawsuits ensued.

Surgeons and teaching programs shied away from TMJ surgery and almost overnight the TMJ turned into the "surgically ignored" joint. However, TMJ surgery forged on and refocused on using other TMJ implant systems and various autologous grafts and techniques, which had problems and downfalls of their own, but none as severe as the Proplast/Teflon disaster.

We, the editors, are grateful to the *Oral and Maxillofacial Surgery Clinics of North America* for dedicating this issue solely to the TMJ. With so many subspecialties in Oral and Maxillofacial Surgery, we are proud to be given this platform in an effort to advance science, health, and education. It is our duty as teachers to devote our time and attention to the study and treatment of the TMJ, to continue the research, and to provide treatment protocols now proven to be successful, despite its torturous history.

We also welcome the young oral and maxillofacial surgeons, as the articles presented in this issue are new collaborations from some of the finest TMJ surgeons worldwide. As our specialty has moved on from the 1980s and 1990s, we embrace ever-improving technologies such as the MRI, the single most important tool for TMD diagnosis or surgical navigation and virtual planning. New implant systems and treatment methods, likewise, have come available despite the increased involvement and monitoring of the FDA.

It's an exciting time to be an oral and maxillofacial surgeon today. We hope to stimulate other oral and maxillofacial surgeons to develop an interest in TMJ and provide this aspect of patient care. There is always more to learn, and hopefully, our knowledge will continue to increase as we further study the most interesting of all joints: the TMJ.

Daniel E. Perez, DDS
Department of Oral and Maxillofacial Surgery
University of Texas Health Science Center
San Antonio
7703 Floyd Curl Drive, MC 7908
San Antonio, TX 78229, USA

Larry M. Wolford, DMD
Departments of Oral and Maxillofacial Surgery
and Orthodontics Texas
A&M University Health Science Center
Baylor College of Dentistry
Baylor University Medical Center
3409 Worth St. Suite 400
Dallas, TX 75246, USA

E-mail addresses:
perezd5@uthscsa.edu (D.E. Perez)
lwolford@drlarrywolford.com (L.M. Wolford)

Juvenile Idiopathic Arthritis Overview and Involvement of the Temporomandibular Joint
Prevalence, Systemic Therapy

Ruy Carrasco, MD

KEYWORDS

- Rheumatoid arthritis • Juvenile idiopathic arthritis • Juvenile rheumatoid arthritis
- Juvenile chronic arthritis • Temporomandibular joint • JIA • TMJ

KEY POINTS

- In the past decade there have been significant advances in the care of patients with inflammatory arthritis.
- Arthritis of the temporomandibular joint (TMJ) has benefited from these advances; yet recognition, evaluation, and management of TMJ arthritis differ significantly between adult and pediatric rheumatologists.
- Orthopantomogram and computed tomography scans have a role in evaluation of TMJ disease and are easily obtained; MRI with and without contrast using a TMJ coil is the preferred modality to determine active versus chronic disease.
- Intra-articular steroids, arthrocentesis, biologic therapies (intra-articular and systemic), and surgery have a role in preventing long-term adverse effects.

The temporomandibular joint (TMJ) is one of the many joints involved in the inflammatory arthritides. As imaging of joints has developed, so have the data regarding extent and prevalence of TMJ involvement in these diseases. TMJ disease is especially prevalent in juvenile arthritis. The adult and pediatric inflammatory arthritides share common pathophysiology but are still markedly different. The preponderance of TMJ arthritis research exists in juvenile arthritis.

CLASSIFICATION OF JUVENILE IDIOPATHIC ARTHRITIS

Arthritis in children affects approximately 300,000 in North America. Approximately half of these children have juvenile idiopathic arthritis (JIA). The prevalence of JIA in developed countries varies from 10 to 150 per 100,000. JIA is the most common chronic rheumatologic disease in the pediatric population. JIA was formerly known as juvenile rheumatoid arthritis (JRA) or juvenile chronic arthritis (JCA) in North America and Europe, respectively (**Table 1**).[1,2]

The clinical features of JIA are morning stiffness, joint swelling, and joint tenderness with changes in range of motion. It often has an insidious onset in the younger population, and its inflammatory nature, as well as the medications used to treat it, contributes to the morbidity and mortality of the disease. The current biologic medications have helped to change the extent of disability and

Division of Rheumatology, Rheumatology, Dell Children's Medical Center of Central Texas, 1301 Barbara Jordan Boulevard, #200, Austin, TX 78723, USA
E-mail address: rcarrasco@sfcaustin.com

Oral Maxillofacial Surg Clin N Am 27 (2015) 1–10
http://dx.doi.org/10.1016/j.coms.2014.09.001

Table 1
Juvenile arthritis aomenclature

Classification	ACR (1972)	ILAR (1997)
Nomenclature	Juvenile rheumatoid arthritis (JRA)	Juvenile idiopathic arthritis (JIA)
Arthritis onset	<16 y old	<16 y old
Arthritis duration	≥6 wk	≥6 wk

Subtypes, %	Pauciarticular	Oligoarticular (50%)
		  Extended
		  Persistent

	Polyarticular	Polyarticular
		  RF negative (15%–25%)
		  RF positive (5%–10%)

	Systemic	Systemic (5%–10%) Enthesitis-related arthritis (5%–10%) Psoriatic arthritis (5%–10%) Undifferentiated (10%)

Abbreviations: ACR, American College of Rheumatology; ILAR, International League of Associations for Rheumatology; RF, rheumatoid factor.

need for major surgeries and joint replacement in JIA; however, the full extent of improvement in morbidity and mortality is not well defined and is a moving target, given the growth of biologic and small molecule treatments.

The term "rheumatoid" in JRA meant a swollen joint, but was interpreted by some as adult rheumatoid arthritis (RA). The term "chronic" was introduced to help alleviate some of the issues with the American College of Rheumatology (ACR) classification of JRA, but the JCA classification system had its own limitations.[3] To help alleviate some of the confusion and shortcomings of the JRA and JCA classification, the International League of Associations for Rheumatology (ILAR) developed the JIA classification system that we use today. This classification system points out exclusion and inclusion criteria, while demonstrating the unique nature of each subtype of JIA.

The JIA nomenclature includes the latest clinical, laboratory, and genomics data; however, it is not without its own limitations.[4,5] As more advances occur in genomics, proteomics, and metabolomics, the utility and need to modify current classification schemes for autoinflammatory and autoimmune conditions will be clearer.

JIA in the ILAR classification system indicates individuals with disease onset before 16 years of age in whom the arthritis is persistent for at least 6 weeks. The ILAR JIA classification system delineates 7 onset categories: oligoarticular (persistent and extended), polyarticular rheumatoid factor (RF)-negative, polyarticular RF-positive, systemic, psoriatic arthritis, enthesitis-related arthritis, and undifferentiated. The undifferentiated category

refers to patients who do not meet criteria for any subtype or meet more than one subtype.

The most common of the subtypes is oligoarticular JIA, making up approximately 50% of patients with JIA. The peak age of onset is 2 years with a female predilection of 5:1 female:male. By definition, patients with oligoarticular JIA have 1 to 4 joints affected in the first 6 months of disease. After the first 6 months, 2 categories exist to define the type: extended oligoarticular JIA or persistent oligoarticular JIA. Extended oligoarthritis encompasses individuals with more than 4 affected joints after the first 6 months of disease. Persistent oligoarthritis is involvement of no more than 4 joints throughout the disease. Children are excluded from this classification if they have psoriasis or a first-degree relative with psoriasis; are HLA-B27 positive or RF positive; or have ankylosing spondylitis, Reiter syndrome, sacroiliitis with inflammatory bowel disease, or systemic JIA features. The antinuclear antibody (ANA) test is positive in up to 80% of oligoarticular JIA. The oligoarticular JIA population does not typically have a positive RF. Up to 30% of oligoarticular JIA children develop uveitis, which is sometimes called iritis or iridocyclitis.

Patients with polyarticular JIA make up 4 in 10 children with JIA. Polyarticular JIA indicates arthritis in 5 or more joints during the first 6 months of disease. Five percent to 10% of children with JIA have RF-positive polyarticular JIA. A positive RF must be demonstrated 2 or more times at least 3 months apart in the initial 6 months of disease onset.

Children with RF-positive polyarticular JIA are the subtype most similar (genotype and phenotype) to RF-positive adult RA. They demonstrate similar positive serology, such as RF and antibodies against citrullinated peptide antigens, namely the anticyclic citrullinated peptide (anti-CCP). Approximately 5% to 10% of children in this subset have a positive RF and similar numbers may be noted with anti-CCP testing. Similar to a positive RF in polyarticular JIA, there is a correlation between anti-CCP and disease severity in JIA.[6,7] Children in this category are older at onset (adolescent), are predominantly female, and have symmetric polyarticular disease.

RF-negative polyarticular JIA is heterogeneous, has at least 2 subtypes, and is not as well defined as RF-positive polyarticular JIA. Overall, patients are younger in disease onset, predominantly female, and have asymmetric arthritis. In contrast to RF-positive polyarticular JIA, the RF-negative polyarticular JIA group has a subgroup with higher percentage of positive ANA and uveitis. This subgroup of ANA-positive, RF-negative polyarthritis most closely resembles oligoarticular JIA.[5]

Systemic JIA forms one of the least common categories, but often with the most significant morbidity and mortality. Systemic JIA does not have a predilection for a gender nor pediatric age of onset. The adult version of systemic JIA is known as adult-onset Still disease. Diagnosis of systemic JIA may be difficult at onset because these children may not have arthritis at onset or the illness may mimic an acute infection, Kawasaki disease, coagulopathy, malignancy, or similar profoundly ill child. Classification of this subtype requires the presence of arthritis preceded or accompanied by fever of at least 2 weeks' duration, and at least 3 days of the fever must be quotidian and have one or more of the following: evanescent rash, generalized lymphadenopathy, hepatomegaly and/or splenomegaly, or serositis (pericarditis, pleuritis, and/or peritonitis).

Individuals with systemic JIA, as the name implies, have systemic features such as fevers, rash, arthritis, leukocytosis with anemia, and very elevated acute-phase reactants. Approximately 5% to 8% of children with systemic JIA may develop macrophage activation syndrome (MAS).[8] MAS is a potentially life-threatening complication characterized by fevers, hepatosplenomegaly, coagulopathy, profoundly elevated ferritin levels, increased triglyceride, and increased aspartate transaminase and alanine transaminase due in part to phagocytosis of hematopoietic components by macrophages and pathogenic T cells.[9]

Enthesitis-related arthritis (ERA) indicates children with arthritis and enthesitis. Individuals may also fit criteria for ERA by having enthesitis or arthritis with at least 2 of the following criteria:

a. HLA-B27 antigen
b. History or presence of sacroiliac tenderness and/or inflammatory lumbosacral pain (morning stiffness)
c. Male with arthritis after 6 years of age
d. Anterior uveitis
e. History of ankylosing spondylitis, Reiter syndrome, sacroiliitis with inflammatory bowel disease, acute anterior uveitis in first-degree relative

Enthesitis indicates inflammation at an enthesis (site of insertion of tendon, ligament, joint capsule, or fascia into bone), often demonstrated by tenderness and/or swelling. These individuals may not have psoriasis or psoriasis in a first-degree relative, be RF-positive, or have systemic JIA.

Psoriatic arthritis indicates presence of arthritis and psoriasis. Individuals also may be classified as having psoriatic arthritis by having arthritis and 2 or more of the following: dactylitis (profound digit swelling beyond the joint margin), nail pits or onycholysis, or psoriasis in a first-degree relative. This category excludes male individuals with HLA-B27–positive onset after 6 years of age; those who are RF-positive; and those with ankylosing spondylitis, Reiter syndrome, sacroiliitis with inflammatory bowel disease, or systemic JIA features.

A positive ANA is a risk factor for uveitis; however, it is not used to diagnose arthritis or uveitis.[10] The onset of uveitis in JIA is often insidious, asymptomatic, and bilateral in 70% of individuals. Uveitis is discovered in more than 90% at the time of JIA diagnosis or shortly after the onset of arthritis. The disease activity of uveitis occurs independent of the disease activity of arthritis and vice-versa. The RF test, similar to the ANA test, is not used to diagnose arthritis but contributes to risk stratification of JIA.

TEMPOROMANDIBULAR JOINT INVOLVEMENT IN JUVENILE IDIOPATHIC ARTHRITIS
Prevalence and Clinical Manifestations of Temporomandibular Joint Arthritis

One of the most commonly involved joints in JIA is the TMJ. Prevalence of TMJ arthritis in JIA is reported between 17% and 87% depending on the modality for evaluation, the changes on imaging classified as arthritis, and subtype of JIA.[11–13] The clinical manifestations and subsequent clinical and radiographic evaluation of TMJ involvement has demonstrated wide variability.

Several studies have looked into the utility of signs and symptoms of TMJ disorder in JIA. There is a lack of clear correlation between the clinical manifestations of temporomandibular disorders (TMD) and the extent of arthritis.[12,13] One study developed a total clinical score and total MRI score and did not demonstrate correlation between the 2 studies.[14] Part of the lack of clarity with symptomatology and imaging is that healthy children may have similar presentation of TMD,[15] the TMJs are not easily accessible to palpate to evaluate pain or swelling and children with JIA have wide variation in pain manifestation.[16,17] Thus, clinical manifestations may not provide a consistently reliable method to assess presence of arthritis, response to therapy, or change in joint morphology or disease activity.

Imaging Investigations in Diagnosis

Use of radiographs, including orthopantomogram (OPG) and cephalometric views, computed tomography (CT), ultrasonography, and specifically MRI have allowed for determination of presence and delineation of extent of involvement of the TMJ arthropathy in the arthritides. OPG is one of the most commonly used modalities for TMJ evaluation. OPG is readily available, easily performed, and relatively low cost. Asymptomatic TMJ arthritis has been noted in up to 69% in one study with the use of OPG imaging.[18] Unfortunately, OPG is not able to evaluate for effusions, pannus formation, synovial thickening, and subsequently whether changes noted are active disease or old changes (chronic).

Compared with OPG, CT scans are able to provide more detailed images of the condyles and surrounding structures. CT scans have shortcomings similar to OPG in the limited ability to evaluate active versus old chronic changes of arthritis and soft tissue changes. CT scans provide the advantage of short imaging times compared with MRIs.

Ultrasonography has demonstrated a consistent role in finding symptomatic and asymptomatic synovitis, erosions, and disease activity in non-TMJ joints in JIA and other arthritides. Ultrasound is not as sensitive for early changes and even in skilled hands may not correlate well with MRI findings.[19]

With MRIs, articular structures may be assessed, such as the cartilage, bone, ligaments, tendons, synovium, and tendon sheaths. MRI in inflammatory arthritis allows for qualitative and quantitative evaluation for the presence or status of synovitis and its sequelae: bone marrow edema, synovial enhancement, synovial thickening, erosions, effusions, cartilage damage, articular disc involvement, and ligamentous involvement. MRI is thus considered the gold standard for evaluation of inflammatory arthritis.[20,21] MRI has been demonstrated to be consistently sensitive for evaluation of arthritis in TMJs of children with JIA.

A study by Kuseler and colleagues[14] found that MRI was able to follow the alterations of TMJ disease over time. This study unfortunately compared MRI of TMJs in JIA with those of adults and not age-matched children. Two studies have obtained MRIs of TMJs of healthy children to develop baseline data.[22,23] Gadolinium uptake in TMJs was noted in healthy children, but its clinical significance is unknown. Nonetheless, MRI has the particular advantage of demonstrating acute versus chronic or acute on chronic changes in TMJ arthritis. A recent study outlined MRI findings of acute (synovial enhancement, synovial effusion, synovial thickening, bone marrow edema) and chronic (TMJ arthritis, pannus, condylar flattening, bony erosions and articular disc changes or displacement) changes.[20]

A thorough MRI evaluation of the TMJs must be done without and with gadolinium contrast.[20] Postgadolinium sequences improve visualization of synovial tissue, erosions, and cartilage changes. The high-field standard for MRIs is 1.5 T. Now 3-T MRIs exist, which provide increased detail of normal and pathologic changes and allow for shorter scan times. The proper coil also must be selected when evaluating the TMJs. Multipurpose coils exist for different sizes including for TMJs. Disadvantages of the MRI modality include cost, need for contrast, extended imaging time, and some patients may require sedation.

Treatment: the Rheumatologist's Viewpoint

The goals of therapy for the adult and pediatric arthrides hold a common thread: early recognition, prevention of damage, halting damage if present, suppressing disease, and finally remission off medications. TMJ arthritis should be no different in terms of goals for the treating team members, oral and maxillofacial surgeons, orthodontists, general dentists, and rheumatologists. Treatment of autoimmune arthritis and similarly TMJ arthritis combines physiotherapy, psychosocial support, anti-inflammatory medications, immunomodulatory medications, and surgery (**Table 2**).

TMJ arthritis, if not recognized early, could cause irreversible damage to the TMJ and masticatory system, requiring surgical correction, such as mandibular advancements or TMJ replacement surgery to correct, for example, micrognathia, malocclusion, retrognathia, overjet.

The medical treatments often engaged by rheumatologists include nonsteroidal anti-inflammatory drugs (NSAIDs), corticosteroids

Table 2
Treatments in temporomandibular joint arthritis

Method	Preferred Medication	Dose	Time Between Administration	Improvement	Note
Intra-articular steroids	THA	5 to 10 mg per TMJ	Minimum 4 mo[a]	$\frac{1}{2}$ on MRI	Can be done blind vs CT or ultrasound guided
Iontophoresis	Dexamethasone sodium phosphate	1.5 mL of dexamethasone sodium phosphate (total dose 6 mg per TMJ per session)	1–3 d, with a total of 8–10 sessions	MIO 68%, MLE 69%, TMJ pain resolution 73%	Bipolar electrodes used for iontophoresis machine; drug delivered over 15–30 min
TNF inhibitor	Infliximab	0.5–1 mL of 10 mg/mL	Unknown	6/48 TMJs had resolution of arthritis based on MRI	23-gauge needle and normal saline lavage
Arthrocentesis with or without THA	THA	0.5 mL of 20 mg/mL		Both had significant improvement 3 and 8 mo later in PIO, MIO and pain; No differences between 2 groups	Arthrocentesis: push and pull solution of vitamin B 12 and physiologic salt

Abbreviations: CT, computed tomography; MIO, maximum incisal opening; MLE, maximal lateral excursion; PIO, pain incisal opening; THA, triamcinolone hexacetonide; TNF, tumor necrosis factor.

[a] If less than 4-month improvement, consider change in therapy.

(oral, intravenous, intra-articular), conventional disease-modifying antirheumatic drugs (DMARDs), and biologic DMARDs.

The ACR published recommendations for treatment of JIA in 2011 and 2013. The ACR recommendations took into account the severity of disease activity, features of prognosis, sacroiliac joint involvement, number of joints, and systemic arthritis.[24,25] These recommendations separate disease activity into low, moderate, and high.

NSAIDs are effective for JIA in one-fourth to one-third of patients, but primarily in oligoarticular disease.[26] Their goal in TMJ disease would be for modifying pain and stiffness. NSAIDs have been tried with some success in TMJ arthritis.[27] There is insufficient evidence to recommend topical NSAIDs in TMJ disorders. NSAIDs may be tried as monotherapy in patients with low disease activity, but with close monitoring. NSAIDs should be considered as adjunctive or bridge therapy to more definitive interventions in patients with more extensive disease. If there is evidence of joint damage, joint contracture, or worsening disease, then NSAIDs should not be used as monotherapy.

The DMARDs help halt or prevent arthritis progression and its sequelae. The most commonly used DMARDs are sulfasalazine, methotrexate, and leflunomide. Other DMARDs, D-penicillamine, gold, azathioprine, mycophenolate, and cyclosporine, are not commonly used in JIA with the exception of hydroxychloroquine. The 2011 ACR task force did not recommend hydroxychloroquine as monotherapy in JIA. Methotrexate is the most commonly used DMARD in JIA. The dose of methotrexate in JIA is 10 to 25 mg/m^2 per week oral or subcutaneous routes, not to exceed 30 mg per week. Folic acid 1 mg per day is often given concurrently with methotrexate to help minimize the side effects of methotrexate. Methotrexate is the only conventional DMARD with any significant evidence in TMJ arthritis.[28] The study was limited to patients with pauciarticular and polyarticular JRA and did not include the use of MRIs for evaluation of efficacy or disease activity.

Arthrocentesis has been evaluated in TMJ osteoarthritis, with or without injection of sodium hyaluronate.[29] This method of arthrocentesis has not been evaluated in JIA. A recent prospective study evaluated TMJ arthrocentesis in 21 patients with JIA and TMJ disease.[30] Patients were randomized to TMJ arthrocentesis alone or TMJ arthrocentesis with injection of triamcinolone. Triamcinolone hexacetonide was used in the study. Improvements in TMJ function (pain incisal opening and maximum incisal opening) and symptoms were noted in both groups up to 8 months later. There was no statistical difference between the 2 groups.

Intra-articular steroids (IAS) for TMJs have been used with success in the adult arthritides, but the best evidence comes from the pediatric arthritides.[31,32] Triamcinolone hexacetonide (THA) has been found to be superior to triamcinolone acetonide, betamethasone, and methylprednisolone acetate in treatment of arthritis in other joints (non-TMJ).[24,33] Using MRIs to evaluate efficacy, approximately half of patients demonstrate improvement with IAS. In the study by Stoll and colleagues, 18% of patients had complete resolution of TMJ arthritis. Short- and long-term studies have also confirmed the safety and efficacy of IAS.[34,35] THA in TMJs is given in doses of 5 to 10 mg of a 20-mg/mL suspension. THA may be given alone or administered with an anesthetic agent (1% lidocaine) into the superior TMJ space. IAS injections have been traditionally administered under CT or ultrasound guidance. Experienced operators may perform IAS injections without CT or ultrasound guidance.

The expected improvement from IAS should last at least 4 months. If duration of improvement is less than 4 months, other therapies, such as systemic therapy, should be considered. Dexamethasone iontophoresis is a noninvasive physiotherapy for TMJ therapy. Of patients receiving dexamethasone iontophoresis, 68% had improvement in maximal interincisor opening, 69% improved in maximal lateral excursion, and 73% had resolution of TMJ pain.

Concern exists about corticosteroid use in TMJ arthritis. One animal model study in rabbits demonstrated arrest of the mandibular growth plate with IAS.[36] This arrest was not noted in another animal model in goats or in human studies. Documented adverse effects specifically from IAS include one case report of ankylosis in an adult with trauma-related TMJ disorder and a case series of osteoarthritis in adults who suffered damage to the condylar head (fibrous layer, cartilage, bone), hypopigmentation, facial swelling, and lipoatrophy.[32,37,38]

The biologic medications include tumor necrosis factor (TNF)-alpha inhibitors, interleukin (IL)-1 inhibitors, T-cell costimulation inhibitor (CTLA4-Ig), IL-6 inhibitor, and anti-CD20 monoclonal antibody. These medications may be administered subcutaneously or intravenously. An emerging class of medications includes the small molecules sometimes called oral biologics. These include the janus kinase inhibitors (JAK inhibitors or jakinibs), such as tofacitinib. Tofacitinib is approved for use only in adult RA. Data do not exist on the use of tofacitinib in TMJ arthritis or JIA.

There is a wealth of information on the safety, efficacy and adverse effects of the biologic medications in the adult and pediatric autoimmune arthritides. Included in these data are the 16 randomized controlled trials (RCTs) in JIA. Three (etanercept, adalimumab, infliximab) of the 5 commercially available TNF-alpha inhibitors are commonly used in JIA. In general, the TNF-alpha inhibitors are given in combination with methotrexate.

There are 3 IL-1 inhibitors commercially available (anakinra, canakinumab, rilonacept), they are administered subcutaneously. The IL-1 inhibitors are used almost exclusively for systemic JIA. One RCT in JIA exists for abatacept, the fusion protein of cytotoxic T-cell lymphocyte antigen-4 (CTLA4-Ig) fused with the Fc region of human immunoglobulin. Tocilizumab is an IL-6 inhibitor and is effective for systemic JIA and polyarticular JIA. Rituximab is a chimeric monoclonal antibody directed against the CD20 receptor on B cells. Rituximab has limited data, case reports and one case series in JIA, but is used more in adult RA.

The TNF-alpha inhibitors given systemically as monotherapy or in combination with methotrexate have demonstrated efficacy in TMJ movement and pain.[39,40] TNF inhibitors have been administered in non-TMJ joints with some efficacy.[41] Patients in these studies had failed some combination of methotrexate, IAS, or biologic therapy. A recent study demonstrated the safety and efficacy of infliximab given into arthritic TMJs of 24 patients with JIA.[42] These patients had refractory disease and all but one patient had failed at least 2 rounds of IAS. All of the patients were on systemic therapy, with 23 on biologic therapies. Patients received 1 or 2 rounds of infliximab into TMJs. Six TMJs (5 patients) of the 48 TMJs receiving direct infliximab had resolution of disease. No adverse effects were noted, as can be seen in IAS treatment. Intra-articular administration into TMJs of other biologic therapies (non-TNF inhibitors) has not been evaluated.

Biologic therapy is not without its share of morbidity and mortality concerns. The RCTs of biologics in adults and children with arthritis have raised concerns of malignancy risks. The data regarding malignancy risk are difficult to interpret given the increased baseline risk of malignancy in JIA and RA. Rare adverse effects noted in adults and pediatric patients with the TNF-alpha inhibitors include neurologic changes (optic neuritis, multiple sclerosis), psoriasis, and lupuslike disease. Another side effect includes serious infections: bacterial (*Legionella*, *Listeria*), fungal (histoplasmosis, coccidiomycosis, aspergillosis), and mycobacteria (tuberculosis). The safety of TNF inhibitors through pregnancy and breastfeeding has not been established in long-term studies.

Preventive measures before initiating biologic therapy include tuberculosis screening before and while on biologic therapy, hepatitis B virus serologic screening (HBsAg, HBcAb), hepatitis C antibody testing, varicella vaccine if immunity is lacking, or Zoster vaccine in patients older than 60 years. Influenza vaccine is recommended annually for patients on biologic therapy and their close contacts (**Table 3**).

Perioperative infection risks are a natural concern for patients on DMARDs or biologics. The risk of infection for inflammatory arthritis is due in part to the autoimmune nature of the disease, patient comorbidities, and corticosteroid use. Methotrexate does not appear to increase the risk of surgical infections. The data regarding risk of perioperative infection with biologic medications in the arthritides is conflicting. If the determination is made to stop biologic medications before surgery, then consideration should include risk of flare, half-lives, and when to restart therapy (see **Table 3**). Therapy may be restarted after demonstration of proper wound healing and no active infection.

Table 3
NSAIDs, conventional and biologic DMARDs monitoring

Name	Initial Monitoring	Monitoring Laboratory Test Frequency	Half-life
NSAIDs	CBC, serum creatinine, liver enzymes	Every 6 mo	Variable
Methotrexate	CBC, serum creatinine, liver enzymes	1–2 mo after dose change; every 3–4 mo with stable dose	Adults: 3–10 h Children: 1–6 h
TNF inhibitors	CBC, serum creatinine, liver enzymes Tuberculosis screening *before* therapy start Hepatitis B or C antibody testing	Every 3–6 mo Annually	Etanercept: 80 h Infliximab: 8–9.5 d Adalimumab: ∼14 d

Abbreviations: CBC, complete blood count; DMARD, disease-modifying antirheumatic drugs; NSAID, nonsteroidal anti-inflammatory drug; TNF, tumor necrosis factor.

DISCUSSION

More than 90% of bone formation takes places during the first 2 decades of life in pediatrics.[43] Included in this bone formation is that of the TMJ in the chondrogenic zone on the articular surface on the head of the TMJ condyles. Mandibular growth does not stop until 16 to 18 years for girls and boys, respectively. Significant research and clinical data on arthritis of the TMJ is in juvenile arthritis. All of the subtypes of JIA reviewed herein may have TMJ involvement. Similar to juvenile arthritis, various forms of adult arthritis, such as adult RA, osteoarthritis, psoriatic arthritis, and ankylosing spondylitis, also may have TMJ involvement.[44–46] The significant changes that occur in the TMJ during the pediatric years and the lack of randomized, double-blind, placebo-controlled trials for TMJ arthritis point to the need for early recognition, thorough evaluation by the oral and maxillofacial surgeon and rheumatologist for etiology, then determination of optimal therapeutic options, such as physical therapy, splints, medications, or surgical intervention.

In the past decade, there have been significant advances in the care of patients with inflammatory arthritis. Arthritis of the TMJ has benefited from these advances; yet recognition, evaluation, and management of TMJ arthritis differ significantly between adult and pediatric rheumatologists.[47] TMJ arthritis is prevalent in the inflammatory arthritides. Disease activity is difficult to recognize using clinical signs and symptoms as evaluated by rheumatologists. Clinical findings of TMJ arthritis as performed by oral and maxillofacial surgeons needs to be evaluated.

OPG and CT scans have a role in evaluation of TMJ disease and are easily obtained. MRI with and without contrast using a TMJ coil is the preferred modality to determine active versus chronic disease. Various therapies exist for management of TMJ arthritis. A team approach is best used to determine which modalities to entertain at different points in the disease activity of patients. No one size fits all for patients especially in the pediatric population, given the ongoing growth, refractory nature of the disease, and need for continuous monitoring. IAS, arthrocentesis, biologic therapies (intra-articular and systemic), and surgery have a role in preventing long-term adverse effects. There is still a need for more studies to better understand the most efficacious and safe therapies with optimal outcomes.

REFERENCES

1. Petty RE, Southwood TR, Manners P, et al. International League of Associations of Rheumatology classification of juvenile idiopathic arthritis: second revision, Edmonton, 2001. J Rheumatol 2004;31: 390–2.
2. Fink CW, the Taskforce for Classification Criteria. Proposal for the development of classification criteria for idiopathic arthritides of childhood. J Rheumatol 1995;22:1566–9.
3. European League Against Rheumatism. Nomenclature and classification of arthritis in children. EULAR Bulletin No.4. Basel (Switzerland): National Zeitung AG; 1977.
4. Ferrell EG, Ponder LA, Minor L, et al. Limitations in the classification of childhood-onset rheumatoid arthritis. J Rheumatol 2014;41(3):547–53.
5. Martini A. It is time to rethink juvenile idiopathic arthritis classification and nomenclature. Ann Rheum Dis 2012;71:1437–9.
6. Omar A, Abo-Elyoun I, Hussein H, et al. Anti-cyclic citrullinated peptide (anti-CCP) antibody in juvenile idiopathic arthritis (JIA): correlations with disease activity and severity of joint damage (a multicenter trial). Joint Bone Spine 2013;80:38–43.
7. Gilliam BE, Chauhan AK, Low JM, et al. Measurement of biomarkers in juvenile idiopathic arthritis patients and their significant association with disease severity: a comparative study. Clin Exp Rheumatol 2008;26:492–7.
8. Ravelli A, Magni-Manzoni S, Pistorio A, et al. Preliminary diagnostic guidelines for macrophage activation syndrome complicating systemic juvenile idiopathic arthritis. J Pediatr 2005;146:598–604.
9. Grom AA, Mellins ED. Macrophage activation syndrome: advances towards understanding pathogenesis. Curr Opin Rheumatol 2010;22:561–6.
10. Heiligenhaus A, Niewerth M, Ganser G, et al. Prevalence and complications of uveitis in juvenile idiopathic arthritis in a population-based nation-wide study in Germany: suggested modification of the current screening guidelines. Rheumatology 2007; 46(6):1015–9.
11. Arabshahi B, Cron R. Temporomandibular joint arthritis in juvenile idiopathic arthritis: the forgotten joint. Curr Opin Rheumatol 2006;18(5):490–5.
12. Billiau AD, Hu Y, Verdonck A, et al. Temporomandibular joint arthritis in juvenile idiopathic arthritis: prevalence, clinical and radiological signs, and relation to dentofacial morphology. J Rheumatol 2007;34: 1925–33.
13. Pedersen TK, Kuseler A, Gelineck J, et al. A prospective study of magnetic resonance and radiographic imaging in relation to symptoms and clinical findings of the temporomandibular joint in children with juvenile idiopathic arthritis. J Rheumatol 2008;35:1668–75.
14. Kuseler A, Thomas KP, Gelineck J, et al. A 2 year followup study of enhanced magnetic resonance imaging and clinical examination of the

temporomandibular joint in children with juvenile idiopathic arthritis. J Rheumatol 2005;32:162–9.

15. Nielsen L, Melsen B, Terp S. Prevalence, interrelation and severity of signs of dysfunction from masticatory system in 14-16 year old Danish children. Community Dent Oral Epidemiol 1989;17:91–6.

16. Sherry D, Rabinovich CE, Poduval M, et al. Juvenile idiopathic arthritis. Updated April 21, 2014. Available at: http://emedicine.medscape.com/article/1007276-clinical. Accessed August 26, 2014.

17. Twilt M, Mobers SM, Arends LR, et al. Temporomandibular involvement in juvenile idiopathic arthritis. J Rheumatol 2004;31:141.

18. Ringold S, Cron R. The temporomandibular joint in juvenile idiopathic arthritis: frequently used and frequently arthritic. Pediatr Rheumatol Online J 2009;7:11.

19. Weiss PF, Arabshahi B, Johnson A, et al. High prevalence of temporomandibular joint arthritis at disease onset in children with juvenile idiopathic arthritis, as detected by magnetic resonance imaging but not by ultrasound. Arthritis Rheum 2008;58:1189–96.

20. Vaid YN, Dunnavant FD, Royal SA, et al. Imaging of the temporomandibular joint in juvenile idiopathic arthritis. Arthritis Care Res 2014;66:47–54.

21. Meyers AB, Laor T. Magnetic resonance imaging of the temporomandibular joint in children with juvenile idiopathic arthritis. Pediatr Radiol 2013;43(12):163241.

22. Tzaribachev N, Fritz J, Horger M. Spectrum of magnetic resonance imaging appearances of juvenile temporomandibular joints (TMJ) in non-rheumatic children. Acta Radiol 2009;12(10):1182–6.

23. von Kalle T, Winkler P, Stuber T. Contrast-enhanced MRI of normal temporomandibular joints in children–is there enhancement or not? Rheumatology (Oxford) 2013;12(2):363–7.

24. Beukelman T, Patkar NM, Saag KG, et al. 2011 American College of Rheumatology recommendations for the treatment of juvenile idiopathic arthritis: initiation and safety monitoring of therapeutic agents for the treatment of arthritis and systemic features. Arthritis Care Res (Hoboken) 2011;63(4):465–82.

25. Ringold S, Weiss PF, Beukelman T, et al. 2013 Update of the 2011 American College of Rheumatology recommendations for the treatment of juvenile idiopathic arthritis: recommendations for the medical therapy of children with systemic juvenile idiopathic arthritis and tuberculosis screening among children receiving biologic medications. Arthritis Rheum 2013;65(10):2499–512.

26. Hashkes PJ, Laxer RM. Medical treatment of juvenile idiopathic arthritis. JAMA 2005;294:1671–84.

27. Kerins CA, Spears R, Bellinger LL, et al. The prospective use of COX-2 inhibitors for the treatment of temporomandibular joint inflammatory disorders. Int J Immunopathol Pharmacol 2003;16(Suppl 2):1–9.

28. Ince DO, Ince A, Moore TL. Effect of methotrexate on the temporomandibular joint and facial morphology in juvenile rheumatoid arthritis patients. Am J Orthod Dentofacial Orthop 2000;118:75–83.

29. Alpaslan HG, Alpaslan C. Efficacy of temporomandibular joint arthrocentesis with and without injection of sodium hyaluronate in treatment of internal derangements. J Oral Maxillofac Surg 2001;59:613–8.

30. Olsen-Bergem H, Bjørnland T. A cohort study of patients with juvenile idiopathic arthritis and arthritis of the temporomandibular joint: outcome of arthrocentesis with and without the use of steroids. Int J Oral Maxillofac Surg 2014;43(8):990–5.

31. Stoustrup P, Kristensen KD, Verna C, et al. Intraarticular steroid injection for temporomandibular joint arthritis in juvenile idiopathic arthritis: a systematic review on efficacy and safety. Semin Arthritis Rheum 2013;12(1):63–70.

32. Stoll ML, Good J, Sharpe T, et al. Intra-articular corticosteroid injections to the temporomandibular joints are safe and appear to be effective therapy in children with juvenile idiopathic arthritis. J Oral Maxillofac Surg 2012;70(8):1802.

33. Zulian F, Martini G, Gobber D, et al. Comparison of intra-articular triamcinolone hexacetonide and triamcinolone acetonide in oligoarticular juvenile idiopathic arthritis. Rheumatology (Oxford) 2003;42:1254–9.

34. Vallon D, Akerman S, Nilner M, et al. Long-term follow-up of intra-articular injections into the temporomandibular joint in patients with rheumatoid arthritis. Swed Dent J 2002;26:149–58.

35. Goldzweig O, Carrasco R, Hashkes PJ. Systemic adverse events following intraarticular corticosteroid injections for the treatment of juvenile idiopathic arthritis: two patients with dermatologic adverse events and review of the literature. Semin Arthritis Rheum 2013;43(1):71–6.

36. Stoustrup P, Kristensen KD, Kuseler A, et al. Reduced mandibular growth in experimental arthritis in the temporomandibular joint treated with intra-articular corticosteroid. Eur J Orthod 2008;12(2):111–9.

37. Haddad IK. Temporomandibular joint osteoarthrosis. Histopathological study of the effects of intra-articular injection of triamcinolone acetonide. Saudi Med J 2000;21:675–9.

38. Hugle B, Laxer RM. Clinical images: Lipoatrophy resulting from steroid injection into the temporomandibular joint. Arthritis Rheum 2009;60:3512.

39. Moen K, Grimstvedt K, Hellem S, et al. The long-term effect of anti TNF-a treatment on temporomandibular joints, oral mucosa, and salivary flow in patients with active rheumatoid arthritis: a pilot study. Oral Surg Oral Med Oral Pathol Oral Radiol Endod 2005;100:433–40.

40. Kopp S, Alstergren P, Ernestam S, et al. Reduction of temporomandibular joint pain after treatment with a combination of methotrexate and infliximab is associated with changes in synovial fluid and plasma cytokine in rheumatoid arthritis. Cells Tissues Organs 2005;180:22–30.

41. Bliddal H, Terslev L, Qvistgaard E, et al. Safety of intra-articular injection of etanercept in small-joint arthritis: an uncontrolled, pilot-study with independent imaging assessment. Joint Bone Spine 2006; 73:714–7.

42. Stoll ML, Morlandt AB, Teerwattanapong S, et al. Safety and efficacy of intra-articular infliximab therapy for treatment resistant temporomandibular joint arthritis in children in children: a retrospective study. Rheumatology (Oxford) 2013;52(3):554–9.

43. Theintz G, Buchs B, Rizzoli R, et al. Longitudinal monitoring of bone mass accumulation in healthy adolescents: evidence for a marked reduction after 16 years of age at the levels of lumbar spine and femoral neck in female subjects. J Clin Endocrinol Metab 1992;75:1060–5.

44. Gynther GW, Holmlund AB, Reinholt FP, et al. Temporomandibular joint involvement in generalized osteoarthritis and rheumatoid arthritis: a clinical, arthroscopic, histologic, and immunohistochemical study. Int J Oral Maxillofac Surg 1997;26(1):10–6.

45. Alstergren P, Larsson PT, Kopp S. Successful treatment with multiple intra-articular injections of infliximab in a patient with psoriatic arthritis. Scand J Rheumatol 2008;37:155–7.

46. Major P, Ramos-Remus C, Suarez-Almazor ME, et al. Magnetic resonance imaging and clinical assessment of temporomandibular joint pathology in ankylosing spondylitis. J Rheumatol 1999;26(3): 616–21.

47. Ringold S, Tzaribachev N, Cron RQ. Management of temporomandibular joint arthritis in adult rheumatology practices: a survey of adult rheumatologists. Pediatr Rheumatol Online J 2012;10:26.

Orthognathic Surgery in the Presence of Temporomandibular Dysfunction: What Happens Next?

 CrossMark

Mohammed Nadershah, BDS, MSc[a,b],
Pushkar Mehra, BDS, DMD[b,*]

KEYWORDS

- Orthognathic surgery • Internal derangement • Temporomandibular dysfunction
- Temporomandibular joint

KEY POINTS

- Temporomandibular joints (TMJs) must be thoroughly evaluated before and after orthognathic surgery using universally accepted criteria.
- TMJs must be stable for predictable orthognatic surgery outcomes. Proposed methods for stabilizing the joints include nonsurgical management (splints, pharmaceutical therapy) or surgery (disk repositioning or joint replacement).
- Orthognathic surgery can result in improvement, no change, or deterioration of preexisting temporomandibular dysfunction signs and symptoms.
- Both sagittal split and intraoral vertical ramus osteotomies are acceptable techniques for mandibular setback in patients with TMJ dysfunction.
- Avoiding prolonged maxillomandibular fixation after orthognathic surgery should decrease the incidence of postoperative mandibular hypomobility.
- Counterclockwise rotation of the maxillomandibular complex and large mandibular advancements increase stress and loading of the TMJ and should be used with caution in patients with preexisting internal derangement.

INTRODUCTION

It is essential to define temporomandibular dysfunction (TMD) before discussing its relationship with orthognathic surgery. There are many definitions of TMD in the literature, which adds to the complexity of this topic. Luther[1] defined TMD as the variety of signs and symptoms assigned to the temporomandibular joint (TMJ) and its related structures. These signs and symptoms include joint noises (clicking and popping), tenderness of the muscles of mastication, headaches, TMJ pain, facial and neck pain, limitation of mouth opening, jaw locking, wear of dentition, parafunctional habits (clenching and grinding), and otalgia. The need for a standardized index was first addressed by Helkimo, who developed a clinical index to quantify the severity of TMD.[1,2] In 1992, the research diagnostic criteria (RDC) for TMD

[a] Department of Oral and Maxillofacial Surgery, Faculty of Dentistry, King Abdul Aziz University, PO Box 80200, Jeddah 21589, Saudi Arabia; [b] Department of Oral and Maxillofacial Surgery, Boston University Henry M. Goldman School of Dental Medicine, 100 East Newton Street, Suite G-407, Boston, MA 02118, USA
* Corresponding author.
E-mail address: pmehra@bu.edu

Oral Maxillofacial Surg Clin N Am 27 (2015) 11–26
http://dx.doi.org/10.1016/j.coms.2014.09.002
1042-3699/15/$ – see front matter © 2015 Elsevier Inc. All rights reserved.

index was introduced, with the hope of establishing a common ground for clinical research. It was based on physical findings (axis 1) and psychosocial assessment (axis 2).[3] The RDC/TMD was further revised in 2010, and a second version was proposed.[4–6] Recently, a diagnostic criteria (DC) for TMD tool has been recommended for use in both clinical and laboratory research.[7]

Internal derangement (ID) includes clinical or radiologic disk displacement, and it is often associated with pain in the TMJ or its surrounding tissues, functional limitations of the mandible, or clicking in the joint during motion. The cause of TMJ ID remains unclear, but it is likely multifactorial. Abnormal dentoskeletal occlusion, parafunctional habits (eg, bruxism), stress, anxiety, trauma, systemic factors like hormonal imbalances, or autoimmune disease are some of the known likely causes described in the literature. Wilkes described a commonly cited classification for the stages of ID based on the clinical, radiographic, and anatomic disk-fossa relations.[8] However, there are no controlled prospective studies relating detailed analysis of TMJ-related clinical symptoms and orthognathic surgery with appropriate radiologic correlation, specifically through MRI.

Jaw deformities requiring orthognathic surgery often coexist with TMJ disease. Unrecognized or untreated TMJ diseases are one of the primary factors leading to postsurgical complications, resulting in poor-quality and unpredicted unfavorable outcomes. Although esthetic and psychosocial factors may be the primary motivation for some patients who seek orthognathic surgery, it is often the correction of the functional disability that determines success or failure in this type of treatment. Most research and publications evaluating the relationship between orthognathic surgery and TMD have used nebulous definitions of TMD instead of universally accepted ones.[9]

DOES MALOCCLUSION CAUSE TEMPOROMANDIBULAR DYSFUNCTION?

The cause of TMD remains unknown, but it is thought to be multifactorial. There are many conflicting data in the literature as to whether malocclusion contributes to TMD.[9] McNamara and colleagues[10] reported that malocclusion is suggested to play only a minor role in the development of TMD. These investigators estimated that approximately 10% to 20% of TMD is related to occlusal factors; however, it is clearly not a simple cause-and-effect relation. Other possible causes of TMD include trauma, habits, psychological factors, stress, bruxism, and systemic factors.[9] Proffit

and colleagues[11] reported that the prevalence of TMD in the general population is 5% to 30%, whereas it is higher among people with moderate malocclusion (50%–75%), but these investigators concluded that it is unlikely that occlusal patterns are the only causative factor of TMD. Some studies have correlated certain types of malocclusion (class III, deep bites, and open bites) with the prevalence of TMD.[12,13] Contrastingly, multiple other studies have reported that TMD and TMJ ID are more prevalent in patients with class II skeletal malocclusion.[14–17] Moreover, orthodontic treatment relation to the development of TMD is also controversial, with studies suggesting both improvement and worsening of TMD after orthodontic treatment.[18–20] In our personal experience, although both class II and III patients often complain of some TMJ signs and symptoms (eg, pain, clicking, locking, headaches), most patients presenting with significant functional disability are those with mandibular retrognathism with or without open bites. It is not uncommon to see class III patients with asymptomatic TMJ clicking or mild TMJ dysfunction; in contrast, the high-angle, class II patients often complain of more significant symptoms.

Summary

The literature reports a significant variation in prevalence of TMD in patients with skeletal malocclusion. Many studies report higher incidence of TMD in patients with retrognathic mandibles; these patients usually have steep occlusal and mandibular planes (high angle). Other studies report higher incidence in class III patients, most of whom have flat occlusal but steep, high mandibular planes (low angle). This finding is likely a reflection of the multifactorial causes of TMJ disease. In our experience, we have noticed a higher incidence of TMD in patients with retrognathic mandibles and in those with steep occlusal planes, as mentioned earlier. Even so, most of the published literature in TMD incidence is limited by small sample sizes and selection bias.

WHAT IS THE EFFECT OF ORTHOGNATHIC SURGERY ON TEMPOROMANDIBULAR DYSFUNCTION?

The literature studying the effect of orthognathic surgery in patients with preexisting TMD is similarly inconclusive because of lack of consistency in methods and measured outcomes.[9] There is still controversy as to the ideal management of patients with preexisting ID of the TMJ who require orthognathic surgery for correction of dentofacial deformity.

Historically speaking, there have been 2 different philosophic approaches in the management of orthognathic patients with preexisting TMD.

Orthognathic Surgery Aids in the Reduction of Temporomandibular Joints Dysfunction or Does Not Aggravate the Current Temporomandibular Dysfunction

Proponents of this more common philosophy recommend that orthognathic surgery be routinely attempted if the patient can tolerate presurgical orthodontics for functional improvement of TMD signs and symptoms.[21–24]

Let us first review some of the published research articles supporting this philosophy. Karabouta and Martis[21] evaluated the TMJ in 280 patients who underwent bilateral sagittal split osteotomy (SSO) for the correction of various dentofacial deformities. These investigators reported that the TMD incidence improved from 40.8% preoperatively to 11.1% postoperatively, but there were new TMD symptoms after surgery in 3.7% of previously asymptomatic patients. The average follow-up time was only 6 months (inadequate for long-term results), and only 23 patients had mandibular advancement surgery. Magnusson and colleagues[22] followed 20 patients with TMD for 1 to 2.5 years postoperatively and reported improvement in TMD symptoms after mandibular surgery. However, the type of movement (advancement vs setback) was not described. Upton and colleagues[23] conducted a questionnaire-based study asking patients to rate their TMJ symptoms before and after orthognathic surgery. Fifty-five patients completed the survey and reported 78% with improvement in TMJ symptoms after surgery, 16% with no change, and 3% with new TMD symptoms. However, these investigators neither measured any objective date nor mentioned the length of follow-up. White and Dolwick[15] evaluated 75 patients, 49.3% of whom had symptomatic TMD. These investigators found that 89.1% of this group improved with orthognathic surgery, 2.7% unchanged, and 8.1% experienced worsening of their TMD symptoms. New-onset TMD was noted in only 7.9% of preoperatively asymptomatic patients after orthognathic surgery.[15] Hackney and colleagues[25] did not find an increase in TMD after bilateral SSO by measuring the intercondylar width and angle, indicating the excellent adaptive capacity of the TMJ. Onizawa and colleagues[26] compared TMD incidence in 30 patients who underwent bilateral SSO with a control group of 30 healthy volunteers and found no significant difference, concluding that the alteration in TMD symptoms after orthognathic surgery is not always a direct result of the correction of malocclusion.

Orthognathic Surgery Causes Further Deleterious Effect on the Temporomandibular Joints

In contrast to group I, this philosophy is supported by literature showing poor clinical outcomes after orthognathic surgery in patients with preexisting ID.[26,27] Moore and colleagues[28] reported condylar resorption in 5 patients after mandibular advancement; 3 of the 5 individuals had presurgical TMD. Crawford and colleagues[29] similarly reported 7 cases of condylar resorption after orthognathic surgery. These investigators noted a predilection for females with preexisting TMJ disease, especially after large mandibular advancements.

Wolford and colleagues have been studying this issue for a long period and have presented a lot of literature over many years supporting this philosophy. In a widely quoted study,[27] they reported that preexisting TMJ dysfunction worsens after orthognathic surgery. In this study, they retrospectively reviewed the records of 25 patients with ID who underwent only orthognathic surgery. The incidence of TMJ pain increased from 36% to 84% after surgery, and 24% of the patients developed postoperative condylar resorption. Based on their experience, these investigators advocated surgical correction of the anatomic TMJ disease (ID) using disk repositioning procedures before, or at the time of (this is their preference), orthognathic surgery procedures for all (symptomatic or asymptomatic) patients with preexisting TMJ ID.[30] The investigators also advised against using conservative TMJ therapy (eg, splint, arthroscopy, arthrocentesis), because these therapies do not reposition the TMJ disk into an anatomically correct position, which in their opinion is critical for ensuring predictable orthognathic surgery outcomes.[30]

When this study is analyzed in depth, despite its being one of few, if any, standard publications reviewing the debatable relationship between orthognathic surgery outcomes and preexisting TMJ ID, it has certain drawbacks. Some of these drawbacks include a small patient sample, retrospective design, and lack of postoperative MRI findings to document anatomic disk position. In addition, most patients underwent mandibular advancement surgery with counterclockwise rotation of the maxillomandibular complex (MMC) and lowering of the occlusal plane. Although this particular surgical movement has been repeatedly shown to be stable,[31,32] it causes overloading of the TMJs both by lengthening the class III lever arm of the mandible and TMJ and by lowering the occlusal plane angle. Performing counter-clockwise mandibular advancements in the presence of less than anatomically ideal TMJs may have been a (co)factor in the high incidence of postoperative complications encountered in this study patient sample.

Summary

This is a difficult area to study and research because of multiple, varying differences in the classification, diagnosis, and treatment of TMJ ID. When the existing literature is critically evaluated, it becomes evident that the inferences are often based more on anecdotal opinion(s) and clinician experience. Recommendations have been rationalized on less than optimal or flawed, retrospective, chart review–type research protocols. There are no randomized, prospective, multicenter clinical trials studying this complex relationship. If one were to pick a subgroup of patients who could possibly have adverse outcomes after orthognathic surgery relative to preexisting TMJ signs and symptoms, it is likely to be high-angle, class II patients undergoing counterclockwise rotation or large mandibular advancement procedures.

WHAT IS THE EFFECT OF ORTHOGNATHIC SURGERY ON MANDIBULAR RANGE OF MOTION?

Orthognathic surgery aims to improve esthetic and function. However, mandibular hypomobility after orthognathic surgery has been reported in multiple studies.[33–37] The mechanism remains debatable and could be multifactorial. Preexisting TMD, postoperative maxillomandibular fixation,[38] surgical technique, and myotomy of the suprahyoid muscles have all been implicated in postoperative mandibular hypomobility.[33,35] Zimmer and colleagues[36] reported that the mandibular hypomobility after maxillary advancement, mandibular setback, or double jaw surgery was temporary. Postoperative physical rehabilitation was also shown to improve mandibular range of motion.[33] Al-Riyami and colleagues[39] systematically reviewed this issue and concluded that the mandibular range of motion is often decreased in the short-term after orthognathic surgery, but most patients fully regain the full range of motion within 2 years.

Summary

For most patients, orthognathic surgery should have no long-term beneficial or adverse effects relative to mandibular mobility. The maximum interincisal opening is expected to decrease in the immediate, short-term postsurgery interval in almost all patients, with a greater decrease in patients who are kept in maxillomandibular fixation postoperatively.

WHAT IS THE EFFECT OF ORTHOGNATHIC SURGERY ON THE MAXIMUM BITE FORCE?

Bite force changes after orthognathic surgery are a multifactorial process. Finn and colleagues[40] described a biomechanical model to study the effect of different orthognathic surgery movements. They concluded that mandibular setback would result in a mechanical gain for the mandibular adductor muscles and predicted that this would result in an increase in the bite force.[41] However, human studies showed mixed results. Proffit and colleagues[42] reported the effect of mandibular setback in 21 patients; 6 patients showed a significant increase, 9 had no change, and 6 had a significant decrease in the bite force. These investigators also found similar mixed results with maxillary superior repositioning and isolated mandibular advancement. Moreover, they calculated the mechanical advantage of the masticator muscles and found it to be a poor predictor of the change in bite force. Ellis and colleagues[43] found that the bite force in patients with mandibular prognathism was lower than control individuals but approached normal values 2 to 3 years after mandibular setback. On the other hand, mandibular advancement did not increase the bite force, possibly because of lengthening of the lever arm.[44,45] Kim and Oh[46] found an inverse relation between the duration of maxillomandibular fixation after orthognathic surgery and the time needed to recover the bite force. Using miniplates or bicortical screws after SSO did not show a difference in the recovery of masticatory function.[47]

Summary

The maximum bite force changes after orthognathic surgery are affected by multiple factors and cannot be solely explained based on mechanics. Despite variability in the literature, multiple studies indicate that mandibular setback increases the bite force, and mandibular advancement did not improve the masticatory function.

DO DIFFERENT SURGICAL ORTHOGNATHIC TECHNIQUES AND MOVEMENTS HAVE VARIABLE EFFECT ON TEMPOROMANDIBULAR DYSFUNCTION?

The 2 most common mandibular osteotomies used are the SSO and the intraoral vertical ramus osteotomy (IVRO). Each technique has its inherent advantages and disadvantages, and there exists controversy over the best technique for the correction of mandibular prognathism.[48,49] An IVRO,[50,51] or modified condylotomy,[52] has shown favorable effect on the TMJ because of the anterior-inferior repositioning of the condyle resulting from the pull of the lateral pterygoid muscles. This technique allows for an increase in the joint space and for recapturing an anteriorly displaced disk, which may improve TMD symptoms, especially those related to pain. In contrast, some clinicians believe that the SSO may create a greater change in the condylar position, with an especially higher chance of development of TMD with rigid fixation.[53,54] This situation has led to varying recommendations regarding the optimal method for fixing these osteotomies (eg, monocortical plates, positional bicortical screws). Kawamata and colleagues[55] evaluated postoperative condylar position using three-dimensional computed tomography (CT) scans after orthognathic surgery. These investigators found that in SSO patients, lateral tilting of the condyles was predominant, in contrast to IVRO patients, in whom medial tilting of the condyles was more prevalent.

Adequate fixation of SSO can be achieved using bicortical screws (positional or lag) or monocortical plates. Lag screws cause a lateral torque of the condyle as a result of compression of the segments and should be avoided.[56] On the other hand, positional screws avoid this problem without compromising the fixation. However, positional screws are less forgiving than monocortical miniplates in regard to condylar seating. Yamashita and colleagues[47] found a higher incidence of TMD with bicortical positional screws compared with monocortical plates 5 years after SSO.

Summary

Existing literature is inconclusive relative to the superiority of an IVRO or SSO for mandibular setback procedures. In our opinion, an experienced clinician can obtain stable results with both procedures. The choice should be based on factors like personal experience or patient preference. There is no substitute for sound surgical technique. Removing all bony interferences between the proximal and distal segments, passive seating of the

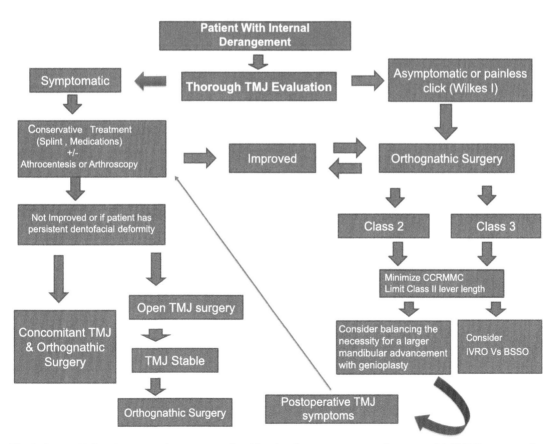

Fig. 1. Boston University protocol: treatment algorithm for the management of patents with TMJ ID or resorption who present for orthognathic surgery.

condyles intraoperatively, and use of positional screws rather than compression or lag screws for fixation should minimize the displacement of the condyles after SSO.[25,57] Miniplates are considered more forgiving than bicrotical screws for SSO fixation as they permit condylar seating with lesser potential for torque and/or sag.

WHAT IS THE EFFECT OF THE ROTATION OF THE OCCLUSAL PLANE ON THE TEMPOROMANDIBULAR JOINTS?

Rotation of the occlusal plane, also known as rotation of the MMC, was first described by Wolford and colleagues[58] in 1984. Clockwise rotation

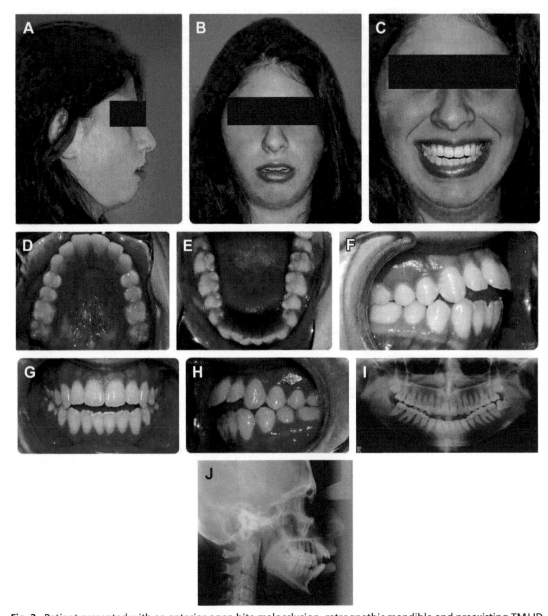

Fig. 2. Patient presented with an anterior open bite malocclusion, retrognathic mandible and preexisting TMJ ID. She had TMJ arthritis and pain with recurrent locking. The patient was managed by maxillary orthognathic surgery only for correction of open bite and camouflage genioplasty. The aim of this treatment approach was to minimze postsurgical TMJ loading by not increasing the lever arm of the mandible, which would have occurred with a SSO advancement. (*A–H*) Presurgical clinical pictures. (*I, J*) Presurgical radiographs showing advanced TM arthritis, steep mandibular and occlusal planes and open bite. (*K–T*) Postsurgical results showing stability of surgery and acceptable facial esthetics without SSO surgery.

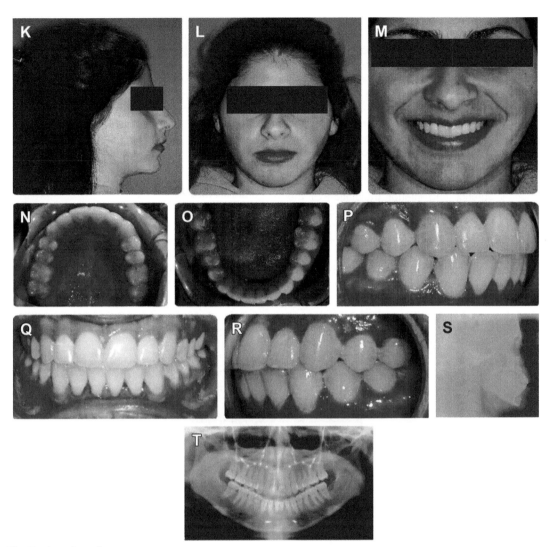

Fig. 2. (*continued*)

(CR) of the MMC refers to increasing the occlusal plane angle. This procedure should not be confused with mandibular plane rotation as in open bite cases, in which the maxillary and mandibular occlusal planes do not coincide. This distinction is critical, because a single jaw surgery to superiorly affect the maxilla with auto counter-clockwise rotation of the mandibular plane is one of the most stable orthognathic movements. On the other hand, counterclockwise rotation (CCR) of the MMC during a double jaw orthognathic surgery was believed to be unstable, mainly because of the rotation of the distal mandibular segment, resulting in lengthening of the pterygomasseteric muscles and stretching of the soft tissues.[59] As this movement theoretically increases TMJ loading biomechanically, it has often been described as a predisposing factor for causing worsening of TMD and as responsible for relapse after orthognathic surgery.[59]

It is imperative to determine the center of rotation for MMC, which affects the percent of posterior and anterior vertical lengthening or shortening. Drawing a triangular shape between the posterior nasal spine, the anterior nasal spine, and the pogonion on the cephalometric tracing may aid in presurgical planning and prediction of the impact of different rotation points during CR and CCR MMC.[60] With the improvement in surgical technique and rigid fixation, CCR MMC has been repeatedly shown to be stable, especially if the TMJs are healthy preoperatively.[31,61,62] Reyneke and colleagues[63] compared both CR and CCR MMC with conventional treatment (no alteration in the occlusal plane) and found no significant difference in stability. However, these investigators did not report on the clinical TMJ status before or after surgery. In patients with preexisting TMD, CCR MMC may aggravate the problem if the TMJ was not addressed beforehand.[27]

Sequencing of bimaxillary surgery plays an important role, especially when the occlusal plane is altered. The mandible-first approach is advantageous during CCR MMC, because using the maxilla-first approach with this movement results in a thick intermediate splint. Moreover, the maxillary molars are inferiorly repositioned, which requires the mandible to rotate open, resulting in a potential anterior and inferior translation of the condyles down the articular eminence.[64] Similarly, the maxilla-first approach may be advantageous during CR MMC, especially in less experienced hands.[65]

Sequencing is also critical when there is a functional shift or a large difference between centric relation and centric occlusion. The maxilla-first approach requires accurate preoperative centric relation record and precise replication of any centric relation–centric occlusion difference during model surgery. On the contrary, an inaccurate interocclusal record is of no consequence when the mandibular surgery is performed first. This finding results from the dissipation of the centric relation–centric occlusion discrepancy in the mandibular osteotomy gap during condylar seating.[64]

Summary

With proper surgical technique, both CR and CCR MMC are stable and predictable orthognathic surgical movements if the TMJs are able to withstand the postsurgical loading and stress. CCR MMC leads to greater loading on the TMJs compared

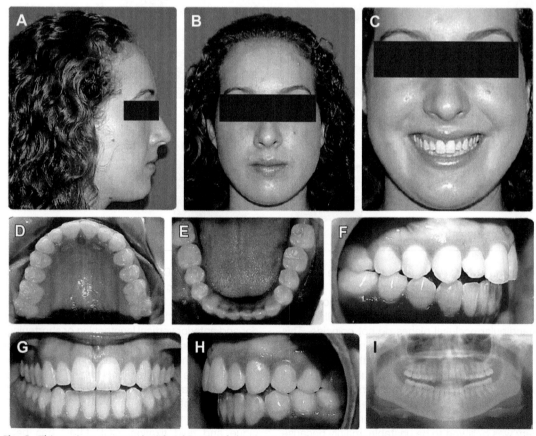

Fig. 3. This patient presented with a history of development of an anterior open bite secondary to progressive mandibular retrusion due to TMJ condylar resorption. The work-up was negative for known etiology for condylar resorption and she was observed for 2 years. Her occlusion was found to be stable for more than one year from initial exam and thus, she was managed by maxillary and mandibular orthognathic surgery only without TMJ surgery. (*A–H*) Presurgical clinical pictures. (*I, J*) Presurgical panoramic radiograph. (*K–N*) Presurgical MRI examination demonstrating bilateral condylar anterior disc displacement without reduction. (*O-R*) 5-year postsurgical clinical and radiographic results demonstrating stability of occlusal results after 2-jaw orthognathic surgery with rigid fixation.

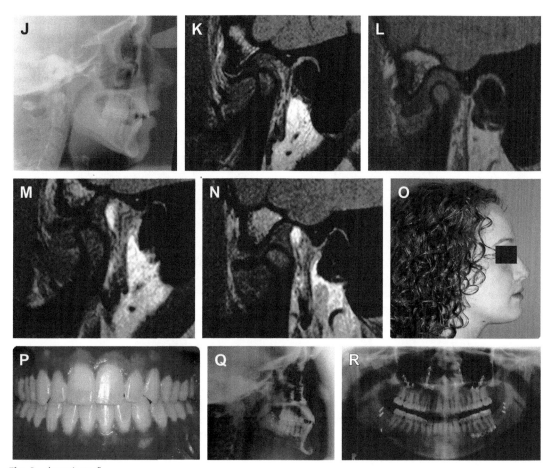

Fig. 3. (*continued*)

with CR MMC after double jaw orthognathic surgery. Sequencing of bimaxillary surgery plays a critical role in seating the condyles in bimaxillary surgery, especially when the occlusal plane is altered. The mandible-first approach may have multiple advantages, when large, complex movements are planned in patients with TMJ disorders that may interfere with optimal and accurate presurgical record obtaining, perioperative treatment planning, or intraoperative surgical execution.

CONTEMPORARY CONCEPTS AND FUTURE DIRECTIONS

Combined surgical-orthodontic treatment via orthognathic surgery is a common and well-accepted management approach for patients with dentofacial deformity. It aims to produce more harmonious facial skeletal relationships, with an objective to prevent long-term deleterious effects on the TMJs and dentition. The improvement criteria of TMJ symptoms after orthognathic

surgery are often based on lack of pain or clicking and popping of TMJ.

Clinical Considerations

Most practitioners have long agreed that orthognathic surgery benefits TMD. How and why are unproved, but it is believed to be caused by normalization of anatomic skeletal patterns and balancing of osseous, articular, and neuromuscular structures of the maxillofacial region. Current research is focusing on 2 specific areas:

1. Patients with preexisting TMJ condylar resorption: this area relates to orthognathic surgical treatment options for patients with active or arrested condylar resorption
2. Patients with preexisting TMD/TMJ ID: this area attempts to preoperatively identify a group of patients who are prone to complications after orthognathic surgery (postoperative relapse caused by new-onset TMJ condylar resorption

or suboptimal improvement in TMJ signs and symptoms after jaw surgery).

TMJ condylar resorption can occur as a result of a multitude of causes including but not limited to local or systemic arthritide and trauma; it can also be idiopathic.[66] It has been proposed that although the root cause of condylar resorption can be variable between the diagnoses, all bone loss involves a common resorptive pathway, which is inflammation related: cytokine-activated osteoblasts promote the recruitment and activity

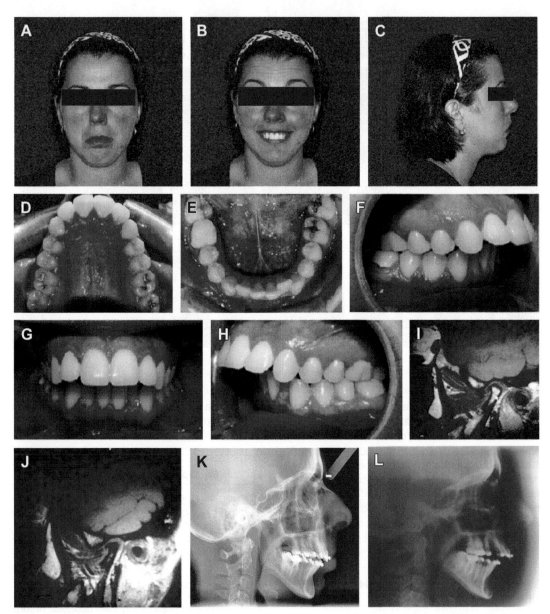

Fig. 4. This patient presented with severe TMJ and myofascial pain, headaches, locking, restricted jaw function, and arthritis. She was initially managed by splint therapy followed by maxillary and mandibular orthognathic surgery without TMJ surgery. (A–H) Presurgical clinical pictures showing Class I skeletal and dental relationship. (I–J) Presurgical MRI scans showing anterior disk displacement, osteophyte formation and flattening of condylar heads bilaterally. (K, L) Presurgical cephalometric radiographs demonstrating CO-CR discrepancy. This patient had a habit of posturing her mandible anteriorly (see K) and splint therapy for utilized to successfully obtain a stable CO-CR position and eliminate pain prior to surgery. (M–U) Postsurgical results. 2-jaw orthognathic surgery was performed successfully in the presence of advanced TMJ Disease using principles of: 1) Stabilize TMJ non-surgically, and, 2) avoiding overloading of TMJ postoperatively (judicious mandibular advancement, avoid CCRMC).

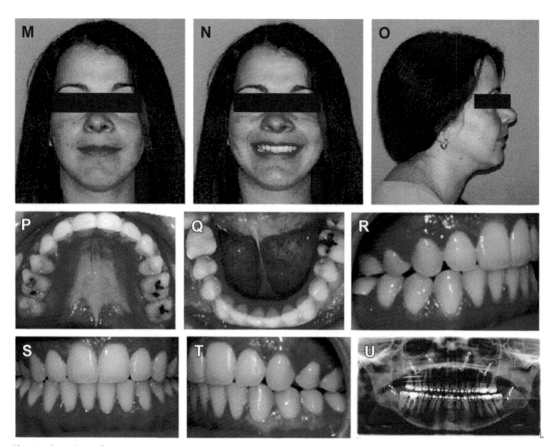

Fig. 4. (*continued*)

of osteoclasts, which, in turn, result in secretion of enzymes that are responsible for breakdown of hydroxyapatite and collagen. Certain factors may predispose an individual to develop condylar resorption. These factors include gender, nutritional status, genetics, and oral habits, including parafunction and iatrogenic compression.[66] Broadly speaking, resorption is likely to occur when loading of the TMJ exceeds the adaptive capacity of the TMJ.

Radiographic Considerations

A precise evaluation of joint structures is of major importance in the diagnostic assessment of abnormalities, because clinical examination alone does not always provide a complete understanding of the changes in intra-articular anatomy.[67–69] Thus, an accurate diagnostic assessment with MRI is indispensable. The importance of MRI in the diagnosis of TMD has been confirmed in numerous studies.[67,70] Emshoff and Rudisch[71] evaluated the clinical diagnostic criteria for TMJ disorders against the MRI diagnosis of TMJ ID

and osteoarthritis in a patient group, and it was observed that the classification system of the clinical diagnostic criteria for TMJ disorders is not sufficiently reliable for determining TMJ ID and osteoarthritis. It was further determined that a clinical diagnosis of ID type 3 may need to be supplemented by evidence from an MRI to determine functional disk-condyle relationship.

Improvement of the quality of TMJ MRI could be achieved with the use of higher field strengths as a result of their higher signal-to-noise ratios.[72] Benefits of higher field strengths have already been shown for the examinations of various joints. In comparative studies of smaller joints, including TMJ, field strengths of 3.0 T provided for superior quality versus a field strength of 1.5 T.[73–75] The high-resolution radiologic changes in disk relationship with the joint both before and after surgery have not been studied in an evidence-based manner in the literature using MRI scans. Thus, it is expected that clinicians will continue to face some unanswered questions as to why some patients' TMJ symptoms improve whereas others do not after the orthognathic surgery.

Table 1
Preliminary results of the pilot project studying changes in TMJ function and signs and symptoms after orthognathic surgery has been performed in patients with preexisting TMJ ID or TMD

Group	Age (y)	Follow-up (mo)	Headache		TMJ Pain		Jaw Function Restriction		Dietary Restrictions		Disability		MIO Without Pain (mm)		Lateral Excursion (mm)	
			T1	T3	T1	T3	T1	T3	T1	T3	T1	T3	T1	T3	T1	T3
Wilkes I (n = 62) Asymptomatic click	32 (18–53)	68.23 (20–81)	0.1	0.1	0.0	0.2	1.5	1.0	4.0	1.9	0.7	0.0	33.5	42.5	5.2	5.8
Wilkes II (n = 57) Symptomatic click	26.3 (15–43)	68.5 (22–84)	3.5	1.7	5.5	0.8	5.8	2.1	7.8	1.0	3.6	1.3	22.5	40.6	5.1	6.2
Wilkes III (n = 46) No click Frequent locking	45.4 (19–56)	53.87 (24–88)	6.7	2.1	6.2	0.7	4.9	2.4	5.0	2.7	4.3	1.8	28.7	41.6	7.1	7.4
Wilkes IV (n = 50) No click Bony changes Stable mandible	45.4 (16–62)	26.7 (14–34)	5.7	2.4	6.1	1.5	5.7	1.4	7.1	2.9	6.3	2.1	22.7	34.4	7.7	6.3

Data from Wilkes CH. Structural and functional alterations of the temporomandibular joint. Northwest Dent 1978;57(5):287–94.

PERSONAL EXPERIENCE AND RESEARCH

As is evident from this article, the relationship between the TMJ and orthognathic surgery is complex and debatable. There is no consensus and often more questions than answers. At our center, when a patient with TMJ ID and TMD is referred for orthognathic surgery, a standard protocol is followed for diagnosis and management (**Fig. 1**).

The initial step involves a thorough preoperative TMJ evaluation followed by conservative (nonsurgical) therapy in symptomatic patients. If the patient improves, we proceed with orthognathic surgery using principles that minimize intraoperative and postoperative increase in TMJ loading. This surgery includes avoiding CCR of the MMC, carefully assessing the necessity for large mandibular advancements, considering using IVRO in some cases instead of bilateral SSO for mandibular setback if the surgeon deems acceptable, and using maxillary surgery to replace or minimize mandibular movement if possible.

Use of this management strategy has the advantage of enhancing success and predictability and balancing function and esthetics without the need for surgical management of the TMJ (**Figs. 2–4**). Concomitant TMJ and orthognathic surgery is usually reserved only for patients who (1) fail the above conservative protocol (approximately 2%–3 % in our experience), (2) patients with advanced TMJ condylar resorption who require TMJ replacements, and (3) patients with active TMJ pathologic conditions like condylar hyperplasia, osteochondroma, who require treatment of the TMJ disease via surgery.

Our initial results are promising, with more than 95% of patients reporting significant improvement postoperatively relative to TMD symptoms (**Table 1**). At the time of submission of this article, of a total of 165 patients, only 1 patient (<1%) has developed worsening of TMJ signs and symptoms postoperatively, and 2 patients (<2%) have developed condylar resorption postoperatively after orthognathic surgery.

We are also initiating another study to first analyze the TMJ intra-articular soft tissue relationship with the mandibular condyle both preoperatively and postoperatively using MRI, and then correlate the radiographic results with differences in clinical signs and symptoms, both preoperatively and postoperatively. This study has the potential to clarify some key ambiguities on this topic and to serve as a platform to introduce findings that will lead to better clinical understanding of the indications for surgery. The objective is to promote more evidence-based clinical management of such patients in the future. The specific aims of this study proposal include (1) correlating TMJ dysfunction symptoms with MRI findings in patients with dentoskeletal deformities, (2) recording TMJ anatomic and morphologic changes during various phases of combined surgical-orthodontic treatment, and (3) assessing the effects of varying orthognathic surgery procedures on the intra-articular and periarticular TMJ anatomy.

REFERENCES

1. Luther F. Orthodontics and the temporomandibular joint: where are we now? Part 1. Orthodontic treatment and temporomandibular disorders. Angle Orthod 1998;68(4):295–304. http://dx.doi.org/10.1043/0003-3219(1998)068<0295:OATTJW>2.3.CO;2.
2. Helkimo M. Studies on function and dysfunction of the masticatory system. II. Index for anamnestic and clinical dysfunction and occlusal state. Sven Tandlak Tidskr 1974;67(2):101–21.
3. Dworkin SF, LeResche L. Research diagnostic criteria for temporomandibular disorders: review, criteria, examinations and specifications, critique. J Craniomandib Disord 1992;6(4):301–55.
4. Look JO, Schiffman EL, Truelove EL, et al. Reliability and validity of axis I of the research diagnostic criteria for temporomandibular disorders (RDC/TMD) with proposed revisions. J Oral Rehabil 2010;37(10):744–59. http://dx.doi.org/10.1111/j.1365-2842.2010.02121.x.
5. Anderson GC, Gonzalez YM, Ohrbach R, et al. The research diagnostic criteria for temporomandibular disorders. VI: future directions. J Orofac Pain 2010;24(1):79–88.
6. Schiffman EL, Truelove EL, Ohrbach R, et al. The research diagnostic criteria for temporomandibular disorders. I: overview and methodology for assessment of validity. J Orofac Pain 2010;24(1):7–24.
7. Schiffman E, Ohrbach R, Truelove E, et al. Diagnostic criteria for temporomandibular disorders (DC/TMD) for clinical and research applications: recommendations of the International RDC/TMD consortium network* and Orofacial Pain Special Interest Group†. J Oral Facial Pain Headache 2014;28(1):6–27.
8. Wilkes CH. Structural and functional alterations of the temporomandibular joint. Northwest Dent 1978;57(5):287–9.
9. Al-Riyami S, Moles DR, Cunningham SJ. Orthognathic treatment and temporomandibular disorders: a systematic review. Part 1. A new quality-assessment technique and analysis of study characteristics and classifications. Am J Orthod Dentofacial Orthop 2009;136(5):624.e1–15. http://dx.doi.org/10.1016/j.ajodo.2009.02.021 [discussion: 624–5].
10. McNamara JA, Seligman DA, Okeson JP. Occlusion, orthodontic treatment, and temporomandibular disorders: a review. J Orofac Pain 1995;9(1):73–90.

11. Proffit WR, Fields HW Jr, Sarver DM. Contemporary orthodontics. Philadelphia: Elsevier Health Sciences; 2006.

12. Mohlin B, Ingervall B, Thilander B. Relation between malocclusion and mandibular dysfunction in Swedish men. Eur J Orthod 1980;2(4):229–38.

13. Mohlin B, Thilander B. The importance of the relationship between malocclusion and mandibular dysfunction and some clinical applications in adults. Eur J Orthod 1984;6(1):192–204. http://dx.doi.org/10.1093/ejo/6.1.192.

14. De Clercq CA, Abeloos JS, Mommaerts MY, et al. Temporomandibular joint symptoms in an orthognathic surgery population. J Craniomaxillofac Surg 1995;23(3):195–9.

15. White CS, Dolwick MF. Prevalence and variance of temporomandibular dysfunction in orthognathic surgery patients. Int J Adult Orthodon Orthognath Surg 1992;7(1):7–14.

16. Kerstens H, Tuinzing DB. Temporomandibular joint symptoms in orthognathic surgery. J Craniomaxillofac Surg 1989;17(5):215–8.

17. Link JJ, Nickerson JW. Temporomandibular joint internal derangements in an orthognathic surgery population. Int J Adult Orthodon Orthognath Surg 1992;7(3):161–9.

18. Egermark I, Carlsson GE, Magnusson T. A prospective long-term study of signs and symptoms of temporomandibular disorders in patients who received orthodontic treatment in childhood. Angle Orthod 2005;75(4):645–50. http://dx.doi.org/10.1043/0003-3219(2005)75[645:APLSOS]2.0.CO;2.

19. Mohlin BO, Derweduwen K, Pilley R, et al. Malocclusion and temporomandibular disorder: a comparison of adolescents with moderate to severe dysfunction with those without signs and symptoms of temporomandibular disorder and their further development to 30 years of age. Angle Orthod 2004;74(3):319–27. http://dx.doi.org/10.1043/0003-3219(2004)074<0319:MATDCO>2.0.CO;2.

20. Sadowsky C, Theisen TA, Sakols EI. Orthodontic treatment and temporomandibular joint sounds–a longitudinal study. Am J Orthod Dentofacial Orthop 1991;99(5):441–7. http://dx.doi.org/10.1016/S0889-5406(05)81577-X.

21. Karabouta I, Martis C. The TMJ dysfunction syndrome before and after sagittal split osteotomy of the rami. J Maxillofac Surg 1985;13(4):185–8.

22. Magnusson T, Ahlborg G, Finne K, et al. Changes in temporomandibular joint pain-dysfunction after surgical correction of dentofacial anomalies. Int J Oral Maxillofac Surg 1986;15(6):707–14.

23. Upton LG, Scott RF, Hayward JR. Major maxillomandibular malrelations and temporomandibular joint pain-dysfunction. J Prosthet Dent 1984;51(5):686–90.

24. Stavropoulos F, Dolwick MF. Simultaneous temporomandibular joint and orthognathic surgery: the case against. J Oral Maxillofac Surg 2003;61(10):1205–6.

25. Hackney FL, Van Sickels JE, Nummikoski PV. Condylar displacement and temporomandibular joint dysfunction following bilateral sagittal split osteotomy and rigid fixation. J Oral Maxillofac Surg 1989;47(3):223–7.

26. Onizawa K, Schmelzeisen R, Vogt S. Alteration of temporomandibular joint symptoms after orthognathic surgery: comparison with healthy volunteers. J Oral Maxillofac Surg 1995;53(2):117–21 [discussion: 122–3].

27. Wolford LM, Reiche-Fischel O, Mehra P. Changes in temporomandibular joint dysfunction after orthognathic surgery. J Oral Maxillofac Surg 2003;61(6):655–60. http://dx.doi.org/10.1053/joms.2003.50131 [discussion: 661].

28. Moore KE, Gooris PJ, Stoelinga PJ. The contributing role of condylar resorption to skeletal relapse following mandibular advancement surgery: report of five cases. J Oral Maxillofac Surg 1991;49(5):448–60.

29. Crawford JG, Stoelinga PJ, Blijdorp PA, et al. Stability after reoperation for progressive condylar resorption after orthognathic surgery: report of seven cases. J Oral Maxillofac Surg 1994;52(5):460–6.

30. Wolford LM. Concomitant temporomandibular joint and orthognathic surgery. J Oral Maxillofac Surg 2003;61(10):1198–204.

31. Chemello PD, Wolford LM, Buschang PH. Occlusal plane alteration in orthognathic surgery–part II: long-term stability of results. Am J Orthod Dentofacial Orthop 1994;106(4):434–40. http://dx.doi.org/10.1016/S0889-5406(94)70066-4.

32. Wolford LM, Chemello PD, Hilliard F. Occlusal plane alteration in orthognathic surgery–part I: effects on function and esthetics. Am J Orthod Dentofacial Orthop 1994;106(3):304–16. http://dx.doi.org/10.1016/S0889-5406(94)70051-6.

33. Storum KA, Bell WH. Hypomobility after maxillary and mandibular osteotomies. Oral Surg Oral Med Oral Pathol 1984;57(1):7–12.

34. Aragon SB, Van Sickles JE, Dolwick MF, et al. The effects of orthognathic surgery on mandibular range of motion. J Oral Maxillofac Surg 1985;43(12):938–43.

35. Boyd SB, Karas ND, Sinn DP. Recovery of mandibular mobility following orthognathic surgery. J Oral Maxillofac Surg 1991;49(9):924–31.

36. Zimmer B, Schwestka R, Kubein-Meesenburg D. Changes in mandibular mobility after different procedures of orthognathic surgery. Eur J Orthod 1992;14(3):188–97.

37. Al-Belasy FA, Tozoglu S, Dolwick MF. Mandibular hypomobility after orthognathic surgery: a review article. J Oral Maxillofac Surg 2013;71(11):1967.e1–11. http://dx.doi.org/10.1016/j.joms.2013.06.217.

38. Ueki K, Marukawa K, Hashiba Y, et al. Assessment of the relationship between the recovery of maximum mandibular opening and the maxillomandibular fixation period after orthognathic surgery. J Oral Maxillofac Surg 2008;66(3):486–91. http://dx.doi.org/10.1016/j.joms.2007.08.044.

39. Al-Riyami S, Cunningham SJ, Moles DR. Orthognathic treatment and temporomandibular disorders: a systematic review. Part 2. Signs and symptoms and meta-analyses. Am J Orthod Dentofacial Orthop 2009;136(5):626.e1–16. http://dx.doi.org/10.1016/j.ajodo.2009.02.022.

40. Finn RA, Throckmorton GS, Bell WH, et al. Biomechanical considerations in the surgical correction of mandibular deficiency. J Oral Surg 1980;38(4):257–64.

41. Throckmorton GS, Finn RA, Bell WH. Biomechanics of differences in lower facial height. Am J Orthod 1980;77(4):410–20.

42. Proffit WR, Turvey TA, Fields HW, et al. The effect of orthognathic surgery on occlusal force. J Oral Maxillofac Surg 1989;47(5):457–63.

43. Ellis E, Throckmorton GS, Sinn DP. Bite forces before and after surgical correction of mandibular prognathism. J Oral Maxillofac Surg 1996;54(2):176–81.

44. van den Braber W, van der Glas H, van der Bilt A, et al. Masticatory function in retrognathic patients, before and after mandibular advancement surgery. J Oral Maxillofac Surg 2004;62(5):549–54. http://dx.doi.org/10.1016/j.joms.2003.06.016.

45. Zarrinkelk HM, Throckmorton GS, Ellis E, et al. A longitudinal study of changes in masticatory performance of patients undergoing orthognathic surgery. J Oral Maxillofac Surg 1995;53(7):777–82 [discussion: 782–3].

46. Kim YG, Oh SH. Effect of mandibular setback surgery on occlusal force. J Oral Maxillofac Surg 1997;55(2):121–6 [discussion: 126–8].

47. Yamashita Y, Otsuka T, Shigematsu M, et al. A long-term comparative study of two rigid internal fixation techniques in terms of masticatory function and neurosensory disturbance after mandibular correction by bilateral sagittal split ramus osteotomy. Int J Oral Maxillofac Surg 2011;40(4):360–5. http://dx.doi.org/10.1016/j.ijom.2010.11.017.

48. Ghali GE, Sikes JW. Intraoral vertical ramus osteotomy as the preferred treatment for mandibular prognathism. J Oral Maxillofac Surg 2000;58(3):313–5.

49. Wolford LM. The sagittal split ramus osteotomy as the preferred treatment for mandibular prognathism. J Oral Maxillofac Surg 2000;58(3):310–2.

50. Bell WH, Yamaguchi Y. Condyle position and mobility before and after intraoral vertical ramus osteotomies and neuromuscular rehabilitation. Int J Adult Orthodon Orthognath Surg 1991;6(2):97–104.

51. Bell WH, Yamaguchi Y, Poor MR. Treatment of temporomandibular joint dysfunction by intraoral vertical ramus osteotomy. Int J Adult Orthodon Orthognath Surg 1990;5(1):9–27.

52. Werther JR, Hall HD, Gibbs SJ. Disk position before and after modified condylotomy in 80 symptomatic temporomandibular joints. Oral Surg Oral Med Oral Pathol Oral Radiol Endod 1995;79(6):668–79.

53. Timmis DP, Aragon SB, Van Sickels JE. Masticatory dysfunction with rigid and nonrigid osteosynthesis of sagittal split osteotomies. Oral Surg Oral Med Oral Pathol 1986;62(2):119–23.

54. Paulus GW, Steinhauser EW. A comparative study of wire osteosynthesis versus bone screws in the treatment of mandibular prognathism. Oral Surg Oral Med Oral Pathol 1982;54(1):2–6.

55. Kawamata A, Fujishita M, Nagahara K, et al. Three-dimensional computed tomography evaluation of postsurgical condylar displacement after mandibular osteotomy. Oral Surg Oral Med Oral Pathol Oral Radiol Endod 1998;85(4):371–6.

56. Ochs MW. Bicortical screw stabilization of sagittal split osteotomies. J Oral Maxillofac Surg 2003;61(12):1477–84.

57. Spitzer W, Rettinger G, Sitzmann F. Computerized tomography examination for the detection of positional changes in the temporomandibular joint after ramus osteotomies with screw fixation. J Maxillofac Surg 1984;12(3):139–42.

58. Wolford LM, Hilliariard FW, Dugan DJ. Surgical treatment objective: systematic approach to the prediction tracing. St Louis (MO): CV Mosby; 1984.

59. Schendel SA, Epker BN. Results after mandibular advancement surgery: an analysis of 87 cases. J Oral Surg 1980;38(4):265–82.

60. Reyneke JP. Essentials of orthognathic surgery. Hanover Park (IL): Quintessence; 2010.

61. Wolford LM, Chemello PD, Hilliard FW. Occlusal plane alteration in orthognathic surgery. J Oral Maxillofac Surg 1993;51(7):730–40. http://dx.doi.org/10.1016/S0278-2391(10)80410-0.

62. Rosen HM. Occlusal plane rotation: aesthetic enhancement in mandibular micrognathia. Plast Reconstr Surg 1993;91(7):1231–40 [discussion: 1241–4].

63. Reyneke JP, Bryant RS, Suuronen R, et al. Postoperative skeletal stability following clockwise and counterclockwise rotation of the maxillomandibular complex compared to conventional orthognathic treatment. Br J Oral Maxillofac Surg 2007;45(1):56–64. http://dx.doi.org/10.1016/j.bjoms.2005.12.015.

64. Perez D, Ellis E. Sequencing bimaxillary surgery: mandible first. J Oral Maxillofac Surg 2011;69(8):2217–24. http://dx.doi.org/10.1016/j.joms.2010.10.053.

65. Turvey T. Sequencing of two-jaw surgery: the case for operating on the maxilla first. J Oral Maxillofac

Surg 2011;69(8):2225. http://dx.doi.org/10.1016/j.joms.2010.10.050.

66. Gunson MJ, Arnett GW, Milam SB. Pathophysiology and pharmacologic control of osseous mandibular condylar resorption. J Oral Maxillofac Surg 2012; 70(8):1918–34. http://dx.doi.org/10.1016/j.joms.2011.07.018.

67. Limchaichana N, Nilsson H, Ekberg EC, et al. Clinical diagnoses and MRI findings in patients with TMD pain. J Oral Rehabil 2007;34(4):237–45. http://dx.doi.org/10.1111/j.1365-2842.2006.01719.x.

68. Briedl JG, Robinson S, Piehslinger E. Correlation between disk morphology on MRI and time curves using electronic axiography. Cranio 2005;23(1):22–9.

69. Tognini F, Manfredini D, Montagnani G, et al. Is clinical assessment valid for the diagnosis of temporomandibular joint disk displacement? Minerva Stomatol 2004;53(7–8):439–48.

70. Katzberg RW, Tallents RH. Normal and abnormal temporomandibular joint disc and posterior attachment as depicted by magnetic resonance imaging in symptomatic and asymptomatic subjects. J Oral Maxillofac Surg 2005;63(8):1155–61. http://dx.doi.org/10.1016/j.joms.2005.04.012.

71. Emshoff R, Rudisch A. Validity of clinical diagnostic criteria for temporomandibular disorders: clinical versus magnetic resonance imaging diagnosis of temporomandibular joint internal derangement and osteoarthrosis. Oral Surg Oral Med Oral Pathol Oral Radiol Endod 2001;91(1):50–5.

72. Hansson LG, Westesson PL, Katzberg RW, et al. MR imaging of the temporomandibular joint: comparison of images of autopsy specimens made at 0.3 T and 1.5 T with anatomic cryosections. AJR Am J Roentgenol 1989;152(6):1241–4. http://dx.doi.org/10.2214/ajr.152.6.1241.

73. Wieners G, Detert J, Streitparth F, et al. High-resolution MRI of the wrist and finger joints in patients with rheumatoid arthritis: comparison of 1.5 Tesla and 3.0 Tesla. Eur Radiol 2007;17(8):2176–82. http://dx.doi.org/10.1007/s00330-006-0539-0.

74. Stehling C, Vieth V, Bachmann R, et al. High-resolution magnetic resonance imaging of the temporomandibular joint: image quality at 1.5 and 3.0 Tesla in volunteers. Invest Radiol 2007;42(6):428–34. http://dx.doi.org/10.1097/01.rli.0000262081.23997.6b.

75. Schmid-Schwap M, Drahanowsky W, Bristela M, et al. Diagnosis of temporomandibular dysfunction syndrome–image quality at 1.5 and 3.0 Tesla magnetic resonance imaging. Eur Radiol 2009;19(5):1239–45. http://dx.doi.org/10.1007/s00330-008-1264-7.

Management of Temporomandibular Joint Ankylosis

Reza Movahed, DMD[a],*, Louis G. Mercuri, DDS, MS[b]

KEYWORDS

- Temporomandibular joint • Ankylosis • Total joint replacement • Autologous fat grafting

KEY POINTS

- Trauma is the most common cause of TMJ ankylosis, followed by infection.
- TJR should be considered as the initial treatment modality for management of TMJ ankylosis.
- The use of patient-fitted or stock prostheses reduces operative time, there is no potential donor site morbidity, and the patient can immediately return to function.
- Consider TJR in children with failed, overgrown, or ankylosed CCG grafts.
- Autologous fat grafting is a very useful adjunct to alloplastic TMJ TJR, which can reduce the chance of heterotopic bone formation around the fossa.

INTRODUCTION

Temporomandibular joint (TMJ) ankylosis is a pathologic condition where the mandible is fused to the fossa by bony or fibrotic tissues. This interferes with mastication, speech, oral hygiene, and normal life activities, and can be potentially life threatening when struggling to acquire an airway in an emergency. Attempting to open the mouth, stretching the periosteum, can also result in pain.[1]

There are multiple factors that can result in TMJ ankylosis, such as trauma, arthritis, infection, previous TMJ surgery, congenital deformities, idiopathic factors,[2] and iatrogenic causes. Trauma is the most common cause of TMJ ankylosis, followed by infection.[3,4] TMJ ankylosis in growing patients can result in dentofacial deformity.[5]

Diagnosis of TMJ ankylosis is usually made by clinical examination and imaging studies, such as plain films, orthopantomograms, computed tomography (CT) scans, MRI, and three-dimensional reconstruction.[6] Sawhney[7] and He

and colleagues[8] proposed classification systems for TMJ ankylosis (**Fig. 1**).

The management goal in TMJ ankylosis is to increase the patient's mandibular function, correct associated facial deformity, decrease pain, and prevent reankylosis. Multiple surgical modalities have been proposed to manage TMJ ankylosis including gap arthroplasty, interpositional arthroplasty, and total joint reconstruction (TJR). Autogenous tissues, such as ear cartilage, temporalis muscle flap, dermis, fat, and bone, have been used or after gap arthroplasty (**Fig. 2**).(refs?) Alloplastic materials, such as Proplast Teflon (Vitek, Houston, TX) and Silastic (Dow, Corning, Midland, MO), have also been used, but with high failure rates.[9–12]

TJR can be divided into autogenous replacement, such as costochondral (CCG) and sternoclavicular grafts (SCG); microvascular reconstruction; or alloplastic replacement (**Fig. 3**).[13–17] CCG has been reported to have unpredictable results in TMJ reconstruction.[18–21] The common postoperative complications include reankylosis, resorption,

[a] Private practice, Orthodontics, Saint Louis University, St Louis, Missouri, USA; [b] Department of Orthopedic Surgery, Rush University Medical Center, West Harrison Street, Chicago, IL 60612, USA
* Corresponding author.
E-mail address: movaheddmd@gmail.com

Oral Maxillofacial Surg Clin N Am 27 (2015) 27–35
http://dx.doi.org/10.1016/j.coms.2014.09.003
1042-3699/15/$ – see front matter © 2015 Elsevier Inc. All rights reserved.

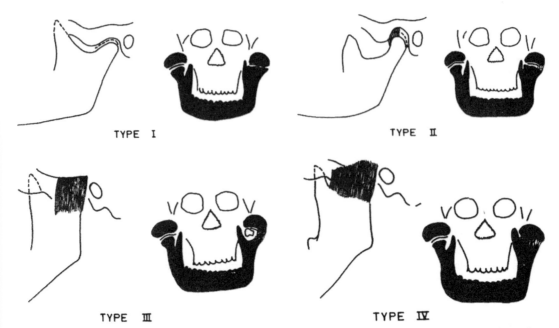

TYPE I

TYPE II

TYPE III

TYPE IV

Fig. 1. (*Type I*) The head was flattened or deformed by lying closely approximated to the upper articular surface. There were dense fibrous adhesions all around the joint, making movement impossible. This probably followed a comminuted fracture of the head of the mandible. (*Type II*) The head was misshaped or flattened, but it was still distinguishable and lay in close approximation to the articular surface. There was, however, bony fusion of the head to the outer edge of articular surface either anteriorly or posteriorly, but this was limited to a small area. Deeper to it, the upper articular surface and the articular disk were undamaged. This probably followed a severe comminuted fracture of the head with associated partial damage to the upper articular surface. (*Type III*) A bony block was seen to bridge across the ramus of the mandible and the zygomatic arch. The upper articular surface and the articular disk on deeper aspect were intact. The displaced head was seen to be atrophic and lying either free or fused with the medial side of the upper end of the ramus. This probably followed a severe injury producing fracture dislocation of the head and neck of the mandible and laceration of capsular ligaments. (*Type IV*) The bony block was wide and deep and extended between the ramus and the upper articular surface, completely replacing the architecture of the joint. This perhaps followed fracture of the neck of the mandible with dislocation of the head and associated injury to the capsular ligaments, articular disk, and even the upper articular surface. This was the most common presentation. (*From* Sawhney CP. Bony ankylosis of the temporomandibular joint: follow-up of 70 patients treated with arthroplasty and acrylic spacer interposition. Plast Reconstr Surg 1986;77(1):32; with permission.)

overgrowth,[22,23] fracture, and pain. SCGs have growth potential similar to the mandibular condyle and a section of the SCG articular disk can be harvested with the SCG providing the potential for improved function.[16] Distraction osteogenesis has also been used to manage TMJ ankylosis with release of ankylosis before and after the distraction process.[24] However, harvesting complications and questionable long-term outcomes must be taken into consideration.

The use of patient-fitted or stock prostheses[11,25,26] reduces operative time, there is no potential donor site morbidity, and the patient can immediately return to function.[27] The disadvantages include cost, difficulty in correction of significant dentofacial deformities, potential material wear, and failure.[28] TMJ TJR is thought to be

more costly than autogenous tissue for TMJ reconstruction, but the extra operating room time, personnel, and resources must be considered in the latter scenarios. Also, in view of the potential for increased autogenous tissue donor site morbidity resulting in an increased length of hospital stay and the unpredictable nature of the results of autogenous tissue grafting, the economic impact of TMJ TJR is likely less overall. Furthermore, because patient-fitted TMJ TJR components are designed "made to fit," manipulation and implantation time are reduced.

In contrast, with stock TMJ TJR components, the surgeon must "make them fit," requiring increased time and incurring added expense. Wolford and colleagues[29] performed a 5-year follow-up of the TMJ Concepts/Techmedica

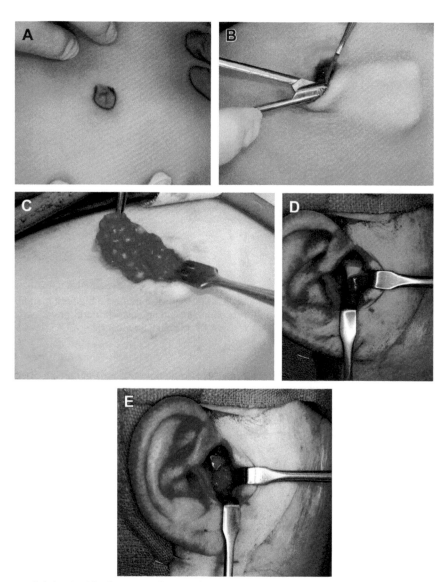

Fig. 2. Images of abdominal fat harvest technique. (*A*) Marked periumbilical incision for harvest of abdominal fat graft. (*B*) Undermining of skin and fat before harvest. (*C*) Composite harvest of abdominal fat. (*D*) Exposure of graft site for circumferential augmentation of fat graft. (*E*) Adaptation of fat graft before closure. (*Courtesy of* Larry Wolford, DMD, Dallas, TX.)

patient-fitted total joint prosthesis (TMJ Concepts Inc., Ventura, CA) with good results. Mercuri and colleagues[30,31] presented a 9- and 14-year follow-up of the same prostheses with good outcomes.

A basic surgical protocol to address TMJ ankylosis is as follows: release the ankylosed joint; remove the heterotopic and reactive bone with thorough debridement (gap arthroplasty of at least 2.0–2.5 cm), replace the TMJ with a patient-fitted total joint prosthesis, place a fat graft around the articulation area of the prosthesis, and perform indicated orthognathic surgery in a single

operation.[32–38] Wolford first used this specific surgical protocol for treatment of TMJ ankylosis in 1992.[35] The basic protocol can also be performed in two or more surgical stages depending on the surgeon's skills, experience, and preference.

TREATMENT OF TEMPOROMANDIBULAR JOINT ANKYLOSIS WITH COSTOCHONDRAL GRAFT

The traditional management of complete bony TMJ ankylosis has been gap arthroplasty and autogenous tissue grafting (**Fig. 4**). Although this

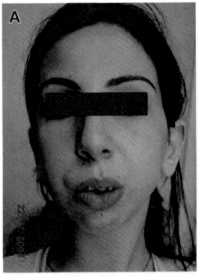
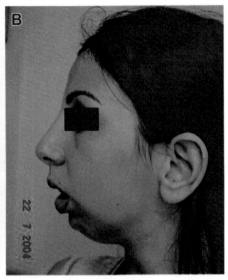

Fig. 3. (*A, B*) A 20-year-old woman, bilateral TMJ ankylosis status post prepubertal bilateral mandibular condyle fractures. Has had five prior unsuccessful bilateral procedures including costochondral grafts twice, temporalis muscle flaps twice, and coronoidectomies. (*Courtesy of* Dr Michael Bowler, Newcastle, New South Wales, Australia.)

restores form, function is delayed, and therefore potentially compromised. This is the case when autogenous bone grafts are used because of the fear that allowing function of the mandible during the graft incorporation period will cause the graft to fail to vascularize properly. In the patient with re-ankylosis, placing autogenous tissue, such as bone, into an area where reactive or heterotopic bone is forming intuitively makes no sense. Orthopedic surgeons always opt for alloplastic joint replacement in similar situations.[36]

It has been reported that capillaries can penetrate a maximum thickness of 180 to 220/μm of tissue, whereas scar tissue surrounding a previously operated joint averages 440/μm in thickness.[27]

This may account for the clinical observation that autogenous tissue grafts, such as CCG and SCG, fail in the patient who has undergone multiple operations. Autogenous grafts require a rich vascular host site to survive. The scar tissue that is found in the patient who has undergone multiple operations does not provide an environment conducive to the predictable success of an autogenous tissue graft.

TEMPOROMANDIBULAR JOINT ANKYLOSIS IN GROWING SUBJECTS

Classically, pathologic, developmental, and functional disorders affecting the TMJ in growing

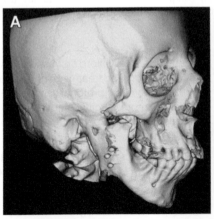
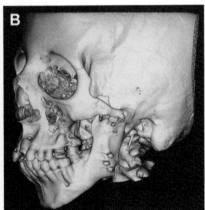

Fig. 4. (*A, B*) Three-dimensional CT scans of patient in **Fig. 2** demonstrating bilateral complete bony TMJ ankylosis. (*Courtesy of* Dr Michael Bowler, Newcastle, New South Wales, Australia.)

patients have been reconstructed with auto-genous tissues. Autogenous CCGs are re-ported as the gold standard for these TMJ reconstructions.[37–41]

In theory, in growing patients, autogenous (eg, costochondral) allografts "grow with the patient." However, often this so-called growth potential has been reported to be unpredictable or to result in ankylosis. These complications can occur either as the result of the allograft and/or fixation failure or because of the uncooperative nature of the young patient with physical therapy after reconstruction.[15,37,38,42,43]

Recent studies have even questioned the necessity for using a cartilaginous graft to restore and maintain mandibular growth.[44,45] Long-term reports of mandibular growth in children whose TMJs were reconstructed with CCG show that excessive growth on the treated side occurred in 54% of the 72 cases examined and growth equal to that on the opposite side occurred in only 38% of the cases.[46–51] Furthermore, Pelto-mäki and colleagues,[52–55] in an investigation of mandibular growth after CCG, supported previous experiments with regard to the inability of the graft to adapt to the growth velocity of the new environment.

Based on the problems that have been reported with CCG TMJ TJR in children, such as graft fail-ure, unpredictable growth, ankylosis, and potential for donor-site morbidity, and the orthopedic expe-rience and success reported with alloplastic TJR in improving the quality of life of growing patients with severe anatomic and functional joint disor-ders, it seems reasonable to consider examining the feasibility of alloplastic TMJ TJR for the following conditions in children: (1) high inflamma-tory TMJ arthritis unresponsive to other modalities of treatment; (2) recurrent fibrosis and/or bony ankylosis unresponsive to other modalities of treatment; (3) failed tissue grafts (bone and soft tis-sue); and (4) loss of vertical mandibular height and/or occlusal relationship because of bony resorp-tion, trauma, developmental abnormalities, or pathologic lesions.

To continue to reoperate in children with failed, overgrown, or ankylosed CCG with either bony or soft tissue replacements (or both), using the same modalities that failed when there may be an appropriate solution available, seems myopic. These patients are better off undergoing allo-plastic TMJ TJR knowing that, depending on growth, revision and/or replacement surgery may likely be required in the future, rather than incurring continued failures of CCG that will also likely require further surgical intervention in the future.[53]

TREATMENT OF TEMPOROMANDIBULAR JOINT ANKYLOSIS WITH TOTAL JOINT RECONSTRUCTION

For the patient with reankylosis, placing autoge-nous tissue, such as bone, into an area where reactive or heterotopic bone is forming intuitively makes no sense. None of the textbooks of ortho-pedic surgery or any journal articles published recently discuss the use of autogenous bone in the reconstruction of any joint of a nongrowing patient affected by ankylotic disease. Alloplastic joint replacement is the recommended manage-ment modality in orthopedics when total joint replacement is required in such cases.[56,57]

In light of the biologic considerations and the orthopedic experience, total alloplastic replace-ment should be considered in the management of recurrent fibrosis and bony ankylosis involving the TMJ.

The protocol CT scan used to generate the stereolithic model from which patient-fitted TMJ TJR components are designed and manufactured has been reported to have a mean dimensional accuracy of 97.9%. Therefore, in the case of anky-losis/reankylosis a two-staged protocol is required when using a patient-fitted TMJ TJR system.[58]

At stage 1 surgery, the surgeon must remove the ankylotic bone, create an adequate gap (2–2.5 cm), and place a material spacer to prevent the reformation of tissue and/or bone (**Fig. 5**).[59] The patient must be placed into maxillomandibular fixation to prevent movement of the spacer or change in bony architecture and/or occlusion.

A postoperative protocol CT scan is then made and the stereolithic model developed. Patient-fitted TMJ TJR components are designed and manufactured from that model to the specific anatomic circumstances of that case.

At stage 2 surgery, the spacer is removed and the patient-fitted TMJ TJR components are fixated. An autogenous abdominal fat graft is placed around the articulation to inhibit formation of heterotopic bone and development of reankylo-sis.[60] The patient can then begin immediate, active postoperative physical therapy. If necessary concomitant orthognathic surgery can be done during this stage to correct any associated dento-facial deformities.

Pearce and colleagues[61] described the use of preoperatively created templates to obviate the two-stage protocol described previously. Many surgeons agree that to realize all of the benefits afforded by a patient-fitted TMJ TJR device, the best fit for the components is achieved and ensured by using the two-stage protocol. The concern often raised about maintaining

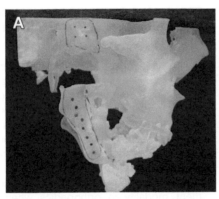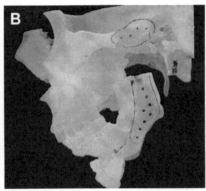

Fig. 5. (*A, B*) Stereolaser design models (ProtoMED, Westminster, CO) following stage 1 bilateral gap arthroplasties, insertion of spacer, and advancement genioplasty of patient in **Fig. 2**. (*Courtesy of* Dr Michael Bowler, Newcastle, New South Wales, Australia.)

maxillomandibular fixation between stages is moot because patients with ankylosis cannot open their mouths before the first-stage procedure.

One-stage surgeries could also be considered but require a more experienced surgeon that can reproduce the stereolithic surgery in the patient to make the prosthesis fit. The benefit includes one surgery for the patient and immediate function with easier and faster rehabilitation (see **Fig. 3**).

IMPORTANCE OF FAT GRAFT IN PREVENTION OF HETEROTOPIC BONE FORMATION

The first reported use of autologous fat graft placement into the TMJ for the treatment of ankylosis was by Blair[62] in 1913 followed by Murphy[63] in 1914. No other references appear in the literature

until the 1990s. In 1992, Wolford developed the technique of placing autogenous fat grafts around the TMJ Concepts to prevent postsurgical heterotopic bone and fibrosis development (**Fig. 3**). The rationale for placing autologous fat grafts around the TMJ TJR was to obliterate the dead space around the joint prosthesis, thus preventing the formation and subsequent organization of a blood clot. Creating this physical barrier serves to minimize the presence of pluripotential cells, and prevents the formation of extensive fibrosis and heterotopic calcification. The fat grafts may be inhibitory to heterotopic bone formation. It may also isolate any residual reactive tissue from previous alloplastic failure or disease to the periphery of the region, minimizing its formation around the joint components (**Fig. 3**).

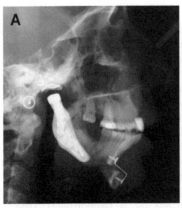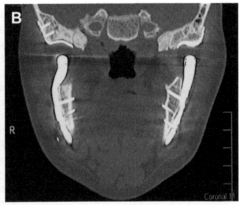

Fig. 6. (*A, B*) Lateral cephalometric and coronal CT post stage 2 implantation of TMJ Concepts (Ventura, CA) patient-fitted prostheses in patient in **Fig. 2**. The articulating aspect of the fossa component is ultra-high molecular weight polyethylene, therefore it is radiolucent. (*Courtesy of* Dr Michael Bowler, Newcastle, New South Wales, Australia.)

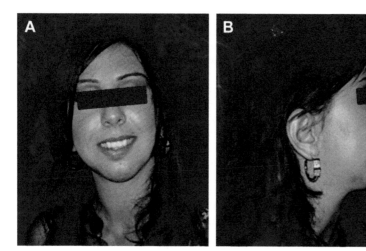
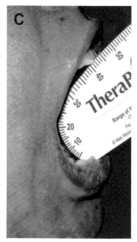

Fig. 7. (*A, C*) The patient in **Fig. 2** after dental rehabilitation, 5 years post bilateral TMJ Concepts patient-fitted replacements. (*A*) Post-surgery frontal view. (*B*) Post-surgery profile view. (*C*) Post-surgery maximum incisal opening of 42 mm with out pain. (*Courtesy of* Dr Michael Bowler, Newcastle, New South Wales, Australia.)

Wolford and Karras[35] published the first study evaluating fat grafts placed around TMJ total joint prostheses. Fifteen patients with 22 joints underwent TMJ reconstruction with TMJ Concepts/Techmedica patient-fitted TMJ TJR devices with autologous fat harvested from the abdomen packed around the articulating portion of the prostheses. There was no radiographic or clinical evidence of heterotopic calcifications in any of the fat grafted group, whereas seven control patients without fat grafts (35%) developed heterotopic bone and required reoperation. This initial study proved that autologous fat transplantation was a useful adjunct to alloplastic TMJ TJR by minimizing the occurrence of joint fibrosis and heterotopic calcification (see **Fig. 2**).

Mercuri and colleagues[60] evaluated 20 patients with 33 reankylosed TMJs managed with patient-fitted TMJ TJR devices and placement of periarticular autogenous abdominal fat grafts. Mean follow-up was 50.4 months. Results showed 52% reduction in pain, and improvement in jaw function (76%), diet (72%), and maximum incisal opening (MIO) (140%) from 11.75 mm to 32.9 mm, whereas 17 of 20 patients (85%) reported improvement in quality-of-life scores.

Autologous fat grafting is a useful adjunct to alloplastic TMJ TJR and may prove to be similarly beneficial in autologous TMJ TJR. Graft procurement is relatively quick and easy, with minimal morbidity.[35,36] The most common complication found in the donor area was seroma or hematoma, which was treated with aspiration and pressure dressing. TMJ reconstruction with TMJ Concepts total joint prostheses and autogenous fat grafts

provides a highly predictable treatment method for patients with nonsalvageable TMJ pathology.

REFERENCES

1. Roychoudhury A, Parkash H, Trikha A. Functional restoration by gap arthroplasty in temporomandibular joint ankylosis: a report of 50 cases. Oral Surg Oral Med Oral Pathol 1999;87:166–9.
2. Erol B, Tanrikulu R, GoÅNrgün B. A clinical study on ankylosis of the temporomandibular joint. J Craniomaxillofac Surg 2006;34:100.
3. Lello GE. Surgical correction of temporomandibular joint ankylosis. J Craniomaxillofac Surg 1990;18:19.
4. Topazian RG. Etiology of ankylosis of temporomandibular joint: analysis of 44 cases. J Oral Surg Anesth Hosp Dent Serv 1964;22:227.
5. Miyamoto H, Kurita K, Ogi N, et al. The role of the disk in sheep temporomandibular joint ankylosis. Oral Surg Oral Med Oral Pathol 1999;88:151–8.
6. Spijkervet FK, de Bont LG, Boering G. Management of pseudoankylosis of the temporomandibular joint: report of cases. J Oral Maxillofac Surg 1994;52:1211–7.
7. Sawhney CP. Bony ankylosis of the temporomandibular joint: follow-up of 70 patients treated with arthroplasty and acrylic spacer interposition. Plast Reconstr Surg 1986;77(1):29–40.
8. He D, Yang C, Chen M, et al. Traunatic temporomandibular joint ankylosis: our classification and treatment experience. J Oral Maxillofac Surg 2011;69:1600–7.
9. Wolford LM, Henry CH, Nikaein A, et al. The temporomandibular joint alloplastic implant problem. In: Sessle BJ, Bryant PS, Dionne RA, editors.

Temporomandibular disorders and related pain conditions. Seattle (WA): IASP Press; 1995. p. 443–7.

10. Wolford LM. Temporomandibular joint devices: treatment factors and outcomes. Oral Surg Oral Med Oral Pathol Oral Radiol Endod 1997;83:143–9.

11. Wolford LM, Cottrell DA, Henry CH. Temporomandibular joint reconstruction of the complex patient with the Techmedica custom-made total joint prosthesis. J Oral Maxillofac Surg 1994;52:2–10.

12. Henry CH, Wolford LM. Treatment outcomes for TMJ reconstruction after Proplast-Teflon implant failure. J Oral Maxillofac Surg 1993;51:352–8.

13. Matukas VJ, Szvmela VF, Schmidt JF. Surgical treatment of bony ankylosis in a child using a composite cartilage-bone iliac crest graft. J Oral Surg 1980;38:903.

14. Dingman RO, Grabb WG. Reconstruction of both mandibular condyles with metatarsal bone grafts. Plast Reconstr Surg 1964;34:441.

15. MacIntosh RB, Henny FA. A spectrum of application of autogenous costochondral grafts. J Maxillofac Surg 1977;5:257–67.

16. Wolford LM, Cottrell DA, Henry CH. Sternoclavicular grafts for temporomandibular joint reconstruction. J Oral Maxillofac Surg 1994;52:119–28.

17. Potter JK, Dierks EJ. Vascularized options for reconstruction of the mandibular condyle. Semin Plast Surg 2008;22(3):156–60.

18. Posnick JC, Goldstein JA. Surgical management of temporomandibular joint ankylosis in the pediatric population. Plast Reconstr Surg 1993;91:791.

19. Pensler JM, Christopher RD, Bewyer DC. Correction of micrognathia with ankylosis of the temporomandibular joint in childhood. Plast Reconstr Surg 1933;91:799.

20. Lindquist C, Pihakari A, Tasanen A, et al. Autogenous costochondral grafts in temporomandibular joint arthroplasty: a surgery of 66 arthroplasties in 60 patients. J Maxillofac Surg 1986;14:143.

21. Munro IR, Chen YR, Park BY. Simultaneous total correction of temporomandibular ankylosis and facial asymmetry. Plast Reconstr Surg 1986;77:517.

22. Perrot DH, Kaban LB. Temporomandibular joint ankylosis in children. Oral Maxillofac Surg Clin North Am 1994;6:187.

23. Kaban LB, Perrot DH, Fisher K. A protocol for management of temporomandibular joint ankylosis. J Oral Maxillofac Surg 1990;48:11.

24. Li J, Zhu S, Wang T, et al. Staged treatment of temporomandibular joint ankylosis with micrognathia using mandibular osteodistraction and advancement genioplasty. J Oral Maxillofac Surg 2012; 70(12):2884–92.

25. Granquist EJ, Quinn PD. Total reconstruction of the temporomandibular joint with a stock prosthesis. Atlas Oral Maxillofac Surg Clin North Am 2011;19: 221–32.

26. Mercuri LG, Wolford LM, Sanders B, et al. Custom CAD/CAM total temporomandibular joint reconstruction system: preliminary multicenter report. J Oral Maxillofac Surg 1995;53:106–15.

27. Mercuri LG. Alloplastic temporomandibular joint reconstruction. Oral Surg Oral Med Oral Pathol 1998;85:631.

28. Loveless TP, Bjornland T, Dodson TB, et al. Efficacy of temporomandibular joint ankylosis surgical treatment. J Oral Maxillofac Surg 2010;68:1276–82.

29. Wolford LM, Pitta MC, Reiche-Fischel O, et al. TMJ concepts/techmedica custom-made TMJ total joint prosthesis: 5-year follow-up study. Int J Oral Maxillofac Surg 2003;32:268.

30. Mercuri LG, Wolford LM, Sanders B, et al. Long-term follow-up of the CAD/CAM patient fitted total temporomandibular joint reconstruction system. J Oral Maxillofac Surg 2002;60:1440–8.

31. Mercuri LG, Edibam NR, Giobbie-Hurder A. Fourteen-year follow-up of a patient-fitted total temporomandibular joint reconstruction system. J Oral Maxillofac Surg 2007;65:1140–8.

32. Wolford LM. Concomitant temporomandibular joint and orthognathic surgery. J Oral Maxillofac Surg 2003;61:1198–204.

33. Wolford LM, Pinto LP, Cardenas LE, et al. Outcomes of treatment with custom-made temporomandibular joint total joint prostheses and maxillomandibular counter-clockwise rotation. Proc (Bayl Univ Med Cent) 2008;21:18–24.

34. Wolford LM. Clinical indications for simultaneous TMJ and orthognathic surgery. Cranio 2007;25: 273–82.

35. Wolford LM, Karras SC. Autologous fat transplantation around temporomandibular joint total joint prostheses: preliminary treatment outcomes. J Oral Maxillofac Surg 1997;55:245–51.

36. Petty W, editor. Total joint replacement. Philadelphia: Saunders; 1991.

37. Ware WH, Taylor RC. Cartilaginous growth centers transplanted to replace mandibular condyles in monkeys. J Oral Surg 1966;24:33.

38. Ware WH, Brown SL. Growth center transplantation to replace mandibular condyles. J Maxillofac Surg 1981;9:50.

39. Poswillo DE. Biological reconstruction of the mandibular condyle. Br J Oral Maxillofac Surg 1987;25:100.

40. MacIntosh RB. Current spectrum of costochondral grafting. In: Bell WH, editor. Surgical correction of dentofacial deformities: new concepts, vol. III. Philadelphia: Saunders; 1985. p. 355–410.

41. MacIntosh RB. The use of autogenous tissue in temporomandibular joint reconstruction. J Oral Maxillofac Surg 2000;58:63.

42. Obeid G, Gutterman SA, Connole PW. Costochondral grafting in condylar replacement and

mandibular reconstruction. J Oral Maxillofac Surg 1988;48:177.

43. Samman N, Cheung LK, Tideman H. Overgrowth of a costochondral graft in an adult male. Int J Oral Maxillofac Surg 1995;24:333.

44. Ellis E, Schneiderman ED, Carlson DS. Growth of the mandible after replacement of the mandibular condyle: an experimental investigation in Macaca mulatta. J Oral Maxillofac Surg 2002;60:1461.

45. Guyot L, Richard O, Layoun W, et al. Long-term radiological findings following reconstruction of the condyle with fibular free flaps. J Craniomaxillofac Surg 2004;32:98.

46. Guyuron B, Lasa CI. Unpredictable growth pattern of costochondral graft. Plast Reconstr Surg 1992; 90:880.

47. Marx RE. The science and art of reconstructing the jaws and temporomandibular joints. In: Bell WH, editor. Modern practice in orthognathic and reconstructive surgery, vol. 2. Philadelphia: Saunders; 1992. p. 1448.

48. Perrot DH, Umeda H, Kaban LB. Costochondral graft/reconstruction of the condyle/ramus unit: long-term follow-up. Int J Oral Maxillofac Surg 1994;23:321.

49. Svensson A, Adell R. Costochondral grafts to replace mandibular condyles in juvenile chronic arthritis patients: long-term effects on facial growth. J Craniomaxillofac Surg 1998;26:275.

50. Ross RB. Costochondral grafts replacing the mandibular condyle. Cleft Palate Craniofac J 1999;36:334.

51. Wen-Ching K, Huang CS, Chen YR. Temporomandibular joint reconstruction in children using costochondral grafts. J Oral Maxillofac Surg 1999;57:789.

52. Peltomäki T, Vähätalo K, Rönning O. The effect of a unilateral costochondral graft on the growth of the marmoset mandible. J Oral Maxillofac Surg 2002; 60:1307.

53. Peltomäki T, Rönning O. Interrelationship between size and tissue-separating potential of costochondral transplants. Eur J Orthod 1991;13:459.

54. Peltomäki T. Growth of a costochondral graft in the rat temporomandibular joint. J Oral Maxillofac Surg 1992;50:851.

55. Mercuri LG, Swift JQ. Considerations for the use of alloplastic temporomandibular joint replacement in the growing patient. J Oral Maxillofac Surg 2009; 67:1979–90.

56. Skinner HB. Current diagnosis and treatment in orthopedics. 2nd edition. New York: Lang Medical Books; McGraw-Hill; 2000.

57. Chapman MW. Chapman's orthopaedic surgery. 3rd edition. Philadelphia: Lippincott Williams & Wilkins; 2001.

58. Mercuri LG. Alloplastic TMJ replacement. Rationale for custom devices. Int J Oral Maxillofac Surg 2012;41:1033–40.

59. Pitta MC, Wolford LM. Use of acrylic spheres as spacers in staged temporomandibular joint surgery. J Oral Maxillofac Surg 2001;59:704–6.

60. Mercuri LG, Alcheikh Ali F, Woolson R. Outcomes of total alloplastic replacement with peri-articular autogenous fat grafting for management of re-ankylosis of the temporomandibular joint. J Oral Maxillofac Surg 2008;66:1794–803.

61. Pearce CS, Cooper C, Speculand B. One stage management of ankylosis of the temporomandibular joint with a custom-made total joint replacement system. Br J Oral Maxillofac Surg 2009;47: 530–4.

62. Blair VP. Operative treatment of ankylosis of the mandible. Trans South Surg Assoc 1913;28:435.

63. Murphy JB. Arthroplasty for intra-articular bony and fibrous ankylosis of the temporomandibular articulation. J Am Med Assoc 1914;62:1783.

Protocol for Concomitant Temporomandibular Joint Custom-fitted Total Joint Reconstruction and Orthognathic Surgery Using Computer-assisted Surgical Simulation

Reza Movahed, DMD[a],*, Larry M. Wolford, DMD[b]

KEYWORDS

- Temporomandibular joint • Total joint reconstruction • Orthognathic surgery
- Computer-assisted surgical simulation

KEY POINTS

- Combined orthognathic and total joint reconstruction cases can be predictably performed in 1 stage.
- Use of virtual surgical planning can eliminate a significant time requirement in preparation of concomitant orthognathic and temporomandibular joint (TMJ) prostheses cases.
- The concomitant TMJ and orthognathic surgery–computer-assisted surgical simulation technique increases the accuracy of combined cases.
- In order to have flexibility in positioning of the total joint prosthesis, recontouring of the lateral aspect of the rami is advantageous.

INTRODUCTION

Clinicians who address temporomandibular joint (TMJ) disorders and dentofacial deformities surgically can perform the surgery in 1 stage or 2 separate stages. The 2-stage approach requires the patient to undergo 2 separate operations and anesthesia, significantly prolonging the overall treatment. However, performing concomitant TMJ and orthognathic surgery (CTOS) in these cases requires careful treatment planning and surgical proficiency in the two surgical areas. This article presents a new treatment protocol for the application of computer-assisted surgical simulation (CASS) in CTOS cases requiring reconstruction with patient-fitted total joint prostheses. The traditional and new CTOS protocols are described and compared. The new CTOS protocol helps decrease the preoperative work-up time and increase the accuracy of model surgery.

INDICATIONS

TMJ disorders and dentofacial deformities commonly coexist. The TMJ disorders may be the causative factor of the jaw deformity, or develop as a result of the jaw deformity, or the two entities may develop independently of each other. The

[a] Orthodontics, Saint Louis University, 40 North Kingshighway Boulevard, Apartment 16A, Saint Louis, MO 63108, USA; [b] Departments of Oral and Maxillofacial Surgery and Orthodontics Texas, A&M University Health Science Center Baylor College of Dentistry, Baylor University Medical Center, 3409 Worth St. Suite 400, Dallas, TX 75246, USA
* Corresponding author.
E-mail address: movaheddmd@gmail.com

Oral Maxillofacial Surg Clin N Am 27 (2015) 37–45
http://dx.doi.org/10.1016/j.coms.2014.09.004
1042-3699/15/$ – see front matter © 2015 Elsevier Inc. All rights reserved.

oralmaxsurgery.theclinics.com

most common TMJ disorders that can adversely affect jaw position, occlusion, and orthognathic surgical outcomes include (1) articular disc dislocation, (2) adolescent internal condylar resorption, (3) reactive arthritis, (4) condylar hyperplasia, (5) ankylosis, (6) congenital deformation or absence of the TMJ, (7) connective tissue and autoimmune diseases, (8) trauma, and (9) other end-stage TMJ disorders.[1] These TMJ conditions are often associated with dentofacial deformities, malocclusion, TMJ pain, headaches, myofascial pain, TMJ and jaw functional impairment, ear symptoms, and sleep apnea. Patients with these conditions may benefit from corrective surgical intervention, including TMJ and orthognathic surgery. Some of the aforementioned TMJ disorders may have the best outcome prognosis using custom-fitted total joint prostheses for TMJ reconstruction.

Using traditional model surgery and treatment planning techniques exposes the outcome to its own subset of error margin. As a result, CTOS requires experience and expertise.

Over the past decade, CASS technology has been integrated into many maxillofacial surgical applications,[2,3] including dentofacial deformities, congenital deformities, defects after tumor ablation, posttraumatic defects, reconstruction of cranial defects,[4] and reconstruction of the TMJ.[5] CASS technology can improve surgical accuracy, provide intermediate and final surgical splints, and decrease surgeons' time input for presurgical preparation compared with traditional methods of case preparation.[6]

PROTOCOL FOR TRADITIONAL CONCOMITANT TEMPOROMANDIBULAR JOINT AND ORTHOGNATHIC SURGERY

Treatment planning for CTOS cases is based on prediction tracing, clinical evaluation, and dental models, which provide the template for movements of the upper and lower jaws to establish optimal treatment outcome in relation to function, facial harmony, occlusion, and oropharyngeal airway dimensions. For patients who require total joint prostheses, a computed tomography (CT) scan is acquired of the maxillofacial region that includes the TMJs, maxilla, and mandible with 1-mm overlapping cuts. Using these CT scan data, a stereolithic model is fabricated, with the mandible as a separate piece.

Using the original cephalometric tracing and prediction tracing (**Fig. 1**A), the mandible on the stereolithic model is placed into its future predetermined position using the planned measurements for correction of mandibular anteroposterior and vertical positions, pitch, yaw, and roll (see **Fig. 1**). The mandible is stabilized to the maxilla with quick-cure acrylic. Many patients with temporomandibular disorders requiring concomitant orthognathic surgery benefit from counterclockwise rotation of the maxillomandibular complex, which requires the development of posterior open bites on the model (see **Fig. 1**B). Because the mandibular position on the stereolithic models is established using hands-on measurements, the operator's manual dexterity and three-dimensional perspective play critical roles in setting the mandible in its proper and final position. This step can predispose the planning process to a certain margin of error.

The next step requires the preparation of the lateral aspect of the rami and fossae (**Fig 2**A, B) for fabrication of the patient-fitted total joint prostheses. The goal of this step is to recontour the lateral ramus to a flat surface in the area where the mandibular component will be placed. The fossa requires recontouring only if heterotopic bone or unusual anatomy is present. The recontouring areas are marked in red for duplication of bone removal at surgery. Because most patients

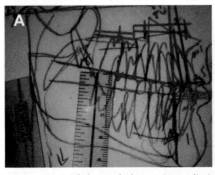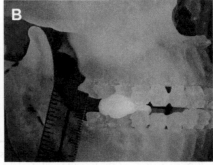

Fig. 1. (*A*) Measurement of the cephalometric prediction tracing for the amount of open bite produced at the second molar after counterclockwise rotation of the mandible into its final position. (*B*) Duplication of the measurement obtained from the prediction tracing to the final mandibular position on the stereolithic model and fixating the mandible to the maxilla with methylmethacrylate. (*From* Movahed R, Teschke M, Wolford LM. Protocol for concomitant temporomandibular joint custom-fitted total joint reconstruction and orthognathic surgery utilizing computer-assisted surgical simulation. J Oral Maxillofac Surg 2013;71(12):2124; with permission.)

with TMJ problems requiring CTOS can benefit from counterclockwise rotation of the maxillomandibular complex, the stereolithic model is likely to be set with posterior open bites, because the maxilla is maintained in its original position.

Once the stereolithic model is finalized, the model is sent to TMJ Concepts (Ventura, CA) to perform the design, blueprint, and wax-up of the custom-fitted total joint prostheses (see **Fig. 2**C), with the design and wax-up sent to the surgeon for approval before manufacture of the prostheses. The period from CT acquisition to the manufacturer's completion of the custom-fitted prostheses is approximately 8 weeks. The surgical procedures are then performed on articulator-mounted dental models. The mandible is repositioned on the articulator, duplicating the movements performed on the stereolithic model, and the intermediate splint is constructed. The maxillary model is repositioned, segmented if indicated, and placed into the maximal occlusal fit. Then, the palatal splint is constructed.

CASS technology and moving the maxilla and mandible into their final position in a computer-simulated environment (**Fig. 3**). Using the computer simulation, the anteroposterior and vertical positions, pitch, yaw, and roll are accurately finalized for the maxilla and mandible based on clinical evaluation, dental models, prediction tracing, and computer-simulation analysis.

Using Digital Imaging and Communications in Medicine (DICOM) data, the stereolithic model is produced with the maxilla and mandible in the final position and provided to the surgeon for removal of the condyles and recontouring of the lateral rami and fossae if indicated (**Fig. 4**A). The stereolithic model is sent to TMJ Concepts for the design, blueprint, and wax-up of the prostheses. Using the Internet, the design is sent to the surgeon for approval. The custom-fitted total joint prostheses are then manufactured (see **Fig. 4**B). It takes approximately 8 weeks to manufacture the total joint custom-fitted prostheses.

Protocol for traditional CTOS preparation

- CT scan including the entire mandible, maxilla, and TMJs
- Fabrication of stereolithic model with the mandible separated
- Surgeon positions the mandible in its final position and fixates it
- Removal of condyles and recontouring the lateral aspect of the rami and fossae if indicated
- Model sent to TMJ Concepts for prostheses design, blueprint, and wax-up
- Approval of total joint prostheses blueprint and wax-up by the surgeon
- Manufacture of custom-fitted total joint prostheses
- Prostheses sent to hospital for surgical implantation

Protocol for traditional CTOS intermediate and palatal splint fabrication

- Acquisition of dental models
- Mounting maxillary and mandibular dental models on an articulator
- Repositioning the mandibular dental model, duplicating the positional changes acquired on the stereolithic model
- Fabrication of intermediate splint
- Repositioning maxillary dental models with segmentation if indicated
- Construction of palatal splint
- Ready for surgery

PROTOCOL FOR CONCOMITANT TEMPOROMANDIBULAR JOINT AND ORTHOGNATHIC SURGERY USING COMPUTER-ASSISTED SURGICAL SIMULATION

For CTOS cases, the orthognathic surgery is planned using Medical Modeling (Golden, CO)

Approximately 2 weeks before surgery, the final dental models are produced, including 2 maxillary models if the maxilla is to be segmented or dental equilibration is required. One of the maxillary models is segmented if indicated, dental equilibration is performed, and the segments are placed in the best occlusion fit with the mandibular dentition and maxillary segments fixed to each other. The dental

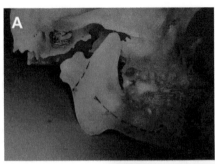
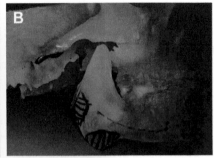
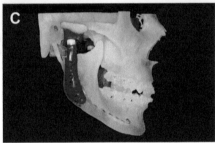

Fig. 2. (*A*) Marking the condylectomy osteotomy and the irregularities of the fossa. (*B*) The stereolithic model after condylectomy and recontouring of the fossae and rami (marked in *red*). (*C*) This stereolithic model demonstrates a prosthesis wax-up for approval by the surgeon. (*From* Movahed R, Teschke M, Wolford LM. Protocol for concomitant temporomandibular joint custom-fitted total joint reconstruction and orthognathic surgery utilizing computer-assisted surgical simulation. J Oral Maxillofac Surg 2013;71(12):2125; with permission.)

models do not require mounting on an articulator. The 3 or 4 models (2 maxillary and 1 mandibular, or 2 mandibular models if equilibrations are done) are sent to Medical Modeling for scanning and simulation into the computer model. Because the authors routinely perform the TMJ reconstruction and mandibular advancement with the TMJ Concepts total joint prosthesis first, the unsegmented maxillary model is simulated into the original maxillary position and the mandible is maintained in the final position. The intermediate splint is constructed (see **Fig. 3**B), and then the segmented maxillary model is simulated into the computer model in its final position, with the maxilla and mandible placed into the best occlusal fit, and the palatal splint is fabricated. The dental models, splints, and images of the computer-simulated surgery are sent to the surgeon for implementation during surgery.

Protocol for CTOS using CASS

- CT scan of entire mandible, maxilla, and TMJs (1-mm overlapping cuts)
- Processing of DICOM data to create a computer model in the CASS environment
- Correction of dentofacial deformity, including final positioning of the maxilla and mandible, with computer-simulated surgery
- Stereolithic model constructed with jaws in final position and sent to surgeon for condylectomy and rami and fossae recontouring if indicated
- Model sent to TMJ Concepts for prostheses design, blueprint, and wax-up
- Surgeon evaluation and approval using the Internet
- TMJ prostheses manufactured and sent to hospital for surgical implantation
- Two weeks before surgery, acquisition of final dental models (2 maxillary, 1 or 2 mandibular models if dental equilibrations are required); 1 maxillary model is segmented and models equilibrated if indicated to maximize the occlusal fit; models sent to Medical Modeling
- Models incorporated into computer-simulated surgery for construction of intermediate and final palatal splints
- Models, splints, and printouts of computer-simulated surgery sent to surgeon

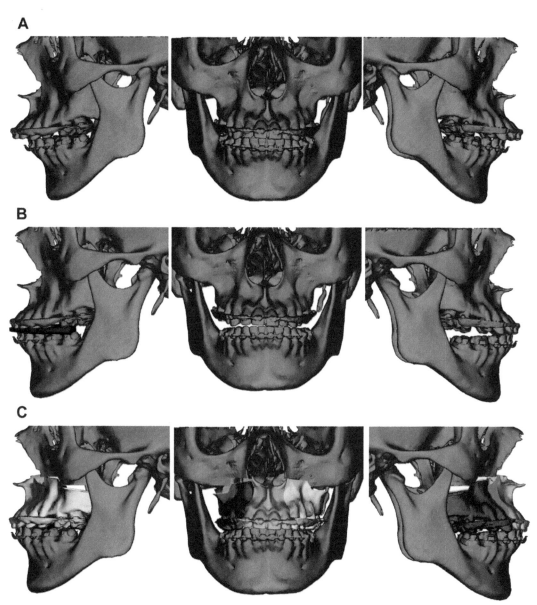

Fig. 3. Staged computer-aided surgical simulation surgical report. (*A*) Simulated preoperative position of the maxilla and mandible. (*B*) The maxilla and mandible in the simulated intermediate position, with the maxilla in its original position, but the mandible in its final position with the mandibular surgery performed first for fabrication of the intermediate splint. (*C*) The final position of maxilla and mandible, after advancement of mandible and segmental osteotomy of the maxilla, for the production of a palatal splint. (*From* Movahed R, Teschke M, Wolford LM. Protocol for concomitant temporomandibular joint custom-fitted total joint reconstruction and orthognathic surgery utilizing computer-assisted surgical simulation. J Oral Maxillofac Surg 2013;71(12):2126; with permission.)

Using CASS technology for CTOS cases eliminates the 'traditional' steps requiring the surgeon to manually set the mandible into its new final position on the stereolithic model, thus saving time and improving surgical accuracy. Although dental model surgery is necessary only if the maxilla requires segmentation, the models do not require mounting on an articulator, which saves

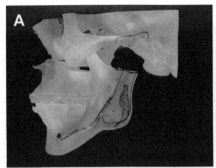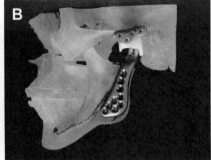

Fig. 4. (*A*) Stereolithic model fabricated after simulated maxillary and mandibular advancement to the final position. Condylectomy and recontouring of the lateral rami and fossae were performed (*red*) and sent to TMJ Concepts for construction of the prostheses. (*B*) Constructed patient-fitted TMJ prosthesis using the computer-aided surgical simulation fabricated stereolithic model. (*From* Movahed R, Teschke M, Wolford LM. Protocol for concomitant temporomandibular joint custom-fitted total joint reconstruction and orthognathic surgery utilizing computer-assisted surgical simulation. J Oral Maxillofac Surg 2013;71(12):2127; with permission.)

considerable time by eliminating the time required to mount the models, prepare the model bases for model surgery, reposition the mandible, construct the intermediate occlusal splint, and make the final palatal splint. With CASS technology, the splints are manufactured by Medical Modeling.

DISCUSSION

Using CASS technology for CTOS cases, the surgeon superimposes the orthognathic computer-simulated surgery into the production of the stereolithic model, hence decreasing the margin of error that can occur with hands-on positioning of the mandible on the stereolithic model. Furthermore, this technique decreases the time taken by the surgeon in the laboratory, by TMJ Concepts for the fabrication of prostheses, and for setting the stereolithic model with increased accuracy in the process.

The remaining areas in which improvement can be made in CASS technology include performing recontouring of the rami and fossae in the simulated environment in an accurate fashion, eliminating the requirement for the acquisition of dental models by using laser scanning technology, and performing accurate maxillary segmentation and equilibration using CASS technology. Further research is necessary to achieve these goals and to move the workflow directly from the CASS environment to the fabrication of custom-fitted TMJ Concepts prostheses, without requiring the surgeon to have 'hands-on' involvement in the process.

Pearls

1. Combined orthognathic and total joint reconstruction cases can be predictably performed in 1 stage.

2. Use of virtual surgical planning can eliminate a significant time requirement in preparation of concomitant orthognathic and TMJ prostheses cases.

3. The CTOS-CASS technique increases the accuracy of combined cases.

4. In order to have flexibility in positioning of the total joint prosthesis, recontouring of the lateral aspect of the rami is advantageous.

CASE

A 32-year-old woman was diagnosed with juvenile idiopathic arthritis in grade school, had orthodontics from 15 to 17 years of age with maxillary first bicuspids extracted, and developed an open bite at age 28 years (**Figs. 5–9**). Over the years she was treated conservatively with occlusal splints and arthroscopic surgeries. Her myofascial pain persisted and worsened before her initial consultation. The maximal incisal opening measured with pain was 36 mm and without pain was 14 mm. Excursion movements to the right were 9 mm and to the left were 10 mm. Her surgery was planned using CTOS-CASS technology:

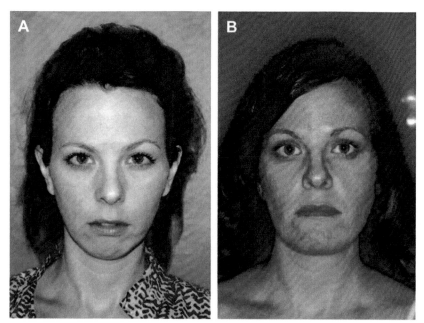

Fig. 5. Frontal view, before surgery (*A*) and 1 year after surgery (*B*).

1. Bilateral TMJ reconstruction and counter-clockwise rotation of the mandible with TMJ Concepts patient-fitted total joint prostheses

2. Bilateral TMJ fat grafts packed around the articulating area of the prostheses, harvested from the abdomen
3. Bilateral coronoidectomies

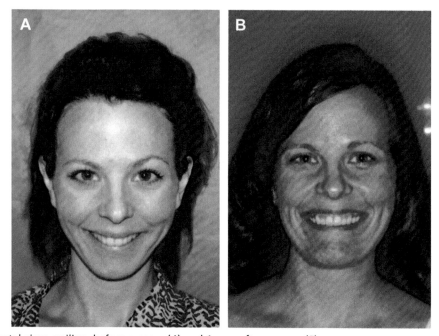

Fig. 6. Frontal view, smiling, before surgery (*A*) and 1 year after surgery (*B*).

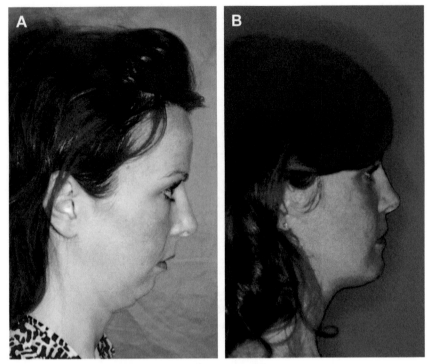

Fig. 7. Profile view, before surgery (*A*) and 1 year after surgery(*B*).

4. Multiple maxillary osteotomies for counter-clockwise rotation and advancement
5. Bilateral partial inferior turbinectomies

One-year after surgery she reported no myofascial, TMJ, or headache pain and her incisal opening improved to 50 mm. Excursion movements were 4 mm to the right and 2 mm to the left. A class I occlusion was obtained and better facial harmony was achieved.

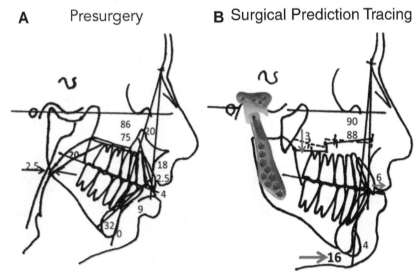

Fig. 8. Cephalometric analysis before surgery (*A*) and Surgical prediction tracing (*B*)

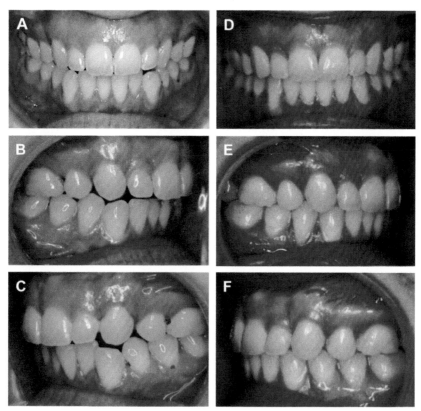

Fig. 9. Presurgery occlusion (*A–C*) and postsurgery occlusion 1 year after surgery (*D–F*).

REFERENCES

1. Wolford LM, Cassano DS, Goncalves JR. Common TMJ disorders: orthodontic and surgical management. In: McNamara JA, Kapila SD, editors. Temporomandibular disorders and orofacial pain: separating controversy from consensus. Craniofacial Growth Series, vol. 46. Ann Arbor (MI): University of Michigan; 2009. p. 159–98.

2. Papadopoulos MA, Christou PK, Athanasiou AE, et al. Three-dimensional craniofacial reconstruction imaging. Oral Surg Oral Med Oral Pathol Oral Radiol Endod 2002;93:382–93.

3. Xia J, Ip HH, Samman N, et al. Computer-assisted three-dimensional surgical planning and simulation: 3D virtual osteotomy. Int J Oral Maxillofac Surg 2000;29:11–7.

4. Rotaru H, Stan H, Florian I, et al. Cranioplasty with custom-made implants: analyzing the cases of 10 patients. J Oral Maxillofac Surg 2012;70:e169.

5. Gateno J, Xia J, Teichgraeber J, et al. Clinical feasibility of computer-aided surgical simulation (CASS) in the treatment of complex cranio-maxillofacial deformities. J Oral Maxillofac Surg 2007;65:728.

6. Movahed R, Teschke M, Wolford LM. Protocol for concomitant temporomandibular joint custom-fitted total joint reconstruction and orthognathic surgery utilizing computer-assisted surgical simulation. J Oral Maxillofac Surg 2013;71(12):2123–9.

Condylar Resorption of the Temporomandibular Joint: How Do We Treat It?

Larry M. Wolford, DMD[a],*,
João Roberto Gonçalves, DDS, PhD[b]

KEYWORDS

- Condylar resorption (CR) • Adolescent internal condylar resorption (AICR)
- Reactive (inflammatory) arthritis • Autoimmune and connective tissue diseases (AI/CT)
- Mitek anchor technique • Patient-fitted total joint prostheses • Periarticular fat grafts
- Orthognathic surgery

KEY POINTS

- There are many different temporomandibular joint (TMJ) pathologic abnormalities that can cause condylar resorption (CR).
- Jaw deformities, malocclusions, TMJ and jaw dysfunction, pain and headaches, and so on commonly accompany TMJ CR pathologic abnormality.
- MRI is an important tool for the diagnosis and treatment planning of TMJ pathologic abnormalities.
- Adolescent internal condylar resorption (AICR) is one of the most common causes of CR, occurs predominately in teenage girls, with onset during their pubertal growth.
- AICR can be predictably treated with disc repositioning using the Mitek anchor and orthognathic surgery performed in one stage, providing that the discs and condyles are salvageable.
- Reactive arthritis is commonly caused by bacterial/viral contamination of the TMJ.
- Patient-fitted total joint prostheses provide the best outcome predictability for TMJ pathologies with non-salvageable discs and condyles.

INTRODUCTION

Condylar resorption (CR) occurs in conditions that cause mandibular condylar bone lysis and loss of condylar volume. There are several suggested causes of CR, including hormonal, neoplasia, metabolic, trauma, inflammation, infection, abnormal condylar loading, aberrant growth factors, connective tissue and autoimmune diseases, and other end-stage temporomandibular joint (TMJ) pathologic abnormalities. Idiopathic condylar resorption (ICR) is a generic term commonly used to identify CR wherein the specific cause is unknown. ICR has been used to encompass several TMJ pathologic abnormalities of different origins. Most of the cases labeled ICR can be categorized into one of the following pathologic processes.

The most common TMJ pathologic abnormalities that cause CR include (1) adolescent internal condylar resorption (AICR), (2) reactive (inflammatory) arthritis, (3) autoimmune and connective

[a] Departments of Oral and Maxillofacial Surgery and Orthodontics Texas, A&M University Health Science Center Baylor College of Dentistry, Baylor University Medical Center, 3409 Worth St. Suite 400, Dallas, TX 75246, USA; [b] Department of Pediatric Dentistry, Faculdade de Odontologia de Araraquara, Univ Estadual Paulista - UNESP Araraquara School of Dentistry, Brazil – Rua Humaita 1680, Araraquara, SP 14801-903, Brazil
* Corresponding author. 3409 Worth Street, Suite 400, Dallas, TX 75246.
E-mail address: lwolford@drlarrywolford.com

Oral Maxillofacial Surg Clin N Am 27 (2015) 47–67
http://dx.doi.org/10.1016/j.coms.2014.09.005

tissue diseases (AI/CT), and (4) other end-stage TMJ pathologic abnormalities. These TMJ conditions may be associated with dentofacial deformities, malocclusion, TMJ pain, headaches, myofascial pain, TMJ and jaw dysfunction, ear symptoms, and, in the more severe cases, speech articulation problems, decreased oropharyngeal airway, sleep apnea, and psychosocial disorders. Patients with these conditions may benefit from corrective surgical intervention, including concomitant TMJ and orthognathic surgery.

Some CR pathologic abnormalities occur more commonly within particular age ranges and gender. Identifying the specific CR pathologic abnormality will provide insight into the nature of the pathologic abnormality; progression if untreated; clinical, imaging, and histologic characteristics; as well as treatment protocols proven to eliminate the pathologic processes and provide optimal functional and esthetic outcomes.

Although patients with TMJ CR commonly have associated TMJ symptoms, approximately 25% of patients with significant TMJ pathologic abnormality will be asymptomatic. These patients are diagnostically challenging when undergoing orthognathic surgery because the TMJ pathologic abnormality may be unrecognized, ignored, or treated inappropriately, resulting in a poor treatment outcome with potential redevelopment of the skeletal and occlusal deformity as further CR occurs, worsening or initiation of pain, headaches, jaw and TMJ dysfunction, and so forth.

The occurrence of TMJ CR has been identified by many authors[1–10] as having association with orthodontic treatment and orthognathic surgery. However, these treatment modalities are usually coincidental with the TMJ pathologic abnormalities and not the specific cause of the problem. The TMJ pathologic abnormality may have been preexisting or developed during treatment and is usually not initiated by orthodontics or orthognathic surgery. However, orthodontics and surgery can exacerbate the CR and TMJ symptoms. Treatment recommendations that have been previously proposed for CR include (1) splint therapy to minimize joint loading; (2) medications to slow down the resorption process; (3) nonloading orthodontic and orthognathic surgical procedures (eg, maxillary surgery only) after 6 to 12 months of disease remission; (4) arthroscopic lysis and lavage; and (5) condylar replacement with a costochondral graft or other autogenous tissues. Although some of these treatment modalities have reported success in some cases, none of these methods of management will provide consistent, predictable, stable functional, occlusal, and esthetic outcomes,

and eliminate pain with all of the various CR pathologic abnormalities.

The literature has clearly demonstrated the adverse affects of performing *only* orthognathic surgery in the presence of displaced TMJ articular discs.[1–5,8–10] Our research studies[1,8,9] show that in the presence of TMJ displaced discs where only orthognathic surgery is performed with the maxilla and mandible surgically advanced, an average anteroposterior (AP) mandibular relapse of 30% can be expected as well as an 84% chance of developing or worsening TMJ pain, myofascial pain, and headaches. A recent study using voxel-based and 3-dimensional (3D) cone beam computed tomography (CBCT) surface analysis showed the protective effect of disc repositioning in condylar morphology maintenance following maxillomandibular advancement (MMA).[11] Accurate diagnosis and proper surgical intervention for the specific TMJ CR pathologic abnormalities that may be present in orthognathic surgery patients will provide highly predictable and stable results.

PATIENT EVALUATION

The authors have previously published detailed methods for clinical, imaging, and dental model analyses as well as TMJ assessment.[12,13] The most dominant facial type that experiences TMJ pathologic abnormality, specifically CR conditions, is the high occlusal plane angle facial morphology[14–22] that exhibits a retruded maxilla and mandible, commonly with a decreased dimension of the oropharyngeal airway. Nasal airway obstruction related to hypertrophied turbinates is also common in these patients.

History

Relative to TMJ pathologic abnormality, the patient history is important and aids in the diagnosis and treatment protocol selected. Important factors are age of onset for TMJ-related symptoms, change in jaw and occlusal relationship, cause, genetic factors, previous treatments (including surgery), habitual patterns such as clenching and bruxism, presence of other symptomatic joints, other disease processes such as connective tissue/autoimmune or metabolic diseases, gastrointestinal problems, recurrent urinary tract infections, diabetes, cardiac conditions, vascular compromises, airway or sleep apnea issues, smoking, alcohol or drug abuse, glandular and hormone imbalances, and others, because these factors may affect TMJ treatment decisions.

MRI Evaluation

MRI is one of the most important diagnostic tools in differentiating the specific TMJ CR pathologic abnormality. In general, T1 MRIs are helpful to identify disc position, the presence of alteration in bone and soft tissue structures, and interrelationships of the bony and soft tissue anatomy. T2 MRIs are helpful to identify inflammatory responses in the TMJ.

Importance of Temporomandibular Joint Disc Position

The importance of disc position cannot be overemphasized. Gonçalves and colleagues[8] evaluated 3 different patient groups that required counterclockwise rotation and advancement of the maxillomandibular complex with either TMJ discs in normal position; displaced discs repositioned with Mitek anchors (Mitek Products Inc., Westwood, MA, USA); or displaced discs left in place. The 3 groups were well matched relative to the amount of advancement at Menton (approximately 13 mm in a counterclockwise direction). At longest follow-up with an average of 31 months, the average relapse at Menton for group 1 with discs in normal position was 5%, or 0.5 mm for every 10 mm of maxillomandibular counterclockwise advancement. Group 2 had salvageable displaced discs repositioned using the Mitek anchor technique and orthognathic surgery with an average relapse of 1%, or 0.1 mm per 10 mm of counterclockwise mandibular advancement. Group 3 had displaced discs where only orthognathic surgery was performed, with the average AP relapse of 28% of the advancement or almost 3 mm for every 10 mm of mandibular advancement, indicating postsurgical CR occurring in group 3. This study conclusively shows the importance of having the articular discs in position for stability in orthognathic surgery, particularly in patients who require mandibular advancement and specifically for those that require counterclockwise rotation of the maxillomandibular complex.

SURGICAL SEQUENCING AND CONSIDERATIONS

CR patients generally have an associated dentofacial deformity. Today, the means exist to accurately diagnose and predictably treat these cases. CR cases can be successfully treated with concomitant TMJ surgery and orthognathic surgery. The 2 most predictable treatment methods for TMJ CR conditions include either articular disc repositioning with a Mitek anchor technique[12,23–27] or patient-fitted total joint prostheses[28–33] in combination with orthognathic surgery. The procedure protocol selected is based on diagnosis, time since onset of TMJ pathologic abnormality, progression of the disease process, presence of polyarthropathies or other systemic issues, and so on. Many TMJ CR patients can benefit from counterclockwise rotation of the maxillomandibular complex to get the best functional and esthetic outcome.[34–36] In this situation, it is easier to address the TMJ pathologic abnormality first followed by repositioning the mandible before performing the maxillary osteotomies.[37] If the surgeon prefers to do the TMJ surgery as a separate operation from the orthognathic surgery, then the TMJ surgery should be done first. The specific treatment protocols are presented as each specific CR pathologic abnormality is discussed.

ADOLESCENT INTERNAL CONDYLAR RESORPTION (AICR)
Cause

AICR, formerly referred to in generic terminology as idiopathic condylar resorption,[6,7,12,13] is one of the most common TMJ conditions affecting teenage girls. AICR is also known as cheerleader syndrome, idiopathic condylysis, condylar atrophy, and progressive CR. AICR is a well-documented disease process occurring with an 8:1 female-to-male ratio; onset is between the ages of 11 and 15 during pubertal growth and development and is rarely initiated before the age of 11 years or after the age of 15 years.[6,7,12,13] There are other local and systemic pathologic abnormalities or diseases that can cause CR, but AICR is a specific disease entity different from all of the other disease processes and can create occlusal and musculoskeletal instability resulting in the development of a dentofacial deformity, TMJ dysfunction, and pain.

Although the specific cause of AICR has not been clearly identified, its strong predilection for teenage girls in their pubertal growth phase supports a theory of hormonal mediation.

Estrogen receptors have been identified in the TMJs of female primates,[38,39] human TMJ tissues,[40] and arthritic knee joints. Estrogen is known to mediate cartilage and bone metabolism in the female TMJ.[41,42] An increase in receptors may predispose an exaggerated response to joint loading from parafunctional activity, trauma, orthodontics, or orthognathic surgery.

The authors' hypothesis for this TMJ pathologic abnormality is as follows: female hormones mediate biochemical changes within the TMJ, causing hyperplasia of the synovial tissues that stimulate the production of destructive substrates that initiate breakdown of the ligamentous structures that normally support and stabilize the articular disc to the condyle, allowing the disc to become anteriorly displaced. The hyperplastic synovial tissue then surrounds the head of the condyle. The substrates penetrate through the outer surface of the condyle and cause thinning of the cortical bone and breakdown of the subcortical bone. The condyle slowly collapses, shrinking in size in all 3 planes as a result of internal condylar bone resorption without clinically apparent destruction of the fibrocartilage on the condylar head and roof of the fossa; unlike the other arthritic conditions, where the fibrocartilage and cortical bone are destroyed by an inflammatory, connective tissue, or autoimmune disease process. AICR can progress for a while and then go into remission or proceed until the entire condylar head has resorbed. In cases where it goes into remission, excessive joint loading (ie, parafunctional habits, trauma, orthodontics, orthognathic surgery) can reinitiate the resorption process. AICR usually occurs bilaterally with symmetric CR, but facial asymmetry can occur if one side resorbs faster than the other or with only unilateral TMJ involvement.

Clinical Features

AICR has classic clinical features that include (1) initiation during pubertal growth (ages 11–15 years) predominately in teenage girls (8:1 female-to-male ratio); (2) progressive worsening skeletal and occlusal deformity, although occurring at a slow rate (average rate of CR is 1.5 mm per year)[6,7]; (3) high occlusal plane angle facial morphology, class II occlusion with or without an anterior open bite; (4) possible association with TMJ symptoms, such as clicking, TMJ pain, headaches, myofascial pain, earaches, tinnitus, vertigo, and others (however, 25% of patients with AICR have no overt symptoms); (5) jaw and jaw joint dysfunction; and (6) no other joint or systemic involvement (**Figs. 1**A–C and **2**A–C).[6,7] Because AICR is normally initiated during pubertal growth, CR that originates before the age of 11 or after the age of 15 is usually not AICR, but a different TMJ pathologic abnormality and may need a different treatment protocol. AICR rarely occurs in low occlusal plane angle (brachiocephalic) facial types or in class III skeletal relationships. All cases are isolated occurrences with no genetic correlation.

Imaging

Radiographic features include (1) progressive decrease of condylar size and volume; (2) some cases having thinning cortex on top of the condyle; (3) some cases presenting with increased, normal,

or decreased superior joint space; (4) some cases presenting with decreased vertical height of the ramus and condyle; (5) high occlusal plane angle facial morphology; and (6) skeletal and occlusal class II relationship (**Fig. 3**A).

A normal MRI is seen in **Fig. 4**A, B. An MRI of AICR (see **Fig. 4**C, D) will show (1) the articular disc anteriorly displacing and commonly becoming nonreducing relatively early in the pathologic process (nonreducing discs have an accelerated rate of deformation and degeneration compared with discs that reduce); (2) condyle getting progressively smaller in 3 dimensions; (3) amorphous-appearing tissue possibly surrounding the condyle, with or without an increased joint space; and (4) no inflammatory process seen.

Treatment Options

When the discs are still salvageable, the authors' treatment protocol has proven to eliminate this TMJ pathologic abnormality and allows optimal correction of the associated dentofacial deformity at the same operation. The protocol includes (1) removing the bilaminar tissue surrounding the condyle; (2) mobilizing, repositioning, and stabilizing the disc to the condyle with a Mitek anchor and artificial ligaments (**Figs. 5** and **6**); (3) performing the indicated orthognathic surgery (usually double jaw) with counterclockwise rotation of the maxillomandibular complex (see **Fig. 3**B); and (4) performing other adjunctive procedures that are indicated.[6,7,12,23–27] Because this high occlusal plane angle facial morphology is commonly associated with decreased oropharyngeal airway space and sleep apnea, the counterclockwise rotation of the maxillomandibular complex will also maximize the AP dimension of the oropharyngeal airway, eliminating sleep apnea symptoms (see **Figs. 1**D–F and **2**D–F). In growing patients, not only will this approach stop the CR but also the mandibular condylar growth will begin again.[6,7] Results are best for AICR if the TMJ surgery is performed within 4 years of the onset of the pathologic abnormality. After 4 years, the discs may become significantly deformed and degenerated so as not to be salvageable; then the indicated treatment would be patient-fitted total joint prostheses (TMJ Concepts Inc., Ventura, CA, USA) to repair the TMJs and advance the mandible.

Although this AICR surgical protocol has been successful for more than 20 years, some controversy still remains in the literature, specifically in regard to the possible side effects related to open joint surgery and condylar changes afterward.[43–45] In an ongoing study, the authors are assessing 3D condylar changes occurring 1-year

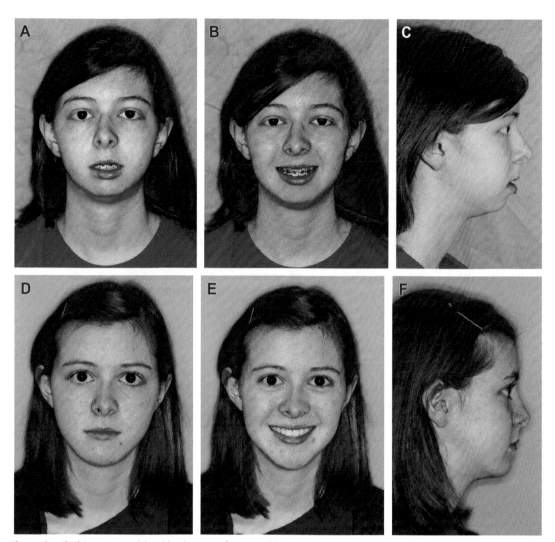

Fig. 1. (*A–C*) This 15-year-old girl had onset of TMJ problems at the age of 12. Her mandible had become progressively more retruded. Her diagnoses included (1) bilateral TMJ AICR; (2) mandibular AP hypoplasia; (3) maxillary anterior vertical hyperplasia as well as AP, posterior vertical and transverse hypoplasia; (4) class II end-on occlusion; (5) anterior open bite of 3 mm, (6) hypertrophied turbinates causing nasal airway obstruction; (7) TMJ pain, myofascial pain, and headaches; and (8) decreased oropharyngeal airway with an AP dimension of 3 mm (normal AP dimension is 11 mm) with sleep apnea symptoms. (*D–F*) Patient is 2 years postsurgery following single-staged procedures: (1) bilateral TMJ articular disc repositioning and ligament repair with Mitek anchors; (2) bilateral mandibular ramus sagittal split osteotomies to advance the mandible in a counterclockwise direction (20 mm); (3) multiple maxillary osteotomies to advance in a counterclockwise direction (7 mm at the incisal tips) and expand; (4) AP augmentation genioplasty (5 mm); and (5) bilateral partial inferior turbinectomies. The patient shows improved facial balance, stable jaw and occlusal relationship, good jaw function, and elimination of pain.

after surgery in 2 patient groups: group 1 consists of young adult patients with normal TMJs; they had MMA only. Group 2 consists of young adult AICR patients with MMA and articular disc repositioning (MMA-Drep). For each patient, CBCTs were segmented in a semi-automatic protocol[46] and registered in a rigid, voxelwise automatic algorithm over the cranial base.[47] Three distinct methods were used to assess the condyles 3-dimensionally: (1) surface shape correspondence using the SPHARM-PDM package[48,49]; (2) subjective analysis of semi-transparent overlays[8,47,50,51]; and (3) condylar volume estimation using ITK-Snap software.[10,11] The values for the voxels in each tomographic image were obtained in Hounsfield units, representing the opacity of the radiographs.

The authors' preliminary results showed that at 1-year following surgery AICR patients (MMA-Drep) had increased condylar volume compared with

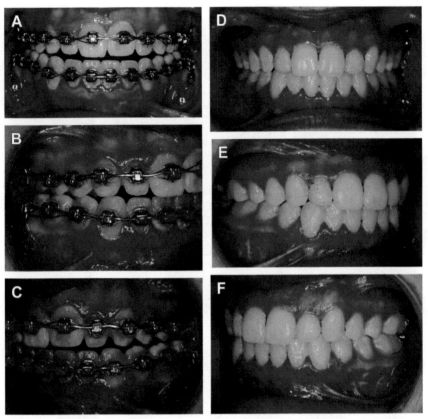

Fig. 2. (A–C) Pretreatment occlusion shows class II end-on with anterior open bite. (D–F) Patient has a class I occlusion and 2-mm overbite 2 years after surgery.

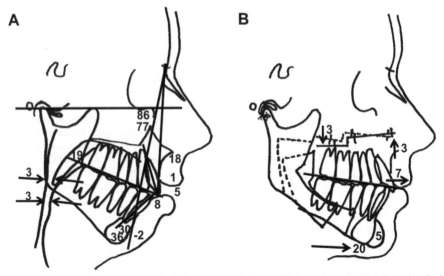

Fig. 3. (A) Pretreatment cephalometric analysis shows retruded mandible and maxilla, high occlusal plane angulation, anterior vertical maxillary hyperplasia, but posterior vertical hypoplasia. *Arrows* and associated numbers indicate the oropharyngeal airway dimension in millimeters (3). (B) The surgical treatment objective demonstrates repositioning the articular discs with the Mitek anchor technique, counterclockwise rotation of the maxillomandibular complex, turbinectomies, and genioplasty, with pogonion advancing 20 mm. *Arrows* and numbers represent the direction of surgical change in millimeters.

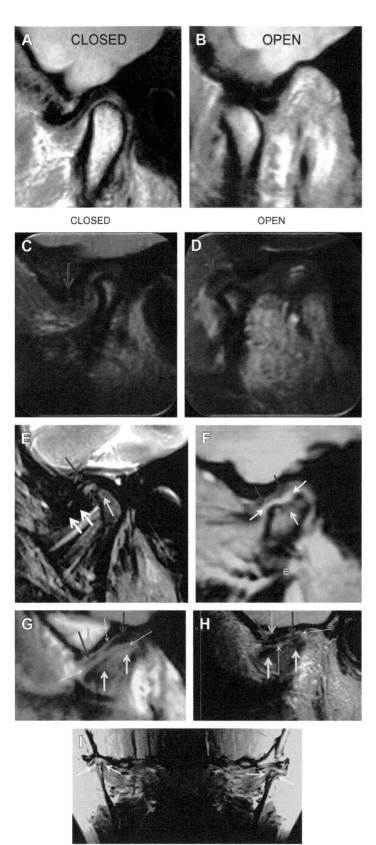

Fig. 4. MRI evaluation. (*A*, *B*) Normal MRI with disc in position in the closed (*A*) and open (*B*) positions. (*C*, *D*) AICR with anteriorly displaced articular disc (*red arrows*) and CR in the closed (*C*) and open (*D*) positions without disc reduction on opening. (*E*) Reactive arthritis showing initiation of arthritic changes of the condyle (*yellow arrow*), moderate inflammation within the joint bilaminar tissues (*red arrows*), and anterior disc displacement (*white arrows*). (*F*) Reactive arthritis with significant inflammation (*white arrows*) between the disc (*red arrows*) and condyle (*yellow arrow*). The condyle has lost vertical height with a relatively large erosive lesion present. (*G*) Advanced JIA with mushrooming of the condyle, loss of condyle vertical height (*yellow arrows*), moderate resorption of the articular eminence (*green arrow*), and reactive pannus (*white arrows*) surrounding the disc (*red arrows*). (*H*) Further advancement of the AI/CT disease process with major erosion of the articular eminence (*green arrow*) and condyle (*yellow arrows*) as well as progressive degeneration of the disc (*red arrows*) with the reactive pannus (*white arrow*) surrounding the disc. (*I*) Coronal imaging shows significant loss of vertical condylar height and transverse width (*yellow arrows*).

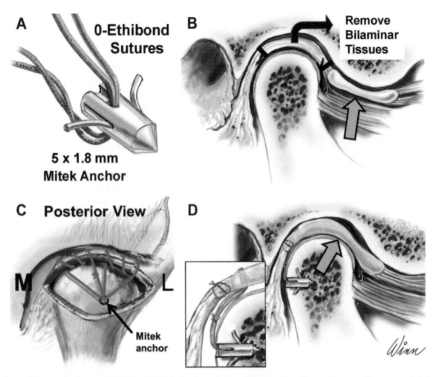

Fig. 5. Mitek anchor technique. (*A*) Mitek Mini Anchor is 5 × 1.8 mm in dimensions with an eyelet to support 2 artificial ligaments (0-Ethibond suture; Ethicon, Inc., Somerville, NJ). (*B*) Bilaminar tissues are excised and anteriorly displaced disc (*green arrow*) is mobilized. (*C, D*) The disc (*green arrow*) is passively positioned over the condyle and Mitek anchor is placed in the lateral aspect of the posterior head, about 8 mm below the top of the condyle; the sutures are attached to the posterior band of the disc and secured. (*Courtesy of* L. Wolford, DMD.)

patients with healthy TMJs with MMA only that experienced a reduction of condylar volume (*P*<.01). The values measured for each anatomic region demonstrated important differences between the 2 groups (**Fig. 7**). The distance maps show the magnitude of changes between 2 point-based correspondent models, while the vector maps provide the directionality of these positional displacements. Positive and negative numbers represent outward and inward displacement, respectively.

REACTIVE (INFLAMMATORY) ARTHRITIS
Cause

Reactive arthritis (also called seronegative spondyloarthropathy) is an inflammatory process in joints commonly related to bacterial or viral factors. This condition reportedly occurs during the third to fourth decade of life, but it can develop at any age. In the TMJ, it more commonly develops in the late teens through the fourth decade. Reactive arthritis commonly is seen in conjunction with a displaced TMJ articular disc, but it also can develop with the disc in position.

Henry and colleagues[52,53] demonstrated that 73% of patients with TMJ articular disc displacements have bacteria in the bilaminar tissues. The bacterial species the authors have identified in the TMJ include *Chlamydia trachomatis* and *Chlamydia psittaci* as well as *Mycoplasma genitalium* and *Mycoplasma fermentans*.[52–55] Other bacteria that have been found in other joints but also may infect the TMJ include *Borrelia burgdorferi* (Lyme disease), *Salmonella* species, *Shigella* species, *Yersina enterocolitica*, and *Campylobacter jejuni*. The authors suspect that other bacterial/viral species may cause reactive arthritis in joints, including *Chlamydia pneumoniae*, *Mycoplasma pneumoniae*, Ureaplasma, Herpes virus, Epstein-Barr virus, Cytomegalovirus, and Varicella zoster, among others. Kim and colleagues[56] analyzed TMJ synovial fluids for specific bacteria and found *M genitalium* and *M fermentans/orale* as well as *Staphlococcus aureus*, *Actinobacillus actinomycetemcomitans*, and *Streptococcus mitis* present in 86%, 51%, 37%, 26%, and 7% of samples, respectively. They did not test for the *Chlamydia* species.

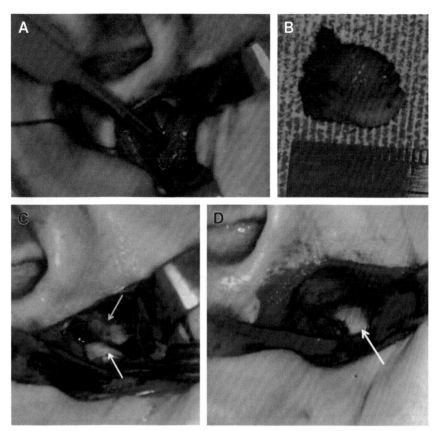

Fig. 6. (*A*) Right TMJ in AICR showing the hyperplastic synovial tissues overlying the condyle. (*B*) Bilaminar/synovial tissues are excised. (*C*) The fibrocartilage is observed covering the condyle (*white arrow*) and fossa (*green arrow*). (*D*) Mitek anchor has been placed and the disc is secured into normal position.

Chlamydia and *Mycoplasma* bacterium species live and function like viruses and, therefore, antibiotics may not be effective in eliminating these bacteria from joints and the body. Antibiotics may affect the extracellular organisms but will not affect the intracellular bacteria, although the microbes may be placed into a dormant state. These bacteria are known to stimulate the production of Substance P, cytokines, and tissue necrosis factor, which are all pain-modulating factors and contribute to the destruction of the bone and cartilage of the joint.[57–59] In addition, these bacterial species have been associated with Reiter syndrome and dysfunction of the immune system.

The authors also have identified specific genetic factors, human leukocyte antigen markers, that occur at a significant greater incidence in TMJ patients than the normal population.[60] These same markers also may indicate an immune dysfunctional problem for these bacterial species, allowing the bacteria to have a greater affect on patients with these markers compared with people without these same markers.

Patients with localized TMJ reactive arthritis may have displaced discs, pain, TMJ and jaw dysfunction, headaches, and ear symptoms. As the disease progresses, CR and/or bony deposition can occur, causing changes in the jaw and occlusal relationships. Patients with moderate to severe reactive arthritis may have other body systems involvement, including the genitourinary, gastrointestinal, reproductive, respiratory, cardiopulmonary, ocular, neurologic, vascular, hemopoietic, immune system, as well as involvement of other joints.[61]

Clinical Features

Although this condition commonly occurs bilaterally, it can occur unilaterally. In some patients, there may not be any significant CR and therefore may not have an adverse affect on facial morphology or occlusion. However, when causing CR, the following features may be observed: (1) mandible may become progressively retruded; (2) jaw and occlusal deformity may progressively

A

Right Posterior Condyle Surface T3/T2

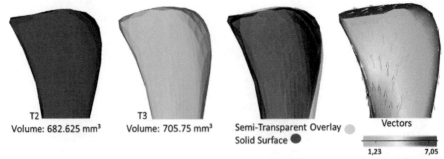

T2	T3	Semi-Transparent Overlay ●	Vectors
Volume: 682.625 mm³	Volume: 705.75 mm³	Solid Surface ●	

1,23   7,05

Measurements: Lateral Pole: -2.76 mm; Medial Pole: -2.69 mm; Superior Condyle: 2.62 mm; Posterior Condyle: 1.12 mm

Left Posterior Condyle Surface T3/T2

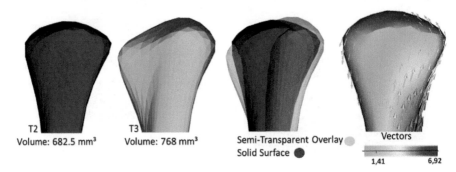

T2	T3	Semi-Transparent Overlay ●	Vectors
Volume: 682.5 mm³	Volume: 768 mm³	Solid Surface ●	

1,41   6,92

Measurements: Lateral Pole: 2.54 mm ; Medial Pole: 1.86 mm; Superior Condyle: -2.59 mm; Posterior Condyle: 2.21 mm

B

Right Posterior Condyle Surface T3/T2

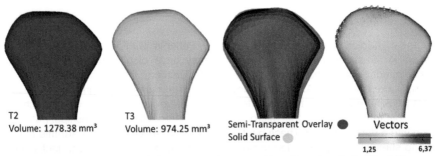

T2	T3	Semi-Transparent Overlay ●	Vectors
Volume: 1278.38 mm³	Volume: 974.25 mm³	Solid Surface ●	

1,25   6,37

Measurements: Lateral Pole: -1.31 mm; Medial Pole: 2,44 mm; Superior Condyle: 2,17 mm; Posterior Condyle: -2,38 mm

Left Posterior Condyle Surface T3/T2

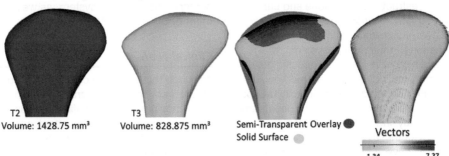

T2	T3	Semi-Transparent Overlay ●	Vectors
Volume: 1428.75 mm³	Volume: 828.875 mm³	Solid Surface ●	

1,34   7,27

Measurements: Lateral Pole: -1,92 mm; Medial Pole: -1,17 mm; Superior Condyle: -2,23 mm Posterior Condyle: -1,41 mm

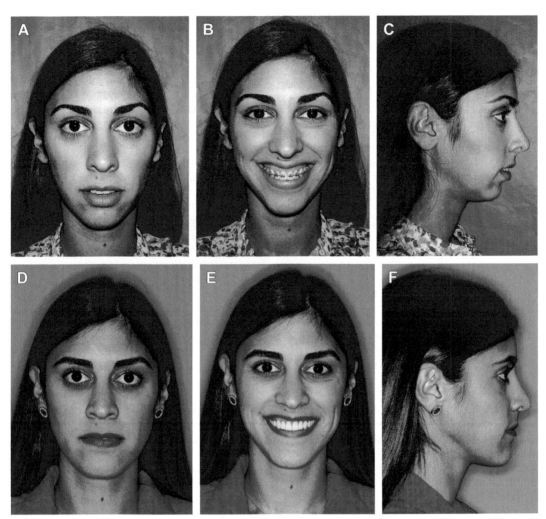

Fig. 8. (*A–C*) This 22-year-old woman had the onset of her TMJ problems at age 18 with the development of a retruded mandible, TMJ pain, and sleep apnea symptoms. She has no other joint involvement or other systemic issues. Her diagnosis was (1) bilateral TMJ reactive arthritis and articular discs anteriorly displaced; (2) mandibular and maxillary hypoplasia; (3) class II end-on occlusion; (4) anterior open bite; (5) high occlusal plane angle; (6) hypertrophied turbinates causing nasal airway obstruction; (7) decreased oropharyngeal airway and sleep apnea symptoms; and (8) TMJ pain. (*D–F*) The patient 3 years after surgery for the following single-stage procedures: (1) bilateral TMJ articular disc repositioning with Mitek anchor technique; (2) bilateral mandibular sagittal split osteotomies with counterclockwise rotation to normalize the occlusal plane angle; (3) multiple maxillary osteotomies to down graft the posterior aspect for counterclockwise rotation of the maxillomandibular complex; (4) bilateral partial inferior turbinectomies. With the above treatment plan, pogonion advanced 18 mm, while sleep apnea symptoms and pain were eliminated.

Fig. 7. (*A*) Left and right condyle surfaces of AICR patient submitted to MMA-Drep. T2 represents the condyle morphology immediately after surgery (*red*) and T3 at 1-year follow-up (*blue*). Right-side and left-side postsurgical condylar volume increased 23.12 mm^3 and 85.5 mm^3, respectively. The directions of bone remodeling/displacement are shown in semi-transparent overlays and at the vectors color map. Specific region changes are shown below the images. (*B*) MMA. Left and right condyle surfaces of patient submitted to MMA and no articular disc repositioning (normal TMJs). T2 represents the condyle morphology immediately after surgery (*red*) and T3 at 1-year follow-up (*blue*). Right-side and left-side after surgical condylar volume decreased 304.13 mm^3 and 599.87 mm^3, respectively. The directions of bone remodeling/displacement are shown in semi-transparent overlays and at the vectors color map. Specific region changes are showed below the images.

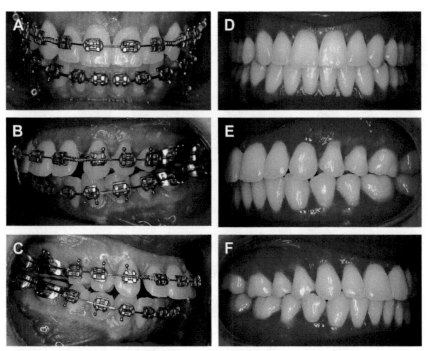

Fig. 9. (*A–C*) Presurgery shows anterior open bite and end-on class II occlusion. (*D–F*) The patient, 3 years after surgery, has good skeletal and occlusal stability.

worsen, although it may occur at a slow rate; (2) class II occlusion and anterior open bite with premature contact on the posterior teeth (**Figs. 8A–C and 9A–C**); (3) common associated TMJ symptoms may include clicking, popping, crepitus, TMJ dysfunction and pain, headaches, myofascial pain, earaches, tinnitus, vertigo; and (4) other joints and body systems may be involved.

Imaging

Radiographic features of reactive arthritis causing CR can include (1) loss of vertical dimension and

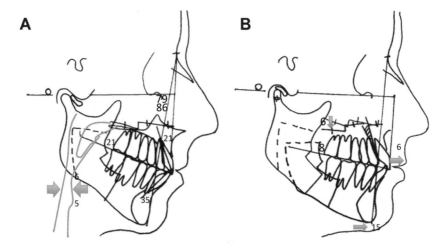

Fig. 10. (*A*) Presurgical cephalometric analysis shows the retruded maxilla and mandible with a high occlusal plane angulation and class II skeletal and occlusal relationship. *Arrows* and associated numbers indicate the oropharyngeal airway dimensions in millimeters (5). (*B*) Surgical treatment objective shows repositioning the articular discs, advancing the mandible, and maxilla with a counterclockwise rotation. Pogonion advanced 15 mm. *Arrows* and numbers represent the direction of surgical change in millimeters.

volume of the condyle; (2) articular surface of the condyle eroded with loss of the fibrocartilage covering the condyle and fossa; (3) retruded mandible; (4) class II occlusion with anterior open bite; and (5) decreased vertical height of the ramus and condyle (**Fig. 10**A).

MRI will commonly show (1) articular disc anteriorly displaced or in normal position; (2) joint effusion and inflammation in T2 imaging; (3) resorbing condyle; and (4) condylar and fossa erosions in advanced conditions (see **Fig. 4**E, F).

Treatment Options

The approach to treating this TMJ pathologic abnormality and associated deformity depends on the length of time that the pathologic abnormality has been present, the amount of destruction to the disc and condyle at the time of surgery, and the presence of other joint involvement (polyarthritis) or other related systemic conditions. If the TMJ condition is identified within the first 4 years of the onset of the disc dislocation, the destruction is not significant, and there are no other joints or systemic conditions present, then removing the bilaminar tissues around the condyle and repositioning the articular disc with the Mitek anchor technique may work well to preserve the normal anatomic structures (see **Fig. 5**).[12,23–27] It is possible that the resection and removal of a large portion of the bilaminar tissue (where it is known that these bacteria reside) during surgery may result in a major reduction of the source of the inflammation. The orthognathic surgery can be done at the same time as the joints are repaired (see **Figs. 8**D–F, **9**D–F, and **10**B).

If there is significant destruction of the condyle and the disc is not salvageable, or polyarthritis or systemic disease is present, then the most predictable treatment procedure is the patient-fitted total joint prosthesis (TMJ Concepts System) (**Fig. 11**) to reconstruct the TMJ as well as reposition the mandible to its proper position (**Figs. 12–14**).[28–33] Fat grafts packed around the total joint prosthesis are an important component to help prevent fibrous tissue and heterotopic bone from forming.[62,63]

AUTOIMMUNE AND CONNECTIVE TISSUE DISEASES
Cause

Conditions included in the classification of AI/CT that can affect the TMJs are rheumatoid arthritis, juvenile idiopathic arthritis (JIA), psoriatic arthritis, ankylosing spondylitis, Sjogren syndrome, systemic lupus erythematosus, scleroderma, and mixed connective tissue disease, among others. The triggers and precise pathophysiology are unknown for most of these disorders. Multiple systems are usually involved. Joint damage may be mediated by cytokines, chemokines, and metalloproteases. Peripheral joints are usually symmetrically inflamed, resulting in progressive destruction of articular structures, commonly accompanied by systemic symptoms.

Clinical Features

Adult onset in some patients may affect the TMJs but not cause significant CR, particularly if caught

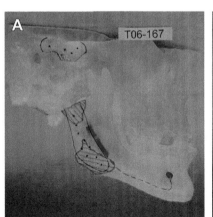
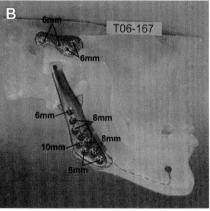

Fig. 11. Patient-fitted total joint prostheses are indicated when the articular discs and condyles are considered nonsalvageable. (A) The 3D stereolithic model of the patient is prepared with the mandible placed into the final predetermined position. A condylectomy has been performed and lateral aspect of the ramus was prepared for construction of the prostheses. (B) The prostheses are manufactured based on the patient's specific anatomic requirements. The numbers represent the length of the 2-mm-diameter screws that are required for bicortical engagement.

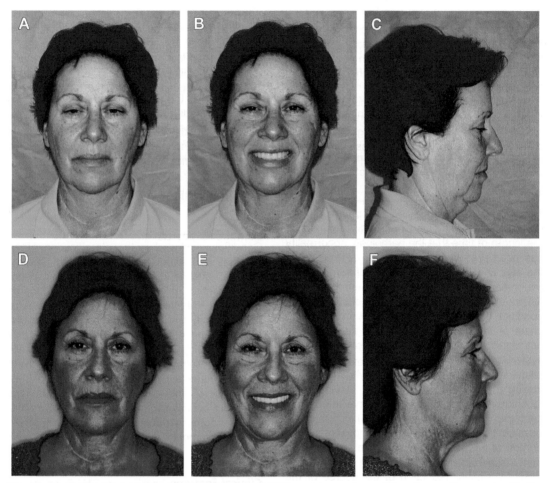

Fig. 12. (*A–C*) This 56-year-old woman had onset of TMJ symptoms at age 39 and was diagnosed with the following: (1) bilateral TMJ reactive arthritis; (2) retruded maxilla and mandible; (3) decreased oropharyngeal airway and sleep apnea requiring continuous positive airway pressure apparatus (CPAP); (4) severe TMJ pain, headaches, myofascial pain; and (5) nonsalvageable TMJs. (*D–F*) The patient is seen 2 years after surgery for (1) bilateral TMJ reconstruction and mandibular counterclockwise rotation advancement (17 mm at pogonion); (2) bilateral TMJ fat grafts harvested from the abdomen; (3) bilateral coronoidectomies; and (4) maxillary osteotomies for counterclockwise rotation. She has no pain, and sleep apnea is eliminated. Incisal opening is improved, and good facial balance is established.

early and placed on appropriate medications. However, when the disease onset is in the first or second decade or adult onset with TMJ involvement and CR, then the following characteristics may be present: (1) progressive retrusion of the mandible with worsening skeletal and occlusal deformity; (2) indirect involvement of the maxilla with posterior vertical hypoplasia particularly when occurring in growing patients; (3) class II occlusion with or without an anterior open bite; (4) TMJ symptoms, which could include clicking, crepitus, TMJ dysfunction and pain, headaches, myofascial pain, earaches, tinnitus, vertigo, and so forth; and (5) other joints and systems commonly involved (**Figs. 15**A–C and **16**A–C).

Imaging

Features may include (1) loss of condylar vertical dimension and volume, residual condyle may become broad in the AP direction, but with significant mediolateral narrowing; (2) in advanced disease, resorption of the articular eminences; (3) residual condyle may function forward beneath the remaining articular eminence; (4) decreased vertical height of the ramus and condyle; (5) skeletal and occlusal class II relationship, high occlusal plane angle facial morphology, with or without anterior open bite; and (6) decreased oropharyngeal airway (**Fig. 17**A).

MRI may show (1) articular discs in position but usually surrounded by a reactive pannus that

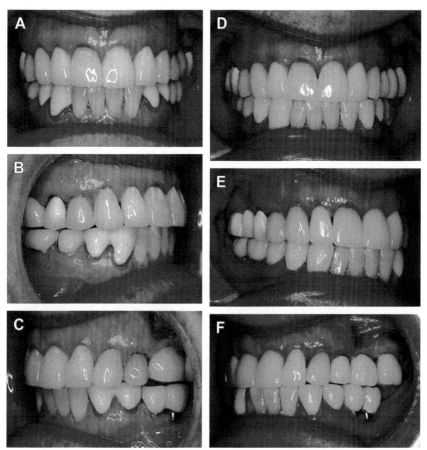

Fig. 13. (*A–C*) Patient has had extensive dental reconstruction that helped correct the malocclusion that developed from the TMJ pathology establishing basically class I occlusion. (*D–F*) At 2 years after surgery, the patient has a stable occlusion.

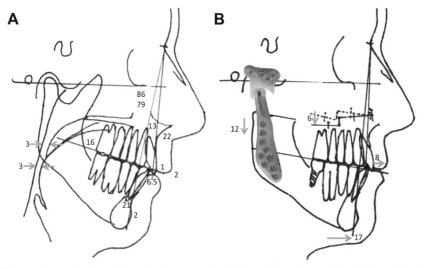

Fig. 14. (*A*) Presurgical cephalometric analysis shows retruded maxilla and mandible, high occlusal plane angle, and decreased oropharyngeal airway. *Arrows* and associated numbers indicate the oropharyngeal airway dimensions in millimeters (3). (*B*) The prediction tracing demonstrates the TMJ reconstruction and counterclockwise mandibular advancement with the TMJ patient-fitted total joint prostheses and maxillary osteotomies with pogonion advancing 17 mm. *Arrows* and numbers represent the direction of surgical change in millimeters.

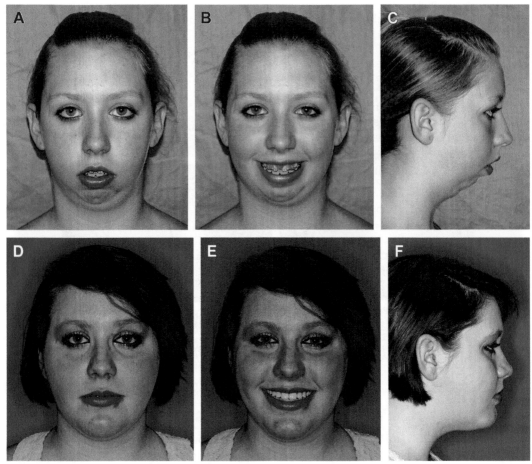

Fig. 15. (*A–C*) This 16-year-old girl presented with progressive retrusion of the mandible and maxilla. She was diagnosed with (1) JIA; (2) significant and progressive CR; (3) progressive retrusion of the mandible and maxilla; (4) class II skeletal and occlusal dentofacial deformity; (5) anterior open bite; (6) decreased oropharyngeal airway with sleep apnea symptoms; (7) hypertrophied nasal turbinates and nasopharyngeal adenoid tissue with nasal airway obstruction; and (8) TMJ pain and headaches. (*D–F*) The patient is seen 2 years after surgery for the following procedures: (1) bilateral TMJ reconstruction and mandibular counterclockwise advancement with patient-fitted TMJ total joint prostheses (TMJ Concepts System); (2) bilateral TMJ fat grafts (harvest from abdomen) packed around the functional component of the prostheses; (3) bilateral coronoidectomies; (4) multiple maxillary osteotomies to down graft the posterior aspect and upright the incisors; (5) bilateral partial inferior turbinectomies and nasopharyngeal adenoidectomy; and (6) chin augmentation with an alloplastic implant.

causes resorption of the condyles and articular eminences and eventually destroy the discs; (2) AP mushrooming of the residual condyle, but narrow medial-lateral width; (3) a possible inflammatory response (see **Fig. 4**G–I).

Treatment

The most predictable treatment of the TMJ affected by AI/CT diseases includes (1) reconstruction of the TMJs and advancement of the mandible in a counterclockwise direction with patient-fitted total joint prosthesis (TMJ Concepts System)[27–33,64]; (2) bilateral coronoidectomy if the rami are significantly

advanced or vertically lengthened with the prostheses; (3) autogenous fat graft packed around the articulation area of the prostheses (harvested from the abdomen or buttock)[62,63]; (4) maxillary osteotomies if indicated; and (5) any additional adjunctive procedures indicated (ie, genioplasty, rhinoplasty, turbinectomies, septoplasty) (see **Figs. 15**D–F, **16**D–F, and **17**B). These diseases can stimulate reactive or heterotopic bone formation around the prostheses. Therefore, it is necessary that fat grafts be packed around the articulating parts of the prostheses to prevent this occurrence and minimize fibrotic tissue formation.[62,63] Orthognathic surgery can be performed

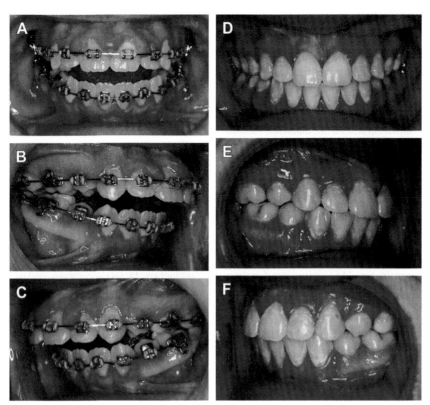

Fig. 16. (*A–C*) The presurgical occlusion demonstrated an anterior open bite and class II end-on cuspid relationship. (*D–F*) The occlusion remains class I with normal overbite at 2 years after surgery.

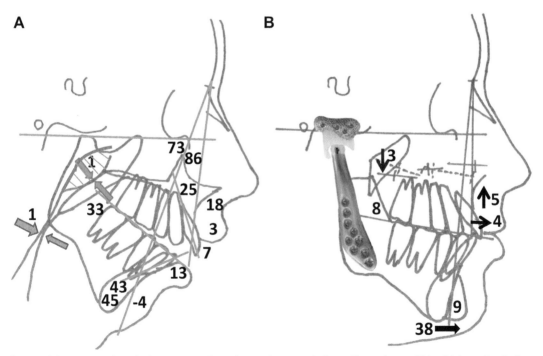

Fig. 17. (*A*) Presurgical cephalometric analysis shows the retruded maxilla and mandible, high occlusal plane angulation, hypertrophied nasopharyngeal adenoid tissue and decreased oropharyngeal airway. *Arrows* and associated numbers indicate the oropharyngeal airway dimensions in millimeters (1). (*B*) Surgical treatment objective illustrates the planned procedures to advance the maxillomandibular complex in a counterclockwise direction, advancing pogonion 38 mm, including the alloplastic chin implant. *Arrows* and numbers represent the direction of surgical change in millimeters.

at the same time as the TMJ is reconstructed or performed at a later surgery, but the TMJ surgery should be performed as the first step in either approach.

Other techniques that have been advocated for TMJ reconstruction in the AI/CT diseases include using autogenous tissues such as temporal fascia and muscle flaps, rib grafts, sternoclavicular grafts, and vertical sliding osteotomy. However, the disease process that created the original TMJ pathologic abnormality can attack the autogenous tissues used in the TMJ reconstruction, causing failure of the grafts.[65] The patient-fitted total joint prosthesis with a fat graft packed around it is a superior technique relative to elimination of the disease process in the TMJ, improved function and esthetics, stability, as well as elimination or decrease in pain.

When treating young growing patients (8–10 years of age or older), the total joint prosthesis is still the best option to eliminate the disease process. However, because there would be no growth potential on the involved side or sides of the mandible, orthognathic surgery will likely be necessary later, but can be delayed until the patient has most of the facial growth complete. Then double jaw surgery can be performed, including the mandibular ramus sagittal split osteotomies (preferable to use an extra-oral approach so as not to contaminate the prostheses) to reposition the jaws into the best alignment, or repositioning of the mandibular components of the prostheses, or manufacturing new longer mandibular components to achieve advancement of the mandible in conjunction with maxillary osteotomies, genioplasty, and others. These secondary procedures are highly predictable when performed at age 14 years or older in girls and 16 years or older in boys. However, the vector of facial growth will change in younger patients to a downward and backward direction as the maxillary and mandibular dentoalveolus continue to grow vertically until growth cessation.[66,67]

The authors' studies[28–31,33,64,65,68] show good outcomes in treating connective tissue/autoimmune diseases affecting the TMJ with custom-fitted total joint prostheses (TMJ Concepts System) for TMJ reconstruction and mandibular advancement, fat grafts, and simultaneous maxillary orthognathic surgery. The authors have evaluated the efficacy of using fat grafts around the prostheses and demonstrated significant improvement in function and decrease in pain for patients when using the fat grafts as compared with patients who did not receive fat grafts.[62,63] After-surgery outcomes of 115 patients that received fat grafts around the prostheses with an average

after-surgery follow-up of 31 months demonstrated significant improvement in jaw opening and function after surgery with no radiographic or clinical evidence of heterotopic bone or significant fibrosis.

OTHER END-STAGE TEMPOROMANDIBULAR JOINT PATHOLOGIC ABNORMALITY

Other conditions that can cause CR include (1) neoplasms; (2) multiple operated joints; (3) failed TMJ autogenous grafts or alloplastic implants; (4) traumatic injuries; (5) avascular necrosis; (6) metabolic diseases; (7) ICR. Some patients with these conditions may have severe pain, TMJ and jaw dysfunction, facial deformities, and major disability issues. Patients with these TMJ pathologic abnormalities, regardless of the severity, may benefit from TMJ reconstruction and mandibular repositioning with patient-fitted total joint prosthesis, as well as simultaneous maxillary orthognathic surgery to achieve the best outcome results relative to function, stability, esthetics, and reduction of pain.

The authors have demonstrated good outcomes using patient-fitted total joint prostheses and orthognathic surgery in treating other TMJ disorders including multiply operated joints, neoplasms, and those having failed alloplastic TMJ implants. However, the quality of results decreases as the number of previous TMJ surgeries increases, particularly in reference to pain relief and function. When the TMJ Concepts total joint prostheses system is used as the first or second TMJ surgery, the success rate is predictable and good relative to jaw function, stability, facial balance, and pain relief.

SUMMARY

During the past 3 decades, major advancements have been made in TMJ diagnostics and the development of surgical protocols to treat and rehabilitate the pathologic, dysfunctional, and painful TMJ as well as the associated dentofacial deformity. Research has clearly demonstrated that TMJ and orthognathic surgery can be safely and predictably performed at the same operation, but it does necessitate the correct diagnosis and treatment protocol as well as requires the surgeon to have expertise in both TMJ and orthognathic surgery. The surgical procedures can be separated into 2 or more surgical stages, but the TMJ surgery should be done first. With the correct diagnosis and treatment protocol, simultaneous TMJ and orthognathic surgical approaches provide complete and comprehensive management of patients with coexisting TMJ pathologic abnormality and dentofacial deformities.

REFERENCES

1. Fuselier C, Wolford LM, Pitta M, et al. Condylar changes after orthognathic surgery with untreated TMJ internal derangement. J Oral Maxillofac Surg 1998;56(Suppl 1):61.

2. Kerstens HC, Tuinzing DB, Golding RP, et al. Condylar atrophy and osteoarthrosis after bimaxillary surgery. Oral Surg Oral Med Oral Pathol 1990; 69:274–80.

3. De Clercq CA, Neyt LF, Mommaerts MY, et al. Condylar resorption in orthognathic surgery: a retrospective study. Int J Adult Orthodon Orthognath Surg 1994;9:233–40.

4. Crawford JG, Stoelinga PJ, Blijdorp PA, et al. Stability after reoperation for progressive condylar resorption after orthognathic surgery: report of seven cases. J Oral Maxillofac Surg 1994;52:460–6.

5. Arnett GW, Tamborello JA. Progressive class II development: female idiopathic condylar resorption. Oral Maxillofac Surg Clin North Am 1990;2:699–716.

6. Wolford LM. Idiopathic condylar resorption of the temporomandibular joint in teenage girls (cheerleaders syndrome). Proc (Bayl Univ Med Cent) 2001;14(3):246–52.

7. Wolford LM, Cardenas L. Idiopathic condylar resorption: diagnosis, treatment protocol, and outcomes. Am J Orthod Dentofacial Orthop 1999; 116(6):667–77.

8. Gonçalves JR, Cassano DS, Wolford LM, et al. Postsurgical stability of counterclockwise maxillomandibular advancement surgery: affect of articular disc repositioning. J Oral Maxillofac Surg 2008; 66(4):724–38.

9. Wolford LM, Reiche-Fischel O, Mehra P. Changes in temporomandibular joint dysfunction after orthognathic surgery. J Oral Maxillofac Surg 2003;61(6): 655–60 [discussion: 661].

10. Moore KG, Gooris PJ, Stoelinga PJ. The contributing role of condylar resorption in orthognathic surgery: a retrospective study. J Oral Maxillofac Surg 1991;49: 448–60.

11. Goncalves JR, Wolford LM, Cassano DS, et al. Temporomandibular joint condylar changes following maxillomandibular advancement and articular disc repositioning. J Oral Maxillofac Surg 2013;71(10): 1759.e1–15.

12. Wolford LM, Dhameja A. Planning for Combined TMJ Arthroplasty and Orthognathic Surgery. Atlas Oral Maxillofac Surg Clin North Am 2011;19:243–70.

13. Wolford L, Fields RJ. Diagnosis and treatment planning for orthognathic surgery. In: Betts N, Turvey T, editors. Oral andmaxillofacial surgery. Philadelphia: WB Saunders Company; 2000. p. 24–55.

14. Kwon HB, Kim H, Jung WS, et al. Gender differences in dentofacial characteristics of adult patients with temporomandibular disc displacement. J Oral Maxillofac Surg 2013;71(7):1178–86.

15. Bertram S, Moriggl A, Neunteufel N, et al. Lateral cephalometric analysis of mandibular morphology: discrimination among subjects with and without temporomandibular joint disk displacement and osteoarthrosis. J Oral Rehabil 2012;39(2):93–9.

16. Emshoff R, Moriggl A, Rudisch A, et al. Cephalometric variables discriminate among magnetic resonance imaging-based structural characteristic groups of the temporomandibular joint. Oral Surg Oral Med Oral Pathol Oral Radiol Endod 2011;112(1):118–25.

17. Emshoff R, Moriggl A, Rudisch A, et al. Are temporomandibular joint disk displacements without reduction and osteoarthrosis important determinants of mandibular backward positioning and clockwise rotation? Oral Surg Oral Med Oral Pathol Oral Radiol Endod 2011;111(4):435–41.

18. Flores-Mir C, Nebbe B, Heo G, et al. Longitudinal study of temporomandibular joint disc status and craniofacial growth. Am J Orthod Dentofacial Orthop 2006;130(3):324–30.

19. Hwang CJ, Sung SJ, Kim SJ. Lateral cephalometric characteristics of malocclusion patients with temporomandibular joint disorder symptoms. Am J Orthod Dentofacial Orthop 2006;129(4):497–503.

20. Lee DG, Kim TW, Kang SC, et al. Estrogen receptor gene polymorphism and craniofacial morphology in female TMJ osteoarthritis patients. Int J Oral Maxillofac Surg 2006;35(2):165–9.

21. Nebbe B, Major PW, Prasad NG. Female adolescent facial pattern associated with TMJ disk displacement and reduction in disk length: part I. Am J Orthod Dentofacial Orthop 1999;116(2):168–76.

22. Saccucci M, Polimeni A, Festa F, et al. Do skeletal cephalometric characteristics correlate with condylar volume, surface and shape? A 3D analysis. Head Face Med 2012;8:15.

23. Wolford LM, Cottrell DA, Karras SC. Mitek mini anchor in maxillofacial surgery. In: SMST-94 First International Conference on shape memory and superelastic technologies. Monterey (CA): MIAS; 1995. p. 477–82.

24. Mehra P, Wolford LM. The Mitek mini anchor for TMJ disc repositioning: surgical technique and results. Int J Oral Maxillofac Surg 2001;30(6):497–503.

25. Wolford LM, Karras S, Mehra P. Concomitant temporomandibular joint and orthognathic surgery: a preliminary report. J Oral Maxillofac Surg 2002; 60:356–62.

26. Wolford LM. Concomitant temporomandibular joint and orthognathic surgery. J Oral Maxillofac Surg 2003;61(10):1198–204.

27. Wolford LM, Cassano DS, Gonçalves JR. Common TMJ disorders: orthodontic and surgical

management. In: McNamara JA, Kapila SD, editors. Temporomandibular disorders and orofacial pain: separating Controversy from Consensus. Ann Arbor (MI): University of Michigan; 2009. p. 159–98.

28. Wolford LM, Cottrell DA, Henry CH. Temporomandibular joint reconstruction of the complex patient with the Techmedica custom-made total joint prosthesis. J Oral Maxillofac Surg 1994;52:2–10 [discussion: 11].

29. Mercuri LG, Wolford LM, Sanders B, et al. Long-term follow-up of the CAD/CAM patient fitted total temporomandibular joint reconstruction system. J Oral Maxillofac Surg 2002;60:1440–8.

30. Wolford LM, Pitta MC, Reiche-Fischel O, et al. TMJ Concepts/Techmedica custom-made TMJ total joint prosthesis: 5-year follow-up study. Int J Oral Maxillofac Surg 2003;32:268–74.

31. Dela Coleta KE, Wolford LM, Gonçalves JR, et al. Maxillo-mandibular counter-clockwise rotation and mandibular advancement with TMJ Concepts total joint prostheses: part I–skeletal and dental stability. Int J Oral Maxillofac Surg 2009;38(2):126–38.

32. Pinto LP, Wolford LM, Buschang PH, et al. Maxillo-mandibular counter-clockwise rotation and mandibular advancement with TMJ Concepts total joint prostheses: part III–pain and dysfunction outcomes. Int J Oral Maxillofac Surg 2009;38(4):326–31.

33. Allen W, Movahed R, Wolford LM. Twenty Year Follow-up of Patient Fitted Total Joint Prostheses for Reconstruction of the Temporomandibular Joint. Abstract presented at Association of Oral and Maxillofacial Surgeons 93rd Annual Meeting, San Diego, CA, September 12-16, 2012.

34. Wolford LM, Chemello PD, Hilliard F. Occlusal plane alteration in orthognathic surgery–part I: effects on function and esthetics. Am J Orthod Dentofacial Orthop 1994;106:304–16.

35. Chemello PD, Wolford LM, Buschang PH. Occlusal plane alteration in orthognathic surgery–part II: long-term stability of results. Am J Orthod Dentofacial Orthop 1994;106:434–40.

36. Wolford LM, Chemello PD, Hilliard FW. Occlusal plane alteration in orthognathic surgery. J Oral Maxillofac Surg 1993;51:730–40 [discussion: 740–1].

37. Cottrell DA, Wolford LM. Altered orthognathic surgical sequencing and a modified approach to model surgery. J Oral Maxillofac Surg 1994;52:1010–20 [discussion: 1020–1].

38. Aufdemorte TB, Van Sickels JE, Dolwick MF, et al. Estrogen receptors in the temporomandibular joint of the baboon (Papio cynocephalus): an autoradiographic study. Oral Surg Oral Med Oral Pathol 1986;61(4):307–14.

39. Milam SB, Aufdemorte TB, Sheridan PJ, et al. Sexual dimorphism in the distribution of estrogen receptors in the temporomandibular joint complex of the baboon. Oral Surg Oral Med Oral Pathol 1987; 64(5):527–32.

40. Abubaker AO, Raslan WF, Sotereanos GC. Estrogen and progesterone receptors in temporomandibular joint discs of symptomatic and asymptomatic persons: a preliminary study. J Oral Maxillofac Surg 1993;51(10):1096–100.

41. Tsai CL, Liu TK, Chen TJ. Estrogen and osteoarthritis: a study of synovial estradiol and estradiol receptor binding in human osteoarthritic knees. Biochem Biophys Res Commun 1992;183(3):1287–91.

42. Koelling S, Miosge N. Sex differences of chondrogenic progenitor cells in late stages of osteoarthritis. Arthritis Rheum 2010;62(4):1077–87.

43. Tzanidakis K, Sidebottom AJ. Outcomes of open temporomandibular joint surgery following failure to improve after arthroscopy: is there an algorithm for success? Br J Oral Maxillofac Surg 2013;51(8): 818–21.

44. Sidebottom AJ. Current thinking in temporomandibular joint management. Br J Oral Maxillofac Surg 2009;47(2):91–4. A.

45. Arnett GW, Gunson MJ. Risk factors in the initiation of condylar resorption. Semin Orthod 2013;19(2):81–8.

46. Yushkevich PA, Piven J, Hazlett HC, et al. User-guided 3D active contour segmentation of anatomical structures: significantly improved efficiency and reliability. Neuroimage 2006;31(3):1116–28.

47. Cevidanes LH, Bailey LJ, Tucker GR, et al. Superimposition of 3D cone-beam CT models of orthognathic surgery patients. Dentomaxillofac Radiol 2005;34(6):369–75.

48. Cevidanes LH, Hajati AK, Paniagua B, et al. Quantification of condylar resorption in TMJ osteoarthritis. Oral Surg Oral Med Oral Pathol Oral Radiol Endod 2010;110(1):110–7.

49. Paniagua B, Cevidanes L, Zhu H, et al. Outcome quantification using SPHARM-PDM toolbox in orthognathic surgery. Int J Comput Assist Radiol Surg 2011; 6(5):617–26.

50. Cevidanes LHS, Bailey LJ, Tucker SF, et al. Three-dimensional cone-beam computed tomography for assessment of mandibular changes after orthognathic surgery. Am J Orthodont Dent Ortho 2007; 131(1):44–50.

51. Cevidanes LH, Styner MA, Proffit WR. Image analysis and superimposition of 3-dimensional cone-beam computed tomography models. Am J Orthod Dentofacial Orthop 2006;129(5):611–8.

52. Henry CH, Hudson AP, Gérard HC, et al. Identification of Chlamydia trachomatis in the human temporomandibular joint. J Oral Maxillofac Surg 1999; 57(6):683–8 [discussion: 689].

53. Henry CH, Hughes CV, Gérard HC, et al. Reactive arthritis: preliminary microbiologic analysis of the human temporomandibular joint. J Oral Maxillofac Surg 2000;58(10):1137–42 [discussion: 1143–4].

54. Hudson AP, Henry C, Wolford LM, et al. Chlamydia psittaci infection may influence development of

temporomandibular joint dysfunction. J Arthritis Rheumatism 2000;43:S174.

55. Henry CH, Pitta MC, Wolford LM. Frequency of chlamydial antibodies in patients with internal derangement of the temporomandibular joint. Oral Surg Oral Med Oral Pathol Oral Radiol Endod 2001; 91(3):287–92.

56. Kim S, Park Y, Hong S, et al. The presence of bacteria in the synovial fluid of the temporomandibular joint and clinical significance: preliminary study. J Oral Maxillofac Surg 2003;61:1156–61.

57. Gérard HC, Carter JD, Hudson AP. Chlamydia trachomatis is present and metabolically active during the remitting phase in synovial tissues from patients with chronic Chlamydia-induced reactive arthritis. Am J Med Sci 2013;346(1):22–5.

58. Paegle DI, Holmlund AB, öStlund MR, et al. The occurrence of antibodies against Chlamydia species in patients with monoarthritis and chronic closed lock of the temporomandibular joint. J Oral Maxillofac Surg 2004;62(4):435–9.

59. Henry CH, Wolford LM. Substance P and mast cells: preliminary histologic analysis of the human temporomandibular joint. Oral Surg Oral Med Oral Pathol Oral Radiol Endod 2001;92(4):384–9.

60. Henry CH, Nikaein A, Wolford LM. Analysis of human leukocyte antigens in patients with internal derangement of the temporomandibular joint. J Oral Maxillofac Surg 2002;60(7):778–83.

61. Wolford LM, Henry CH, Goncalves JR. TMJ and systemic affects associated with Chlamydia psittaci. J Oral Maxillofac Surg 2004;62(Suppl 1):50–1.

62. Wolford LM, Karras SC. Autologous fat transplantation around temporomandibular joint total joint prostheses: preliminary treatment outcomes. J Oral Maxillofac Surg 1997;55(3):245–51 [discussion: 251–2].

63. Wolford LM, Morales-Ryan CA, Morales PG, et al. Autologous fat grafts placed around temporomandibular joint total joint prostheses to prevent heterotopic bone formation. Proc (Bayl Univ Med Cent) 2008;21(3):248–54.

64. Mehra P, Wolford LM, Baran S, et al. Single-stage comprehensive surgical treatment of the rheumatoid arthritis temporomandibular joint patient. J Oral Maxillofac Surg 2009;67(9):1859–72.

65. Freitas R, Wolford LM, Baran S, et al. Autogenous versus alloplastic TMJ reconstruction in rheumatoid-induced TMJ disease. J Oral Maxillofac Surg 2002; 58(Suppl 1):43.

66. Wolford LM, Rodrigues DB. Temporomandibular joint (TMJ) pathologies in growing patients: effects on facial growth and development. In: Preedy VR, editor. Handbook of growth and growth monitoring in health and disease. New York: Springer; 2012. p. 1809–28.

67. Wolford LM, Rodrigues D. Orthognathic considerations in the young patient and effects on facial growth. In: Preedy VR, editor. Handbook of growth and growth monitoring in health and disease. New York: Springer; 2012. p. 1789–808.

68. Coleta KE, Wolford LM, Gonçalves JR, et al. Maxillomandibular counter-clockwise rotation and mandibular advancement with TMJ Concepts total joint prostheses: part II–airway changes and stability. Int J Oral Maxillofac Surg 2009;38(3):228–35.

The Current Role and the Future of Minimally Invasive Temporomandibular Joint Surgery

Raúl González-García, MD, PhD, FEBOMFS[a,b,*]

KEYWORDS

- Minimally invasive temporomandibular joint surgery • Temporomandibular joint arthroscopy
- Temporomandibular joint arthrocentesis

KEY POINTS

- Minimally invasive temporomandibular joint surgery (MITMJS) is a reliable method for the treatment of most internal derangement (ID) of the temporomandibular joint (TMJ), with a relatively low complication rate.
- Arthrocentesis is recommended for the treatment of acute or subacute closed lock of the TMJ for disk displacement without reduction of less than 3 months evolution, whereas arthroscopy is definitively preferred for the treatment of chronic closed lock of the TMJ (>3 months evolution).
- Arthroscopy is indicated for ID of the TMJ, mainly Wilkes stages II, III, and IV, degenerative joint disease, synovitis, painful hypermobility, or recidivist luxation of discal cause, and hypomobility caused by intra-articular adherences.
- With an overall complication rate less than 1.5%, MITMJS seems to be safe, although the surgeon must be aware of any potential complications during or immediately after the procedure.
- In the future, MITMJS may evolve to the combination of arthroscopic and endoscopic techniques with navigation for the treatment of TMJ disease, including ID, TMJ ankylosis, condylar hyperplasia, and TMJ tumors.

INTRODUCTION

As previously reported,[1] some temporomandibular joint (TMJ) diagnoses such as ankylosis, tumors, and growth abnormalities have an absolute indication for TMJ open surgery, whereas most disorders related to temporomandibular disease (TMD) have a relative indication for surgery, because conservative nonsurgical management is often the first approach. Indications for minimally invasive TMJ surgery (MITMJS) seem to be restricted to this second group of patients with relative indications for surgery, because patients with ankylosis, tumors, and growth abnormalities of the TMJ may often need open surgical approaches.

It might be thought that this situation limits MITMJS to secondary or minor indications. However, because most disorders related to TMD with primary involvement of the joint are TMJ internal derangement (ID) and osteoarthrosis, MITMJS becomes a definitive tool for alleviating symptoms in terms of pain and function with minimal expected morbidity. Moreover, MITMJS should be considered early in the management sequence in some cases, even before the failure

[a] Department of Oral and Maxillofacial-Head and Neck Surgery, University Hospital Infanta Cristina, Avenida de Elvas s/n, Badajoz 06080, Spain; [b] University School of Medicine, Avenida de Elvas s/n, Badajoz 06080, Spain
* Calle Los Yébenes 35, 8°C, Madrid 28047, Spain.
E-mail address: raulmaxilo@gmail.com

Oral Maxillofacial Surg Clin N Am 27 (2015) 69–84
http://dx.doi.org/10.1016/j.coms.2014.09.006
1042-3699/15/$ – see front matter © 2015 Elsevier Inc. All rights reserved.

of conservative treatment, to avoid progression of the disease to a more symptomatic stage or to a surgically nonrespondent phase of the disease.

This article focuses on the current role of MITMJS in terms of indications, surgical techniques, clinical outcomes, and complications. Also, the future applications and possible evolution of these techniques for the treatment of TMD are discussed.

HISTORICAL SUMMARY

In 1975, Onishi[2] first reported the use of the arthroscope in the TMJ for diagnostic purposes. In 1982, Murakami and Hoshino[3] developed the nomenclature of TMJ arthroscopic anatomy. In 1983, McCain,[4] in a cadaver study with 67 joints, favored the development of routine TMJ arthroscopy. Holmlund and Hellsing,[5] in a study of 54 cadavers, described anatomic key points to make this technique secure and standardized. Several studies concerning the benefit of arthroscopy for treating TMJ disease begin to appear in the literature. In 1986, Sanders[6] described the benefit of arthroscopy for the treatment of acute closed lock (ACL) or chronic closed lock (CCL) of the TMJ and introduced the term lysis as a distension of the joint with a blunt trocar to eliminate the suction effect of the disk to the fossa, and so lysing or breaking the adherences. In the same year, Murakami and Ono[7] described the arthroscopic removal of intra-articular adherences. In 1989, Israel,[8] Tarro,[9] and Ohnishi[10] independently first described the use of arthroscopic suture for the treatment of anterior disk displacement or recurrent mandibular dislocation. Posteriorly, several techniques for arthroscopic suture were described by McCain and colleagues[11] in 1992, Tarro[12] in 1994, and Goizueta-Adame and Muñoz-Guerra[13] and Yang and colleagues[14] in 2012. Description of each of these techniques and discussion of their advantages and disadvantages are beyond the scope of this article.

Because arthroscopic lysis and lavage (ALL) was already a reliable technique for treating TMJ ID, Murakami and colleagues,[15] in 1987, introduced arthrocentesis of the TMJ, by reporting the recapture of the anteriorly displaced disk by mandibular manipulation after pumping and hydraulic pressure to the upper joint of the TMJ. In 1991, Nitzan and colleagues[16] introduced a modified method, which was based on the insertion of 2 needles in the upper joint space for lavage without direct visualization of the joint.

INDICATIONS OF MINIMALLY INVASIVE TEMPOROMANDIBULAR JOINT SURGERY
Arthrocentesis

- Most of the studies in relation to the use of arthrocentesis for the treatment of ID of the TMJ have investigated its usefulness in ACL. It is also an excellent diagnostic tool for the patient with unclear cause who presents with functional limitations and pain of the TMJ. Several indications have been proposed[17-20]:
  1. ACL of the TMJ: anterior displacement of the disk without reduction of less than a month of evolution that does not respond to passive manipulation of the mandible or conservative treatment
  2. Subacute closed lock (SACL): anterior displacement of the disk without reduction of 1 to 3 months of evolution that does not respond to conservative treatment
  3. Anchored disk phenomenon diagnosed by nuclear magnetic resonance (NMR)
  4. TMJ trauma with chronic pain and capsulitis caused by whiplash
  5. Some cases of painful degenerative joint disease (osteoarthrosis) refractory to conservative treatment
  6. Inflammatory arthropathies: rheumatoid arthritis, juvenile idiopathic arthritis, sclerodermia; metabolic arthropathies: hyperuricemia, chondrocalcinosis, with important articular pain as a temporary way of treating the patient's symptoms
  7. Patients who reject arthroscopy or who cannot be submitted for general anesthesia
- Some contraindications for arthrocentesis have also been proposed:
  1. Psychiatric pathology
  2. Fibrous and osseous ankylosis
  3. Multiply operated joints
  4. Regional infectious disease
  5. Regional tumoral disease

Arthroscopy

- The American Association of Oral and Maxillofacial Surgeons (AAOMS) established 5 main indications for arthroscopy of the TMJ[17-20]:
  1. ID of the TMJ, mainly Wilkes stages II, III, and IV
  2. Degenerative joint disease (osteoarthritis)
  3. Synovitis
  4. Painful hypermobility or recidivist luxation of discal cause
  5. Hypomobility caused by intra-articular adherences

- Some other indications have been proposed:
  1. Inflammatory arthropathies (systemic arthritis)
  2. Articular symptoms subsidiary to orthognathic surgery
  3. Revision of the TMJ in cases of intra-articular implants
- The main contraindications for TMJ arthroscopic procedures are:
  1. Cutaneous, otic, or articular infection
  2. Tumor with risk of extension
  3. Severe fibrous or osseous ankylosis

TMD specifically related to ID of the TMJ closed lock (ie, disk displacement without reduction) has been reported to be effectively treated by MITMJS. According to our research, ACL or SACL of the TMJ (<3 months of evolution) seems to adequately respond to arthrocentesis as well as to arthroscopy, whereas CCL (>3 months of evolution) may need arthroscopy for better control and resolution of the disease. Because arthrocentesis may be less invasive than arthroscopy (particularly, operative arthroscopy [OA]), it is ideal for the treatment of cases of recently established closed lock. Most of the long-standing cases may benefit from the use of instrumentation over the displaced disk and surrounding affected soft tissues, such as the retrodiscal tissue. This process can be accomplished only with operative or advanced arthroscopic techniques. However, some investigators[21] have also reported the benefit of arthrocentesis for the treatment of CCL. The author believes that if arthroscopy can be performed, then CCL of the TMJ is the main scenario for its application. Nevertheless, the results from our group suggest that arthroscopy is a useful technique for the treatment of patients with CCL of the TMJ with minimal complications, showing a significant decrease in pain with a parallel increase in mouth opening from the first month postoperatively; these results were predictable and stable for a minimum period of 2 years.[22]

CLASSIFICATIONS OF TEMPOROMANDIBULAR JOINT INTERNAL DERANGEMENT

The most popular classification for ID of the TMJ is that proposed by Wilkes (**Table 1**).[23] Bronstein and Merrill[24] added arthroscopic findings to the clinical and radiologic findings of previous studies (**Table 2**). Other classifications such as that by Molinari and colleagues[25] have tried to simplify the precedents by evaluating disk displacement in the anterior direction, because it is the most frequently observed. These investigators categorize the classification in 4 clinical

---

Table 1
Clinical and radiologic findings according to Wilkes classification for TMJ ID

Stage	Clinical Findings	Radiologic Findings
I	No significant mechanical symptoms, no pain or limitation of motion	Slight forward displacement and good anatomic contour of disk
II	First few episodes of pain, occasional joint tenderness and related temporal headaches, increase in intensity of clicking, joint sounds later in opening movement, beginning transient subluxations or joint locking	Slight forward displacement and beginning anatomic deformity of disk, slight thickening of posterior edge of disk
III	Multiple episodes of pain, joint tenderness, temporal headaches, locking, closed locks, restriction of motion, difficulty (pain) with function	Anterior displacement with significant anatomic deformity/prolapse of disk, moderate to marked thickening of posterior edge of disk, no hard tissue changes
IV	Characterized by chronicity with variable and episodic pain, headaches, variable restriction of motion, and undulating course	Increase in severity over intermediate stage, early to moderate degenerative remodeling hard tissue changes
V	Crepitus on examination, scraping, grating, grinding symptoms, variable and episodic pain, chronic restriction of motion, difficulty with function	Gross anatomic deformity of disk and hard tissue, essentially degenerative arthritic changes, osteophytic deformity, subcortical cystic formation

Adapted from Wilkes CH. Internal derangements of the temporomandibular joint: pathological variations. Arch Otolaryngol Head Neck Surg 1989;115:469–7.

Table 2
Classification of Bronstein and Merrill of TMJ ID in relation to Wilkes classification

Stage	Roofing (%)	Arthroscopic Findings
I	80–100	Elongation of bilaminar zone, normal synovia and disk, no cartilage involvement
II	50–100	Elongation of bilaminar zone, synovitis with adherences in initial phase, anterolateral prolapse of the capsule
III	25–50	Elongation of bilaminar zone, important synovitis, decrease of lateral recess, decrease of lateral recess, adherences, chondromalacia I–II
IV	0–25	Hyalinization of posterior ligament, synovitis, adherences, chondromalacia III–IV
V	0	Retrodiscal hyalinization, disk perforation, fibrillation of articular surfaces, advanced synovitis, gross adhesions, chondromalacia IV

Adapted from Bronstein SL, Merrill R. Clinical staging for TMJ internal derangement: application to arthroscopy. J Craniomandib Disord 1992;6:7–16.

stages, based on the degree of disk displacement, the reversibility of disk displacement during opening and closing movements, and changes in disk morphology observed by NMR. Despite this simplification, the classifications by Wilkes[23] and Bronstein and Merrill[24] are most frequently used.

ARTHROSCOPIC ANATOMY OF THE TEMPOROMANDIBULAR JOINT

The TMJ is a synovial joint between the temporal bone and the mandibular condyle, which presents both superior and inferior spaces, with an interposed disk between them.[17] The superior joint space (SJS) is cranially limited by an articular surface that covers the articular eminence and the mandibular fossa.[17]

- Within the SJS, 7 areas can be examined (**Fig. 1**). These areas are:
  1. Medial synovial drape
  2. Pterygoid shadow
  3. Retrodiscal synovium:
     a. Zone 1: oblique protuberance
     b. Zone 2: retrodiscal synovial tissue attached to posterior glenoid process
     c. Zone 3: lateral recess of retrodiscal synovial tissue
  4. Posterior slope of articular eminence and glenoid fossa
  5. Articular disk
  6. Intermediate zone
  7. Anterior recess:
     a. Disk synovial crease
     b. Midportion
     c. Medial-anterior corner
     d. Lateral-anterior corner
- Four classic anatomic landmarks have been described:

1. Medial synovial drape with distinct superior to inferior striae
2. Oblique protuberance of the retrodiscal synovium
3. Posterior slope of the articular eminence with distinct anterior to posterior striae
4. Anterior disk synovial crease: juncture of anterior synovium and anterior band of disk

The first area to be arthroscopically examined is the medial synovial drape (**Fig. 2**), which has a gray-white translucent lining and a tense appearance with distinct superior to inferior

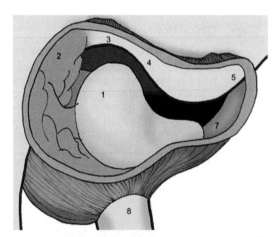

Fig. 1. The TMJ and the arthroscopic areas to be ideally examined. *1*, articular disk; *2*, synovial lining in the posterior recess; *3*, glenoid fossa; *4*, posterior slope of the eminence; *5*, articular eminence; *6*, medial-anterior corner of the anterior recess; *7*, lateral-anterior corner of the anterior recess; *8*, condyle. (*From* González-García R, Gil-Díez Usandizaga JL, Rodríguez-Campo FJ. Arthroscopic anatomy and lysis and lavage of the temporomandibular joint. Atlas Oral Maxillofac Surg Clin North Am 2011;19:132; with permission.)

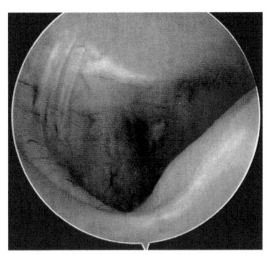

Fig. 2. Medial synovial drape of a right TMJ examined by arthroscopy. Note the oblique protuberance down and focal areas of hyperemia in the medial synovial drape. The posterior band of the disk is visualized at the right side. The temporal fossa is partially appreciated in the upper side of the image.

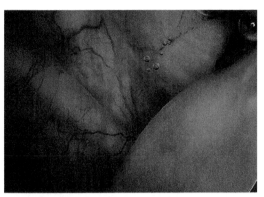

Fig. 4. Retrodiscal synovium and posterior ligament of a right TMJ examined by arthroscopy. Note the prominence of the posterior ligament through the synovia when the disk is anteriorly pulled by the assistant through passive mouth opening during the arthroscopic procedure. Focal areas of hyperemia are observed. Note the milky white and highly reflective disk at the right side of the image.

striae. The second area to be examined is the pterygoid shadow (**Fig. 3**), with a purple appearance, which is located anterior to the medial synovial drape. The third area to be examined is the retrodiscal synovium (**Fig. 4**). Here, the synovial membrane covers the posterior insertion of the disk and is reflected superiorly to the temporal fossa. While the mouth is open, the posterior insertion covered by the synovial lining appears as a crest or crease. This finding is named oblique protuberance. The fourth area of the superior

joint is the posterior slope of the articular eminence (**Fig. 5**). The fibrocartilage is white and highly reflective and is thick in the back slope of the eminence. The articular disk, which is the fifth area to be examined (**Fig. 6**), is milky white, highly reflective, and without striae. Normally, the disk glides fluently along the articular eminence. The concept of roofing evaluates the covering of the articular disk over the condyle. Roofing is graded arthroscopically according to the posterior band of the articular disk and its position relative to the articular eminence. When it is measured with the condyle forward, the disk is in normal position (roofing 100%) if the posterior band of the disk is lying adjacent to the posterior

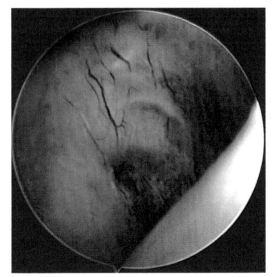

Fig. 3. Pterigoid shadow of a right TMJ examined by arthroscopy. Focal areas of hyperemia are visualized.

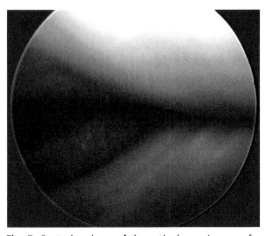

Fig. 5. Posterior slope of the articular eminence of a right TMJ examined by arthroscopy. Note the healthy-appearing area of the examined surfaces.

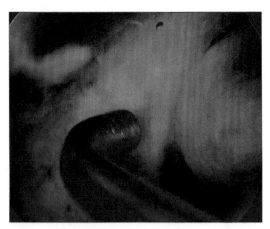

Fig. 6. Articular disk, which in normal conditions is milky white, highly reflective, and without striae, as seen in **Figs. 2–5** and **7**. Here, a perforation of the disk was observed during the arthroscopy. Note that the condylar pole is visualized through the upper joint compartment (*right*), while the margins of the remnant disk are palpated and gently pushed back by a blunt probe through the working cannula (*left*).

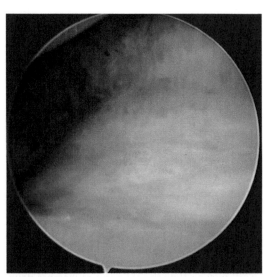

Fig. 8. Anterior recess of a right TMJ examined by arthroscopy. This is the typical area for triangulation and introduction of a working cannula whenever possible. Miotomy of the lateral pterigoid muscle and anterior release may be performed in cases of closed lock with anterior disk displacement.

slope of the articular eminence. With the condyle seated, it is 100% roofed if the posterior band of the disk abuts at approximately the midportion of the glenoid fossa. The intermediate zone is the sixth area to be examined (**Fig. 7**). Without disorders, this area has a white on white appearance, and the concavity of the disk can be observed. The anterior recess (**Fig. 8**) is the seventh area to be examined. It begins with the condyle seated. In this area, the anterior disk synovial crease, which is the fourth classic anatomic landmark, is identified. At the anterolateral site, the union between the lateral synovial capsule and

the anterior disk synovial crease can be observed, and this is the ideal place for insertion of the second or working cannula.

SURGICAL TECHNIQUES
Arthrocentesis

This procedure is usually performed under local anesthesia with or without intravenous sedation. Once the preauricular area is disinfected, the posterolateral puncture site is performed 10 mm ahead of and 2 mm below the canthal-tragal line. At this point, local anesthesia is used to infiltrate the joint by perforating the capsule with an intramuscular needle. Up to 2 cm³ of bupivacaine 0.5% or lidocaine 2% with adrenalin 1:100,000 are infiltrated into the joint. With the patient's mouth gently opened, the syringe must be directed in a 45° angle from posterior to anterior and from downward to upward until the edge of the temporalis fossa at approximately 15 mm from the skin is palpated. Posteriorly, the syringe is directed anteriorly to the eminence until the injected fluid leaks out of the joint into the syringe. A more anterior puncture with an intramuscular needle at 20 mm ahead of and 7 mm below the canthal-tragal line is used for drainage. Instillation of up to 250 to 300 cm³ of Ringer solution is recommended for the entire procedure. After lavage of the upper compartment, substances such as corticoids or sodium hyaluronate can be instilled (**Fig. 9**).

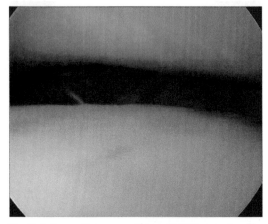

Fig. 7. Intermediate zone of a right TMJ examined by arthroscopy. Note the disk (*bottom*) and the eminence (*top*).

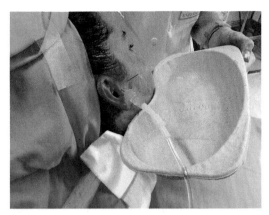

Fig. 9. Arthrocentesis of the TMJ. Continuous irrigation with Ringer solution through a double-puncture technique.

Arthroscopic Lysis and Lavage

ALL can be performed by a single-puncture or a double-puncture technique. If a single-puncture technique is used, lysis is directly performed with the arthroscope. When a double-puncture technique is used, the second cannula is used for the introduction of the instruments that break the adherences, such as hooked probes or biopsy forceps, under direct vision.[25] In contrast to ALL with a double-puncture technique, OA (or advanced arthroscopy) uses 2 or more working cannulas for the introduction of instrumentation to perform procedures other than lysis of adherences, such as debridement, miotomy of the pterigoid muscle for anterior release of the disk, disk reduction, retrodiscal scarification, and suture or rigid disk fixation.

Previously to the insertion of the cannula, an intramuscular G21 green 0.8 × 24 mm needle is introduced in the joint at the same point as the cannula at the most concave point of the glenoid fossa, and insufflation with 2 to 3 mL Ringer lactate is performed. This maneuver allows distension of the joint and facilitates the insertion of the cannula into the joint. According to the description by McCain and de la Rua,[26] the first cannula has to be placed at the maximum concavity of the glenoid fossa, by direct palpation. After the introduction of the sharp trocar through the skin, the ledge of the zygomatic bone at the fossa level must be palpated. Once it has been stepped off, the trocar is directed in a superior and slightly anterior fashion until a resistance is noted. With a controlled pressure and rotational movements in a deeper vector, the capsule of the joint is penetrated.

At this point, the sharp trocar is removed and a blunt trocar is used for further introduction of the cannula. In our experience, most of the patients need the cannula to be introduced up to 25 to 30 mm from the skin surface, although with some very thin patients, it needs to be introduced only up to 20 mm. Immediately, the arthroscope is introduced through the cannula to check if it is effectively placed into the joint space. The structures of the superior joint compartment at the posterior recess have to be clearly visualized in the monitor. If not, the cannula may not be adequately placed into the joint space, and the introduction of the cannula has to be repeated. Once the cannula is adequately placed inside the superior joint, a 22-gauge needle is inserted 5 mm anterior and 5 mm inferior to the fossa puncture site until a continuous irrigation with Ringer lactate solution is obtained. Sweeping is performed with direct visualization for lysis of possible adherences. Lavage with approximately 250 to 300 mL of Ringer solution is performed (**Fig. 10**). Although the introduction of a second cannula is not necessarily accompanied by the performance of any technique over the tissues of the joint other than lysis of the adherences with instrumentation, it is clearly indicated for

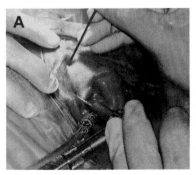
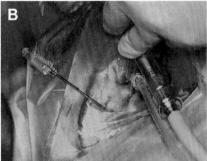

Fig. 10. ALL. (*A*) Introduction of the scope posteriorly and insertion of the 22-gauge needle as a drainage anteriorly to the scope. (*B*) Establishment of a continuous Ringer solution irrigation from the scope to the drainage needle.

OA or advanced arthroscopy, because instrumentation is not usually necessary to eliminate most of the adherences of the joint.

Operative or Advanced Arthroscopy

The first part of the procedure is the same as that for ALL. Whenever possible, the first cannula with the scope must be directed to the anterior recess of the joint under direct visualization. This process can be accomplished with the joint completely seated in the fossa. The working cannula is introduced from an entrance point in the skin at a distance similar to that from the skin to the tip of the first cannula, following the same vector, according to the principles of triangulation, which serve to blindly bring 2 objects together in space (**Fig. 11**).[26] The sharp trocar/cannula penetrates perpendicular to the skin, tracing a triangle with the first cannula, looking for the tip of the scope. Once the sharp trocar is removed and the blunt trocar introduced through the working cannula, both the first and the working cannula have to be moved in a synchronized manner so as not to lose the visualization of the working cannula. At the anterior recess, a miotomy of the lateral pterigoid muscle can be performed by the introduction of a radiofrequency coblation (RFC) terminal through the working cannula in cases in which disk displacement without reduction is observed. Once this procedure has been performed, both cannulas are moved backwards to the posterior recess. RFC can be used for cauterization of areas of synovitis at the retrodiscal tissue (**Fig. 12**).

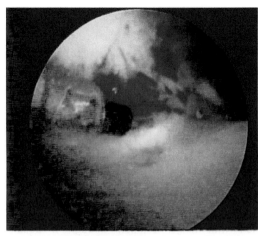

Fig. 12. Use of the RFC instrumentation for treating synovitis of the retrodiscal tissue in the posterior recess of the upper joint compartment.

In cases in which the superior compartment is collapsed because of fibrosis or advanced arthrosis, the entrance point at the skin must be placed at approximately 1 cm ahead of and 1 cm below the entrance point of the first cannula, following the principles of triangulation. Tools can be introduced through the working cannula, such as forceps, scissors, hooks, electric blade, laser (CO_2 laser or holmium yttrium aluminum garnet laser) and RFC terminals. The use of instrumentation for arthroscopic surgery of the TMJ has been reviewed by McCain and Hossameldin.[27] Also, substances such as sodium hyaluronate, corticosteroids, plate-derived growth factors, and nonsteroidal antiinflammatory drugs can be infiltrated in the lumen or subsynovially through the working cannula with direct visual control of the puncture site, in contrast to what is performed by arthrocentesis or ALL with a single-puncture technique.

Miotomy of the lateral pterigoid muscle is performed in the context of arthroscopic discopexy, followed by disk reduction, retrodiscal scarification, and disk fixation. Most of the cases in which discopexy is performed are patients with ID presenting with disk displacement with or without reduction. The aim of the procedure is to restore the normal and functional anatomy of the joint. The author uses RFC for the anterior release of the disk by miotomy of the lateral pterigoid muscle, and also for the treatment of synovitis and scarification or contraction of the retrodiscal tissue (**Fig. 13**). RFC uses a controlled, non–heat-driven process, in which bipolar radiofrequency energy excites the electrodes in a saline solution to generate charged plasma gas.[26] The purpose

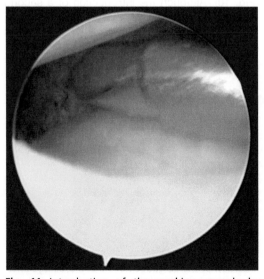

Fig. 11. Introduction of the working cannula by means of the triangulation technique.

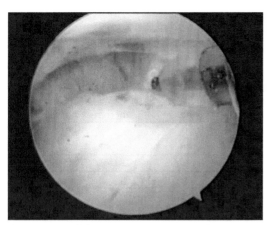

Fig. 13. Use of the RFC instrumentation for anterior release by miotomy of the lateral pterigoid muscle in the anterior recess of the upper joint space.

of scarification is to facilitate the posterior positioning of the disk after anterior release and reduction. Disk fixation may be performed by introducing a second working cannula. Two main methods have been described: (1) suture disk fixation and (2) rigid fixation. Detailed description of each type of fixation is beyond the scope of this article; the reader is referred to McCain and Hossameldin[27] and Yang and colleagues[14] for future reading (**Fig. 14**).

CLINICAL OUTCOMES

Analysis of the literature concerning clinical outcome of MITMJS for the treatment of ID identifies 3 main concerns: (1) most of the studies are retrospective series of cases, and only a few randomized studies comparing different techniques

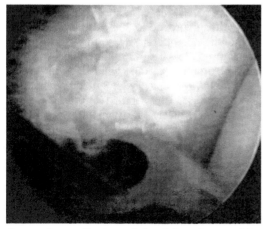

Fig. 14. Suture fixation of the disk with a 2/0 blue nylon for in a case of CCL with disk displacement without reduction.

of MITMJs are available in the literature; (2) inclusion criteria for each technique are not usually well defined; (3) there is no consensus among investigators on the way of measuring success. All these issues make comparison among studies difficult and subjected to bias. Improvement in the severity of pain may be calculated as a relative measure or percentage from the postoperative value in relation to the preoperative one. Another way of measuring results is to establish a success rate. When research is reported, it is desirable to distinguish clearly which method of evaluation was used, so that outcomes can be compared among studies.[28]

Arthrocentesis

Several studies have shown promising results for arthrocentesis, especially when used in cases of acute disk displacement without disk reduction. When compared with ALL, the latter generally had a slightly superior overall success rate. In a review of studies concerning the use of arthrocentesis for the treatment of ID of the TMJ,[29] with evaluation of 612 joints in 586 patients with ACL, a mean success rate up to 83.5% has been reported.

Arthroscopic Lysis and Lavage

Success rates for ALL in the literature according to improvement of maximal interincisal opening (MIO) and decrease of pain in the TMJ are presented in **Table 3**.[4,30–44] The main concern about the data provided in the literature is the absence of homogeneity. Most of the investigators refer to success rate in terms of the percentage of patients presenting with pain reduction or increase of mouth opening. However, few investigators quantify the amount of pain relief or the increase of mouth opening. To alleviate this bias, it is recommended to measure success of ALL and OA according to the criteria of the AAOMS,[45] later modified by Eriksson and Westesson,[46] who considered the technique successful when (1) a visual analogue score (VAS) score of less than 20 and (2) MIO of 35 mm or more were obtained.

Sanders and Buoncristiani,[30] in a series of 137 patients, observed an 82% success rate with patients presenting with MIO more than 40 mm and scarce or complete absence of pain. Indresano[31] reported a 73% global success rate for ALL in a series of 50 patients with TMJ ID. Moses and Poker,[33] in a series of 237 patients (419 joints), reported a 92% success rate for ALL in terms of decrease of pain and a 78% in terms of increase of MIO. Later series[34,36–39,43] have reported an

Table 3
Results in terms of success rate according to pain reduction and increase of mouth opening from most relevant studies in patients with ID of the TMJ undergoing ALL

Author, Year	Number of Patients (Joints)	Global Success Rate (%)	Patients with Pain Reduction/Pain Reduction in VAS/Pain Reduction (%)	Patients with Increase in MIO (%)/MIO Increase (mm)/MIO Increase (%)
Sanders & Buoncristiani,[30] 1987	137	82	—/—/—	—/—/—
Indresano,[31] 1989	50 (80)	73	—/—/—	—/—/—
Moses et al,[32] 1989	92 (152)	92	—/—/—	80/—/—
Moses & Poker,[33] 1989	237 (419)	—	92/—/—	78/—/—
White,[34] 1989	66 (100)	86	—/—/—	—/—/—
Clark et al,[35] 1991	18	81	—/—/57	—/13/67
Moore et al,[36] 1993	63	87	—/—/—	—/—/—
Mosby,[37] 1993	109 (150)	93	—/—/—	—/—/—
Holmlund et al,[38] 1994	42 (42)	50	—/—/—	—/—/—
Nitzan et al,[21] 1997	39 (40)	95	—/from 9.24 to 1.45 (in a 1–15 scale)/84	—/11/—
Kurita et al,[39] 1998	14 (16)	86	—/—/—	—/—/—
Sorel & Piecuch,[40] 2000	22 (44)	91	81/—/—	100/8/—
Dimitroulis,[41] 2002	56	84	66/—/—	—/9.8/—
Kondoh et al,[42] 2003	20	80	—/—/—	—/10/—
Smolka et al,[43] 2008	39 (45)	87	89/—/—	74/—/—
González-García & Rodríguez-Campo,[44] 2011	156	—	75 (WII), 71 (WIII), 71 (WIV)[a] 88 (WII), 86 (WIII), 87 (WIV)[b]	61 (WII), 73 (WIII), 52 (WIV)[a] 74 (WII), 78 (WIII), 66 (WIV)[b]

Abbreviations: WII, Wilkes II; WIII, Wilkes III; WIV, Wilkes IV.
[a] Data at 6 months postoperatively.
[b] Data at 24 months postoperatively.
Data from Refs.[21,30–44]

overall success rate for ALL ranging from 50% to 93% of patients. However, all these series lack information regarding the amount of pain relief or the amount of increase in mouth opening. Clark and colleagues,[35] in a small series of 18 patients, reported a reduction of pain of 57% and a parallel increase in mouth opening of 67% (13 mm). Nitzan and colleagues[21] reported more optimistic results for ALL in terms of overall success, with 95% of patients, 84% pain relief, and a mean increase of 11 mm in mouth opening. More recently, Dimitroulis[41] reported an 84% overall success rate for ALL, with 66% of the patients presenting with decrease of pain and an increase of mouth opening of almost 10 mm. For a better understanding of the influence of Wilkes stages and postoperative follow-up on success rate concerning pain relief and MIO improvement, González-García and Rodríguez-Campo,[44] in a series of 156 patients undergoing ALL for the treatment of

TMJ ID, reported success rates of 75%, 71%, and 71% for pain reduction for Wilkes II, III, and IV, respectively, at 6 months postoperatively; these rates improved to 88%, 86%, and 87% at 24 months postoperatively. In relation to mouth opening greater than 35 mm, success rates changed from 70%, 68%, and 35% for Wilkes II, III, and IV, respectively, at 3 months postoperatively, to 75%, 79%, and 61% for Wilkes II, III, and IV, respectively, at 12 months postoperatively. These data show that it is important to report data in terms of staging and time of evaluation, because of the changing course of the disease and the variability of signs and symptoms according to stage.

The status of the articular surface or the synovial lining may not necessarily improve after ALL, even although a clear improvement in pain and mandibular function was noted. In a series of 30 patients who underwent 2 consecutive ALL, Hamada and colleagues[47] concluded that a clinically verified improvement in patients with ID of the TMJ was not necessarily accompanied by healing of the diseased tissues. According to the study by Moses and Topper[48] of the position of the disk after ALL assessed by MRI, the effect of lysis and lavage is not related to the reposition of the disk in long-term follow-up but to the mobilization of the disk and the removal of degenerative products that produce inflammation.

Operative or Advanced Arthroscopy

Preliminary good results with OA were obtained by McCain and de la Rua,[26] Davis and colleagues,[49] and Tarro,[50] although direct comparison studies between OA and ALL were still absent. In a posterior study by Indresano,[31] 103 of 188 patients who underwent ALL, and 121 of 212 patients who underwent OA, were evaluated and compared in relation to pain and function. Within the group of patients with ALL, followed for 8.3 years, pain was reduced by 71%, and disability was reduced by 66%. In comparison, patients undergoing OA, with a mean follow-up of 4.8 years, showed a pain reduction of 81% and a disability improvement of 86%. In this study, differences were statistically significant. In contrast, in a comparison study of 41 joints treated with ALL and 73 joints treated with OA in patients with advanced ID (Wilkes III–V), Miyamoto and colleagues[51] found similar good results in pain and function for both treatment modalities.

Regarding the success rate according to the stage of ID, variable results have previously been reported in the literature. Bronstein and Merrill[24] observed a success rate of 96% for stage II, 83% for stage III, 88% for stage IV, and 63% for stage V. These investigators used ALL and also OA. Holmlund and colleagues[38] reported a success rate of only 50% for patients suffering CCL with osteoarthrosis, corresponding to Wilkes stage V, whereas Murakami and colleagues[52] reported a success rate of approximately 90% for ALL in stages III and IV and needed OA for a success rate of 93% in stage V. Recently, in a study of 26 joints that underwent ALL, Smolka and colleagues[43] found an overall acceptable success rate of 78.3%, although the treatment was less successful for stages IV and V (71.4% and 75%, respectively) than for stages II and III (80% and 85.7%, respectively). In relation to decrease of pain lower than 20 in the VAS score (0–100) and the increase of mouth opening more than 30 mm, according to the AAOMS criteria,[45,46] González-García and Rodríguez-Campo[44] found

an increasing success rate for both ALL and OA, at each point during follow-up, from the first month to the second year postoperatively. This improvement was also comparable with the increase of mouth opening, for both arthroscopic techniques (**Table 4**).

There is controversy with regards to the position of the disk in relation to the appearance of symptoms in the TMJ. Some investigators have advocated for anatomic reduction of the disk by open surgery or by OA to control the disease, whereas others have reported excellent results with arthrocentesis or ALL. Up to 34% of asymptomatic volunteers have been reported to present with disk displacement, whereas a normal position of the disk has been observed in 16% to 23% of symptomatic patients. In a recent study by our group (unpublished results) of more than 36 TMJ asymptomatic volunteers, ID caused by disk malposition was reported by NMR imaging in 25% of the joints and 30.5% of the individuals; disk displacement with reduction was corrected in 14%, disk displacement without reduction in 9.7%, and anchored disk phenomenon in 1.3% of the TMJs. The investigators conclusions regarding this findings were: (1) a high prevalence of disk displacement of up to approximately 30% (25% of the joints) was observed in asymptomatic patients in our study population; (2) disk and condylar morphology was altered in asymptomatic patients with disk displacement, whereas the glenoid fossa morphology was unaltered independently of the disk position; (3) a reduced angle between the major condylar axis and the temporal fossa reference plane was found to be predictive for disk displacement; and (4) the craniomandibular index was 2.5 times higher in asymptomatic patients with disk displacement than in those with normally positioned disk, thus constituting a clinical tool for differential diagnosis in the daily practice.

COMPLICATIONS AND CONCERNS

Although uncommon, some complications have been reported for MITMJS. Most complications appear during or immediately after the procedure and most of them recover uneventfully. González-García and colleagues,[53] in a series of 500 patients (670 joints) with TMJ ID from Wilkes II to V who underwent arthroscopy, reported an overall 1.34% complication rate. Although not considered as a true complication, bleeding within the SJS was observed in 8.5% of the arthroscopies; it is essential to reduce bleeding by means of adequate instrumentation

Table 4

Evolution of pain and mouth opening and success rate from the preoperative time to the second year postoperatively for ALL and OA or advanced arthroscopy through Wilkes stages II to V. Success rates through the follow-up are reported in terms of percentage (%) of patients who presented with a VAS score less than 20 and MIO higher than 30, according to the AAOMS

Wilkes Stage	Number of Patients/ Joints	Arthroscopic Technique	VAS (0–100)/ MIO	Preoperative	1 mo Postoperative/ Success Rate (%)	3 mo Postoperative/ Success Rate (%)	6 mo Postoperative/ Success Rate (%)	12 mo Postoperative/ Success Rate (%)	24 mo Postoperative/ Success Rate (%)
II	52/72	ALL	VAS (%)	52	30/38	27/61	24/75	35/60	20/88
			MIO (mm)/(%)	39/—	34/58	38/70	37/61	39/75	38/74
		OA	VAS (%)	57	29/43	21/65	18/91	35/74	30/78
			MIO (mm)/(%)	38/—	32/40	36/66	42/91	40/71	43/91
III	132/183	ALL	VAS (%)	55	26/56	25/71	26/71	26/75	23/86
			MIO (mm)/(%)	36/—	32/33	35/68	38/73	38/79	39/78
		OA	VAS (%)	57	32/40	32/59	26/69	22/69	27/74
			MIO (mm)/(%)	34/—	29/20	33/50	36/6	37/74	38/74
IV	252/333	ALL	VAS (%)	53	33/46	28/57	25/71	22/73	17/87
			MIO (mm)/(%)	25/—	30/21	32/35	35/52	35/61	38/66
		OA	VAS (%)	53	35/40	30/61	26/69	20/76	15/86
			MIO (mm)/(%)	24/—	28/11	30/29	35/53	36/62	37/71
V	17/23	ALL	VAS (%)	37	43/—	20/—	17/—	—/—	—/—
			MIO (mm)/(%)	29/—	26/—	29/—	28/—	—/—	—/—
		OA	VAS (%)	61	47/—	32/—	13/—	—/—	—/—
			MIO (mm)/(%)	25/—	28/—	27/—	30/—	—/—	—/—

Adapted from González-García R, Rodríguez-Campo FJ. Arthroscopic lysis and lavage versus operative arthroscopy in the outcome of temporomandibular joint internal derangement: a comparative study based on Wilkes stages. J Oral Maxillofac Surg 2011;69:2513–24; with permission.

and by paying attention to essential points of the surgical technique. Although no definitive paralysis of the facial nerve was observed, temporal paresis of the facial nerve was observed in 0.6% of the series.

Some of the observed complications are included in the following list[27]:

- Hemarthrosis, as a consequence of damage of the superficial temporary artery or vein during entrance of the trocar at the fossa puncture site, or as a consequence of damage of the pterigoid artery during the anterior release of the disk by miotomy
- Infection of the skin area or infectious arthritis (infrequent with adequate sterilization of the surgical field and instrumentation)
- Damage to the seventh cranial nerve and facial palsy by involvement of the frontotemporal or the zygomatic branch
- Damage of the auriculotemporal nerve, which crosses posterior to the fossa puncture site (anesthesia of the zone)
- Damage of the eighth cranial nerve, tympanic disruption, and ossicle disruption with entry in the middle ear, otitis media, and hypoacusia (**Fig. 15**)
- Damage of the maxillary artery and its collaterals with/without arteriovenous fistula, as it crosses laterally to the lateral pterigoid muscle (uncommon)
- Damage of the superficial temporal vessels, as they cross posterior to the puncture site; external compression is needed
- Perforation of the glenoid fossa with entrance into the middle cranial fossa and subsequent cerebrospinal fluid leak: if the leak persists for more than 48 hours, a lumbar drain has to be placed by the neurosurgeon

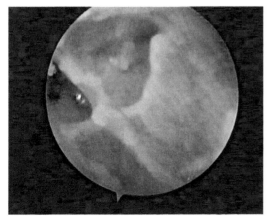

Fig. 15. Complication during the arthroscopic procedure: perforation of the middle ear.

FUTURE TRENDS FOR MINIMALLY INVASIVE TEMPOROMANDIBULAR JOINT SURGERY
Summary

Computer-assisted arthroscopy

- Computer-assisted arthroscopy has been reported as one of the most promising techniques for MITMJS.[54] As an application of what has already been performed in endoscopic sinus surgery or abdominal endoscopy, guiding the movements of the arthroscope or the instruments used in triangulation and OA may be helpful in difficult TMJ cases, such as patients with obesity, tumors, ankylosis, or ID with fibrosis and a severely limited upper joint space.
- With the preliminary idea of showing recalculated MRI or computed tomography (CT) scan sections, Wagner and colleagues[54] developed a system that could visualize both video and CT scans or MRI independently on 2 or more channels, and also to superimpose projected anatomic structures on any online video obtained by the arthroscope.
- Although radiography is not performed intraoperatively, changes in soft tissues such as those caused by synovitis or changes in disk position (ie, disk retroposition after anterior release) may not be detected by CT scans or MRI. Thus, only bony structures in relation to the TMJ act as a reference.
- Although primary goals of this technology are decreasing complication rate and operating time, educational, scientific, and training goals may also be relevant.

Navigation and arthroscopy

- Acquired images of the TMJ (preferably MRI) can be loaded into an intraoperative navigation system to guide joint space manipulation. The navigation system consists of a computer, a monitor, a detector, and a series of emitters or trackers.[55]
- Among its applications: (1) injection and sampling of intra-articular tissue and fluid; (2) other intra-articular more mechanical maniupulations[56] (triangulation and entrance of the working cannula in the upper joint compartment).
- Advantages: (1) decrease of error in access: either by the arthroscope or by the working cannula in the process of triangulation; (2) decrease of the risk of damaging intra-articular tissue and structures by instrumentation; (3) more accuracy in detecting and treating intra-articular disease.

Improvement in cameras and optical lens

- Improvements in camera and optical lens technology will lead to better diagnosis of subjacent tissue damage. Designing smaller and more flexible scopes will allow the surgeon to perform the procedure in a less invasive manner or even under local anesthesia in an office-based setting.[56]

Design of nonhuman synthetic models for training in minimally invasive temporomandibular joint surgery

- Although access to hands-on cadaver courses is scarce and expensive, the development of synthetic models of the TMJ may play a role in the development of educational and training programs for MITMJS. These models must accurately reproduce the anatomy of the joint and must also simulate the surgeon's proprioception for introduction of the arthroscope and additional instrumentation through the triangulation process.
- Virtual models of arthroscopic procedures reproducing normal and pathologic conditions may be added to the synthetic models of the TMJ, so that the surgeon in training may visualize on the monitor the arthroscopic anatomy of normal or affected joints as they practice the movements of the scope and instrumentation through the working cannula.

REFERENCES

1. Dimitroulis G. The role of surgery in the management of disorders of the temporomandibular joint: a critical review of the literature Part 2. Int J Oral Maxillofac Surg 2005;34:231–7.
2. Onishi M. Arthroscopy of the temporomandibular joint. Kokubyo Gakkai Zasshi 1975;42:207–13.
3. Murakami K, Hoshino K. Regional anatomical nomenclature and arthroscopic terminology in human temporomandibular joints. Okajimas Folia Anat Jpn 1982;58:745–60.
4. McCain J. Arthroscopy of the human temporomandibular joint. J Oral Maxillofac Surg 1988;46:648–55.
5. Holmlund A, Hellsing G. Arthroscopy of the temporomandibular joint: an autopsy study. Int J Oral Maxillofac Surg 1985;14:169–75.
6. Sanders B. Arthroscopic surgery of the temporomandibular joint: treatment of internal derangement with persistent closed lock. Oral Surg Oral Med Oral Pathol 1986;62:361–72.
7. Murakami K, Ono T. TMJ arthroscopy by inferolateral approach. Int J Oral Maxillofac Surg 1986;15:410–7.
8. Israel HA. Technique for placement of a discal traction suture during temporomandibular joint arthroscopy. J Oral Maxillofac Surg 1989;47:311–3.
9. Tarro AW. Arthroscopic treatment of anterior disc displacement: a preliminary report. J Oral Maxillofac Surg 1989;47:353–8.
10. Ohnishi M. Arthroscopic surgery for hypermobility and recurrent mandibular dislocation. Oral Maxillofac Surg Clin North Am 1989;1:153–64.
11. McCain JP, Podrasky AE, Zabiegalski NA. Arthroscopic disc repositioning and suturing: a preliminary report. J Oral Maxillofac Surg 1992;50:568–79.
12. Tarro AW. A fully visualized arthroscopic disc suturing technique. J Oral Maxillofac Surg 1994;52:362–9.
13. Goizueta Adame CC, Muñoz-Guerra MF. The posterior double pass suture in repositioning of the temporomandibular disc during arthroscopic surgery: a report of 16 cases. J Craniomaxillofac Surg 2012;40:86–91.
14. Yang C, Cai XY, Chen MJ, et al. New arthroscopic disc repositioning and suturing technique for treating an anteriorly displaced disc of the temporomandibular joint: part I–technique introduction. Int J Oral Maxillofac Surg 2012;41:1058–63.
15. Murakami K, Iizuka T, Matsuki M, et al. Recapturing the persistent anteriorly displaced disk by mandibular manipulation after pumping and hydraulic pressure to the upper joint cavity of the temporomandibular joint. Cranio 1987;5:17–24.
16. Nitzan DW, Dolwick MF, Martinez GA. Temporomandibular joint arthrocentesis: a simplified treatment for severe, limited mouth opening. J Oral Maxillofac Surg 1991;49:1163–7.
17. González-García R, Gil-Díez Usandizaga JL, Rodríguez-Campo FJ. Arthroscopic anatomy and lysis and lavage of the temporomandibular joint. Atlas Oral Maxillofac Surg Clin North Am 2011;19:131–44.
18. Barkin S, Weinberg S. Internal derangements of the temporomandibular joint: the role of arthroscopic surgery and arthrocentesis. J Can Dent Assoc 2000;66:199–203.
19. American Association of Oral and Maxillofacial Surgeons. Position paper on TMJ arthroscopy 1988. In: Thomas M, Bronstein S, editors. Arthroscopy of the temporomandibular joint. Philadelphia: WB Saunders; 1991. p. 347–50.
20. Israel H. Arthroscopy of the temporomandibular joint. In: Peterson L, Indresano T, Marciani R, et al, editors. Principles of oral and maxillofacial surgery. Philadelphia: JB Lippincott; 1992. p. 2015–40.
21. Nitzan DW, Samson B, Better H. Long-term outcome of arthrocentesis for sudden-onset, persistent, severe closed lock of the temporomandibular joint. J Oral Maxillofac Surg 1997;55:151–7.
22. González-García R, Rodríguez-Campo FJ, Monje F, et al. Operative versus simple arthroscopic surgery for chronic closed lock of the temporomandibular

joint: a clinical study of 344 arthroscopic procedures. Int J Oral Maxillofac Surg 2008;37:790–6.

23. Wilkes CH. Internal derangements of the temporomandibular joint: pathological variations. Arch Otolaryngol Head Neck Surg 1989;115:469–77.

24. Bronstein SL, Merrill R. Clinical staging for TMJ internal derangement: application to arthroscopy. J Craniomandib Disord 1992;6:7–16.

25. Molinari F, Gentile L, Manicone P, et al. Interobserver variability of dynamic MR imaging of the temporomandibular joint. Radiol Med 2011;116:1303–12.

26. McCain JP. Principles and practice of temporomandibular joint arthroscopy, St. Louis: Mosby; 1996.

27. McCain JP, Hossameldin RH. Advanced arthroscopy of the temporomandibular joint. Atlas Oral Maxillofac Surg Clin North Am 2011;19:145–67.

28. González-García R. "Improvement" or "success" in arthroscopy for internal derangement of the temporomandibular joint? Br J Oral Maxillofac Surg 2014;52:288–9.

29. Monje F, Nitzan D, González-García R. Temporomandibular joint arthrocentesis. Review of the literature. Med Oral Patol Oral Cir Bucal 2012;17:e575–81.

30. Sanders B, Buoncristiani R. Diagnostic and surgical arthroscopy of the temporomandibular joint: clinical experience with 137 procedures over a 2-year period. J Craniomandib Disord 1987;1:202–13.

31. Indresano AT. Arthroscopic surgery of the temporomandibular joint: report of 64 patients with long-term follow-up. J Oral Maxillofac Surg 1989;47:439–41.

32. Moses JJ, Sartoris D, Glass R, et al. The effect of arthroscopic lysis and lavage of the superior joint space on TMJ disc position and mobility. J Oral Maxillofac Surg 1989;47:674–8.

33. Moses JJ, Poker I. TMJ arthroscopic surgery: an analysis of 237 patients. J Oral Maxillofac Surg 1989;47:790–4.

34. White RD. Retrospective analysis of 100 consecutive surgical arthroscopies of the temporomandibular joint. J Oral Maxillofac Surg 1989;10:1014–21.

35. Clark GT, Moody DG, Sanders B. Arthroscopic temporomandibular joint locking resulting from disc derangement: two-year results. J Oral Maxillofac Surg 1991;49:157–64.

36. Moore LJ. Arthroscopic surgery for the treatment of restrictive temporomandibular joint disease. A prospective longitudinal study. In: Clark GT, Sanders B, Bertolami CH, editors. Advances in diagnostic and surgical arthroscopy of the temporomandibular joint. Philadelphia: WB Saunders; 1993. p. 704–46.

37. Mosby EL. Efficacy of temporomandibular joint arthroscopy: a retrospective study. J Oral Maxillofac Surg 1993;51:17–21.

38. Holmlund A, Gynther G, Axelsson S. Efficacy of arthroscopic lysis and lavage in patients with chronic locking of the temporomandibular joint. Int J Oral Maxillofac Surg 1994;23:262–5.

39. Kurita K, Goss AN, Ogi N, et al. Correlation between preoperative mouth opening and surgical outcome after arthroscopic lysis and lavage in patients with disc displacement without reduction. J Oral Maxillofac Surg 1998;56:1394–7.

40. Sorel B, Piecuch JF. Long-term evaluation following temporomandibular joint arthroscopy with lysis and lavage. Int J Oral Maxillofac Surg 2000;29:259–63.

41. Dimitroulis G. A review of 56 cases of chronic closed lock treated with temporomandibular joint arthroscopy. J Oral Maxillofac Surg 2002;60:519–24.

42. Kondoh T, Dolwick MF, et al. Visually guided irrigation for patients with symptomatic internal derangement of the temporomandibular joint: a preliminary report. Oral Surg Oral Med Oral Pathol Oral Radiol Endod 2003;95:544–51.

43. Smolka W, Yanai C, Smolka K, et al. Efficiency of arthroscopic lysis and lavage for internal derangement of temporomandibular joint correlated with Wilkes classification. Oral Surg Oral Med Oral Pathol Oral Radiol Endod 2008;106:317–23.

44. González-García R, Rodríguez-Campo FJ. Arthroscopic lysis and lavage versus operative arthroscopy in the outcome of temporomandibular joint internal derangement: a comparative study based on Wilkes stages. J Oral Maxillofac Surg 2011;69:2513–24.

45. Dolwick MF, Reid S, Sanders B, et al. Criteria for TMJ meniscus surgery. Chicago: American Association of Oral and Maxillofacial Surgeons; 1984. p. 31.

46. Eriksson L, Westesson PL. Temporomandibular joint diskectomy. No positive effect of temporary silicone implant in a 5-year follow-up. Oral Surg Oral Med Oral Pathol 1992;74:259–72.

47. Hamada Y, Kondoh T, Holmlund AB, et al. Visually guided temporomandibular joint irrigation in patients with chronic closed lock: clinical outcomes and its relationship to intraarticular morphologic changes. Oral Surg Oral Med Oral Pathol Oral Radiol Endod 2003;95:552–8.

48. Moses JJ, Toper DC. A functional approach to the treatment of temporomandibular joint internal derangement. J Craniomandib Disord 1991;5:19–27.

49. Davis CL, Kaminishi RM, Marshall MW. Arthroscopic surgery for treatment of closed lock. J Oral Maxillofac Surg 1991;49:704–7.

50. Tarro AW. TMJ arthroscopic diagnosis and surgery: clinical experience with 152 procedures over a $2^1/_2$-year period. Cranio 1991;9:107–19.

51. Miyamoto H, Sakashita H, Miyata M, et al. Arthroscopic surgery of the temporomandibular joint: comparison of two successful techniques. Br J Oral Maxillofac Surg 1999;37:397–400.

52. Murakami K, Segami N, Okamoto M, et al. Outcome of arthroscopic surgery for internal derangement of

the temporomandibular joint: long-term results covering 10 years. J Craniomaxillofac Surg 2000; 28:64–71.

53. González-García R, Rodríguez-Campo FJ, Escorial-Hernández V, et al. Complications of temporomandibular joint arthroscopic: a retrospective analytic study of 670 arthroscopic procedures. J Oral Maxillofac Surg 2006;64:1587–91.

54. Wagner A, Undt G, Watzinger F, et al. Principles of computer-assisted arthroscopy of the temporomandibular joint with optoelectronic tracking technology. Oral Surg Oral Med Oral Pathol Oral Radiol Endod 2001;92:30–7.

55. Yeung RW, Xia JJ, Samman N. Image-guided minimally invasive surgical Access to the temporal joint: a preliminary report. J Oral Maxillofac Surg 2006;64: 1546–52.

56. Wolf J, Weiss A, Dym H. Technological advances in minimally invasive surgery. Dent Clin North Am 2011;55:635–40.

Disc Repositioning
Does it Really Work?

João Roberto Gonçalves, DDS, PhD[a],*, Daniel Serra Cassano, DDS[a],
Luciano Rezende, DDS, MSc[a], Larry M. Wolford, DMD[b]

KEYWORDS

- Disc repositioning • 3D quantitative findings • Surgical technique and possible pitfalls
- Mitek mini anchor • Treatment alternatives • Lateral cephalometry • Clinical outcomes

KEY POINTS

- The effectiveness of temporomandibular joint (TMJ) disc repositioning is scarce.
- Further guidance for clinicians and patients regarding clinical and surgical options to better treat TMJ internal derangement are needed, especially regarding skeletal malocclusion that requires operative interventions.
- The lack of evidence that TMJ articular disc repositioning is an ineffective procedure points to a future when new TMJ biomarkers will support the technique effectiveness in better studies.
- As a sensitive technique with a wide learning curve, many surgeons have practiced TMJ articular disc repositioning with a large range of outcomes.

INTRODUCTION

Although limited, there is evidence to support the assumption that temporomandibular joint (TMJ) articular disc repositioning indeed works[1–5] and so far there is no evidence that TMJ articular disc repositioning does not work. Despite the controversy among professionals in private practice and academia, TMJ articular disc repositioning is a procedure based on (still limited) evidence; the opposition is based solely on clinical preference and influenced by the ability to perform it or not.

DISC REPOSITIONING AND LEVELS OF EVIDENCE

Evidence in health science can be classified in 6 distinct hierarchical levels according to the US Agency for Healthcare Research and Quality[6]: (1a) Meta-analysis of randomized, controlled trials, (1b) at least 1 randomized controlled trial, (2a) at least 1 well-designed controlled study without randomization, (2b) at least 1 other type of well-designed quasi-experimental study, (3) well-designed, nonexperimental descriptive studies such as comparative, correlation, and case-controlled studies; and (4) expert committee reports or opinions, or clinical experience of respected authorities, or both.

Specialized peered-reviewed journals are also a reasonable source of good scientific evidence. Although they have known limitations, a worldwide accepted metric to evaluate journals' strength is the impact factor, which is calculated by the Institute for Scientific Information[7] as the average number of times published papers are cited up to 2 years after publication. Dental literature has very distinct impact factor compared with the medical literature in most of the specialties. The impact factor of the *Journal of Oral and Maxillofacial Surgery*, *International Journal of Oral and Maxillofacial Surgery*, and *British Journal of Oral and Maxillofacial Surgery* in 2009 were 1.580, 1.444, and 1.327, respectively; the *New England*

[a] Department of Pediatric Dentistry, Faculdade de Odontologia de Araraquara, Universidade Estadual Paulista - UNESP Araraquara School of Dentistry, Araraquara, Brazil; [b] Departments of Oral and Maxillofacial Surgery and Orthodontics Texas, A&M University Health Science Center Baylor College of Dentistry, Baylor University Medical Center, 3409 Worth St. Suite 400, Dallas, Texas
* Corresponding author. Av Dr Gastão Vidigal 295, Araraquara, São Paulo, Brazil.
E-mail address: joaogonc@foar.unesp.br

Oral Maxillofacial Surg Clin N Am 27 (2015) 85–107
http://dx.doi.org/10.1016/j.coms.2014.09.007
1042-3699/15/$ – see front matter © 2015 Elsevier Inc. All rights reserved.

Journal of Medicine, the *Journal of the American Medical Association*, and *The Lancet* were 50.017, 31.171, and 17.457, respectively for the same period.

A recent study that listed the 100 most cited articles in dentistry[8] showed that, among them, only 6 papers that were published in the 2 journals of oral and maxillofacial surgery were included in the list (*Journal of Oral and Maxillofacial Surgery* and *International Journal of Oral and Maxillofacial Surgery*), whereas 41 papers that were published on the 3 journals of periodontology (*Journal of Clinical Periodontology*, *Journal of Periodontology*, and *Journal of Periodontal Research*) were included in the top 100 papers. It was concluded that, in dentistry, there is a predominance of clinical studies, particularly case series and narrative reviews/expert opinions, despite their low evidence level. It is also understandable that randomized, placebo-controlled, prospective clinical trials are not easily executed, mainly in oral surgery, either for ethical reasons or funding issues.[9] In this scenario, scientific evidence levels 2b and 3 should be considered as evidence enough to guide clinical protocols in oral and maxillofacial surgery. A quasi-experimental study is defined as a broad range of nonrandomized intervention studies, usually made when it is not logistically feasible or ethical to conduct a randomized, controlled trial.[10]

The current literature available on the effectiveness of open joint TMJ disc repositioning meets the "patient-oriented evidence that matters" (POEM) criterion. To meet POEM, readers should take advantage "from original research to clinical experience, remembering that each source of medical information is valuable since one learns which source is best for the specific information being sought."[11]

Two meta-analyses about the effectiveness of TMJ management concluded that operative interventions need further evidence for precise conclusions but pointed out some good results for open joint surgery.[3,12]

Mostly, Wolford and coworkers have addressed the outcomes of TMJ articular disc repositioning in several papers that could be classified according to the level of evidence 2b or 3, beside abstracts and expert opinions published by their group in many international scientific meetings held on all continents. The main focus of these studies were orthognathic surgery outcomes in patients with prior TMJ derangements and because of this, most of these studies evaluated patients who underwent TMJ disc repositioning and orthognathic surgery concomitantly.

Wolford and Cardenas in 1993[3] detailed described idiopathic condylar resorption, its possible etiologies and specific treatment options, and showed 12 successfully treated clinical cases of open joint TMJ articular disc repositioning with the aid of a titanium mini anchor used to hold the disc in place with artificial ligaments. All patients showed progressive condylar resorption before the procedure (average of 1.5 mm/y) with progressive steepening of the occlusal plane angle. Operative techniques included removal of the hyperplastic synovial tissue, repositioning of the articular discs, and double jaw surgery for mandibular advancement of 11 mm (range, 2–18 mm) and decrease of the occlusal plane angle an average of 8° (range, 5°–12°). At a postoperative follow-up average of 33 months (range, 18–68) no significant relapses were observed. In fact, 5 young patients (<16 years old) at the time of surgery showed a slight increase in condylar height (average, 0.4 mm; range −0.1 to 1.5).

Two years later, a retrospective clinical study assessed the outcomes of 105 patients who underwent TMJ disc repositioning.[2] At the longest follow-up (minimum of 1 year after surgery), there were no detectable condylar changes or mandibular positional changes. Visual analog scale assessment showed marked reduction of TMJ pain, facial pain, and headaches. TMJ noises, disability, and jaw function; in addition, diet also improved significantly. Interincisal opening improved slightly, whereas lateral excursive movements decreased.

Another retrospective clinical study design was used by Wolford and colleagues[1] in 2002 to evaluate all patients who had undergone concomitant orthognathic and TMJ surgery from 1991 through 1993. All patients who underwent unilateral or bilateral articular disc repositioning with concomitant mandibular ramus osteotomies or double jaw surgery and met the inclusion criteria were included in this study. They compared 70 patients in 3 groups according to mandibular movement: Group 1 had mandibular advancement, group 2 had mandibular setback, and group 3 had the mandibles remain at the original positions. One year after surgery, 20% of patients had pain and 60% reported complete relief of TMJ pain (before surgery, 80% had pain). Pain was assessed on a visual analog scale from 0 (no pain) to 10 (the worst pain imaginable). Severe pain was still present in 7% of the patients 1 year after surgery (before surgery, it was 53%). Concomitant TMJ and orthognathic surgery success based on a greater than 35 mm of maximal interincisal opening and a decrease in pain had an overall success rate of 91.4%.[1]

To our knowledge, there is no single experimental study that showed that articular disc repositioning does not work. No cohort, case-control, retrospective patient data review, single case report, or expert committee report or opinion has described unsuccessful outcomes after TMJ disc repositioning. A few expert opinions (the lowest level of evidence) has expressed against TMJ disc repositioning.[13–15]

ORTHOGNATHIC SURGERY IN THE PRESENCE OF DISC DISPLACEMENT AND CLINICAL OUTCOMES

Controversy surrounds the appropriate management of patients with preexisting internal derangement of the TMJ who need orthognathic surgery for correction of malocclusion and jaw deformities.[16] There are 2 significantly different philosophies; the first posits that orthognathic surgical procedures reduce or eliminate TMJ dysfunction and symptoms,[13,17–20] whereas the second posits that orthognathic surgery causes further harmful effects on the TMJ and thus worsens the symptoms and dysfunction postoperatively.[14,21,22] The second philosophy proposes appropriate operative management of the TMJ pathology in an initial separate operative procedure or concomitantly with the orthognathic surgery.[23]

Some authors[13,17–20] recommend that patients with coexisting TMJ dysfunction and skeletal facial deformities undergo orthodontic preparation followed by orthognathic surgery. For the small number of patients whose TMJ symptoms do not resolve and are too severe to permit orthodontic preparation for orthognathic surgery, TMJ surgery may be performed before orthognathic treatment. However, other studies[1–3,5,23–42] have shown that concomitant surgical correction of TMJ pathology and coexisting dentofacial deformities in a single operation provides high-quality treatment outcomes for most patients relative to function, esthetics, elimination, or significant reduction in pain, and improved patient satisfaction.

Preexisting TMJ pathology (symptomatic or not) that can cause unfavorable outcomes when only orthognathic surgery is performed include: articular disc dislocation, adolescent internal condylar resorption, condylar hyperplasia, osteochondroma, congenital deformities, reactive arthritis, connective tissue/autoimmune diseases, nonsalvageable joints, and others. All of these conditions can be associated with dentofacial deformities, TMJ pain, headaches, myofascial pain, TMJ dysfunction, and other problems.[23]

The most common TMJ pathology is anterior and/or medial displacement of the articular disc, which can initiate a cascade of events leading to arthritis and other TMJ-related symptoms.[23,43] Advancement of the mandible especially, in a counterclockwise direction, in a patient with displaced discs causes the discs to remain displaced as the condyles seek a superoposterior position in the fossa, potentially overloading the joints and causing instability in the long term.[23] Other authors have reported that patients with preoperative TMJ symptoms requiring large mandibular advancement seem to be at increased risk for condylar resorption[44,45]; thus, in these patients, a logical approach would be to return the disc to a normal anatomic and functional position. Concomitant treatment (when the discs are salvageable) may include articular disc repositioning and stabilization using the Mitek anchor (Mitek Surgical Products, Westwood, MA, USA) technique[1,2,23–29] and orthognathic surgery as indicated.[23]

Other factors that may contribute to skeletal relapse and condylar resorption include patient age and gender, a high mandibular plane angle, preoperative orthodontic treatment, bone healing, condylar positioning, neuromuscular adaptation, instability of segments, the degree of mandibular advancement performed, influence of operative technique, and time since onset.[5,16,46]

Several authors have described of TMJ condition that could be possible risk factors for skeletal relapse and condylar resorption after orthognathic surgery, including high mandibular plane angle, shortened posterior facial height, and small posterior/anterior facial height ratio.[16,46,47] However, these same characteristics are commonly seen in patients with TMJ pathology, and those authors apparently did not recognize that the patients who experienced postoperative relapse and condylar resorption likely had preoperative TMJ pathology. Schellhas and colleagues[48] investigated 100 patients clinically and radiographically by computed tomography, and high-field surface-coil MRI to identify risk factors for TMJ degeneration. In their study, 40 patients (52 joints) underwent an open arthroplasty procedure, in which the main surgical and pathologic findings included disc displacement, disc degeneration, and cartilage hypertrophy. TMJ internal derangement was posited to be the main cause of both acquired facial skeleton remodeling and unstable occlusion in patients with intact dentition and without previous mandibular fracture. Similar findings were described previously by Schellhas,[49] who concluded that internal derangement of the TMJ is an irreversible and generally progressive disorder.

The TMJs are the foundation for stable results in orthognathic surgical procedures; if the TMJs are not stable and healthy (pathologic), then orthognathic surgery outcomes may be unsatisfactory relative to function, esthetics, stability, and pain. Orthognathic surgery to correct dentofacial deformities requiring mandibular advancement cannot eliminate coexisting TMJ pathology, and those patients may have unsatisfactory outcomes.[16,21–23,50–54]

Clinical outcomes of TMJ surgery using Mitek mini anchor, including mandibular range of motion, chewing efficiency, pain levels, and disability has been assessed in several papers.[1,2,26,27] Mehra and Wolford[2] evaluated 88 patients with simultaneous TMJ disc repositioning using the Mitek mini anchor and orthognathic surgery and found that this technique provided significant decreases in TMJ pain, facial pain, headaches, TMJ noises, and disability, and significant improvements in jaw function and diet, along with stable occlusal and skeletal results.

Many studies used lateral cephalometry to monitor condylar changes after maxillomandibular advancement and the influence of articular disc repositioning (**Figs. 1** and **2**).[5] Condylar arthritic changes provide mandibular instability and can be detected through lateral cephalometric radiographs.[55] Cranial base superimposition in nongrowing patients can accurately detect condyle remodeling by monitoring mandibular position in a longitudinal basis.

Various methods and devices are currently used to diagnose internal derangement of the TMJ, including radiographic measures, such as arthrography and tomography, and methods that rely on the assessment of jaw movements. More recently, MRI has been used to evaluate the disk position. MRI has gained wide acceptance in evaluating the TMJ and shows a high diagnostic accuracy in determining the articular disk position related to the condyle and the articular eminence. Although arthrography and MRI of the TMJ have become standard in clinical practice and studies involving internal derangement, cephalometric radiography might also be available. Disk displacement has been reported to be associated with reduced posterior facial height, reduced mandibular length, and increased inclination of the mandible relative to the cranial reference planes in adolescents. However, some authors have reported that no cephalometric measurements can clearly distinguish persons with disk displacement of the TMJ from those with normal disk positions. If some characteristic findings from the cephalometric analyses suggest an association with the progression of internal derangement, this is an important implication for orthodontic treatment and patient education

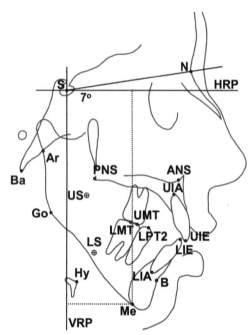

Fig. 1. Landmarks used for cephalometric assessment. The horizontal reference plane (HRP) is constructed at 7° to the SN plane. The vertical reference plane (VRP) is constructed perpendicular to the HRP, through the sella (S). The *dotted lines* indicate the method of measuring the menton (Me) relative to reference planes HRP and VRP. ANS, anterior nasal spine (a point posterior to the tip of the median, sharp bony process of the maxilla, on its superior surface, where the maxilla process first enlarges to a width of 5 mm). Ar, articulare; B, B point; Ba, basion; Go, gonion; Hy, hyoid; LIA, lower incisor apex; LIE, lower incisor edge; LMT, lower molar distal cusp tip; LPT2, lower premolar cusp tip; N, nasion; PNS, posterior nasal spine; S, sella turcica; UIA, upper incisor apex; UIE, upper incisor edge; UMT, upper molar mesial cusp tip; US, upper. (*From* Goncalves JR, Cassano DS, Wolford LM, et al. Postsurgical stability of counterclockwise maxillomandibula advancement surgery: affect of articular disc repositioning. J Oral Maxillofac Surg 2008;66(4):724–38; with permission.)

before treatment. In addition, this might further increase the diagnostic value of cephalometric radiographs.

Goncalves and colleagues[5] reported a retrospective study evaluated the records of 72 patients who underwent maxillomandibular surgical advancement with counterclockwise rotation of the occlusal plane. The sample was divided into 3 groups to address the influence of TMJ health and articular disc surgical repositioning relative to postoperative stability. Group 1, with healthy TMJs, underwent double jaw surgery only. Group 2, with articular disc dislocation, underwent articular disc repositioning using the Mitek anchor technique concomitantly with orthognathic

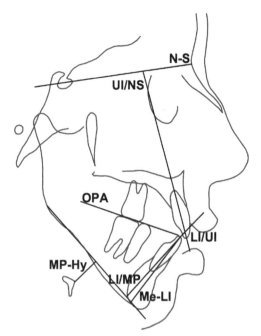

Fig. 2. Distances and planes used to define linear and angular measurements. Linear measurements include the distance from the hyoid to the mandibular plane (MP-Hy) measured on a perpendicular line from the MP; and the distance from the menton to the lower incisor edge (Me-LI). Angular measurements include the angle of the occlusion plane (OPA) to the nasium-sela (N-S line); the angle of the upper incisor to the N-S (UI/NS) line; the angle of the lower incisor to the mandibular plane (LI/MP); and the incisor angle (LI/UI). (*From* Goncalves JR, Cassano DS, Wolford LM, et al. Postsurgical stability of counterclockwise maxillomandibula advancement surgery: affect of articular disc repositioning. J Oral Maxillofac Surg 2008;66(4):724–38; with permission.)

surgery. Group 3, with articular disc dislocation, underwent orthognathic surgery only. Preoperative characteristics included high occlusal plane angle, maxillary and mandibular retrusion, and increased anterior facial height. All 3 patient groups had similar dentofacial deformities and underwent orthognathic operative procedures performed by the same surgeon in the same manner with rigid fixation. Each patient's lateral cephalograms were traced, digitized twice, and averaged to estimate surgical changes and postoperative stability. The maxillomandibular complex was advanced and rotated counterclockwise similarly in all 3 groups (**Fig. 3**). Postoperatively, the occlusal plane angle increased in G3 (37% relapse rate), but remained stable in G1 and G2. Postoperative mandibular changes in the horizontal direction demonstrated a significant relapse in G3 at the menton (28%), the B point (28%), and the lower incisor edge (34%; **Fig. 4**), but remained stable in G1 and G2. Maxillomandibular advancement

with counterclockwise rotation of the occlusal plane is a stable procedure for patients with healthy TMJs and for patients undergoing simultaneous TMJ disc repositioning using the Mitek anchor technique. Those patients with preoperative TMJ articular disc displacement who underwent double jaw surgery and no TMJ intervention experienced significant relapse.

Surgical counterclockwise rotation of the maxillomandibular complex lengthens the functional moment arm (mandible), thereby increasing loading to the TMJs owing to stretch and tension of the suprahyoid muscles, periostium, skin, and other soft tissue elements. It may take several months for the soft tissues to adapt and reestablish a state of equilibrium.[56] Our previous studies[56–58] have shown that maxillomandibular advancement with counterclockwise rotation of the occlusal plane is a stable procedure in patients with healthy TMJs. Goncalves and colleagues[5] showed that the occlusal plane angle was stable postoperatively in patients with healthy TMJs and in articular discs repositioning concomitantly with orthognathic surgery patients, but the patients with articular disc dislocation who underwent only orthognathic surgery relapsed significantly (mean, 2.6°; range, −2.5° to 13.3°). The magnitude of clockwise rotation strongly indicates condylar resorption as the etiologic factor.

Chemello and colleagues[56] and Satrom and colleagues[57] reported that mandibular advancement in double jaw surgery (with or without counterclockwise rotation) using rigid internal fixation with healthy TMJs is a stable procedure over the long term, with a mean anteroposterior relapse at point B of 6% regardless of the amount of surgical advancement performed. On the other hand, Wolford and colleagues[16] evaluated 25 consecutive patients (23 females and 2 males) with jaw deformities and displaced articular discs (confirmed by MRI) who were treated with orthognathic surgery only, including mandibular advancement, and stabilized with rigid fixation. The average postoperative relapse at point B was 36% of the mandibular advancement, and the average distance from the condyle to point B decreased by 34%, indicating condylar resorption. Six patients (24%) demonstrated significant postoperative condylar resorption (3–8 mm), resulting in class II anterior open bite malocclusion. The increased loading of the TMJs as a result of the mandibular advancement most likely stimulated the resorption process. New onset or aggravation of TMJ symptoms (eg, pain, TMJ dysfunction) occurred at an average of 14 months after surgery. At the completion of the study, 48% of patients required TMJ and repeat orthognathic surgery. Before surgery, 36% of the

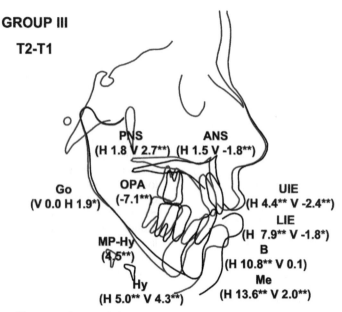

Fig. 3. Mean vertical and horizontal surgical changes (anterior nasal spine [ANS], posterior nasal spine [PNS], upper incisor edge [UIE], lower incisor edge [LIE], B point [B], menton [Me], gonion [Go], hyoid [Hy]), MP-Hy distance, and occlusion plane (OPA) for the 3 groups. The *red lines* indicate presurgery (T1); the *blue lines* indicate immediately postoperatively (T2). (*From* Goncalves JR, Cassano DS, Wolford LM, et al. Postsurgical stability of counterclockwise maxillomandibula advancement surgery: affect of articular disc repositioning. J Oral Maxillofac Surg 2008;66(4):724–38; with permission.)

patients complained of pain or discomfort, but at 2.2 years postoperatively, 84% of the patients reported a 75% increase in pain intensity compared with the preoperative pain. Only 4 of the 25 patients (16%) had a stable outcome without pain. This study clearly demonstrates the problems associated with performing orthognathic surgery only on patients with coexisting TMJ articular disc dislocations.

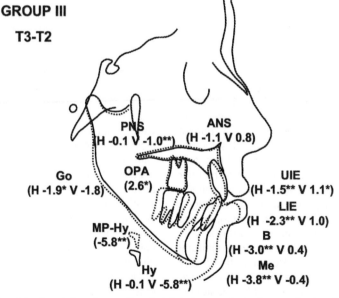

Fig. 4. Mean vertical and horizontal postoperative skeletal changes (anterior nasal spine [ANS], posterior nasal spine [PNS], upper incisor edge [UIE], lower incisor edge [LIE], B point [B], menton [Me], gonion [Go], hyoid [Hy]), MP-Hy distance, and OPA for the 3 groups. The *blue lines* indicate immediately postoperatively (T2); the *dashed lines* indicate long-term postoperatively (T3). (*From* Goncalves JR, Cassano DS, Wolford LM, et al. Postsurgical stability of counterclockwise maxillomandibula advancement surgery: affect of articular disc repositioning. J Oral Maxillofac Surg 2008;66(4):724–38; with permission.)

3-DIMENSIONAL QUANTITATIVE FINDINGS

Our group has studied 3-dimensional (3D) condylar changes after maxillomandibular surgical advancement with and without TMJ articular disc repositioning. We have used 3D quantitative assessment and cranial base voxel-wise automatic registration to compare immediately preoperatively (T1), immediately postoperatively (T2), and at least 11 months follow-up (T3). The first study[4] used iterative closest point rigid deformation to assess condylar changes immediate after surgery (T2–T1) and 1-year follow-up (T3–T2). Although it was not a randomized trial, all patients who met specific criteria were included in this retrospective study. We found that immediately after surgery, condylar displacements differ significantly between the 2 groups. Although patients with normal TMJ submitted to maxillomandibular advancement (MMA) have their condyles displaced up, backward, lateral, or medially (**Fig. 5**), patients with articular disc displacement submitted to maxillomandibular advancement with simultaneous articular disc repositioning (MMA-Drep) have their condyles moved down, forward, lateral,

or medially (**Fig. 6**). One year after surgery, more than one half the patients in the 2 groups presented condylar resorptive changes of at least 1.5 mm and, interestingly, only the MMA-Drep patients showed bone apposition in localized condylar regions.

Articular disc repositioning seemed to promote a protective function that was demonstrated by limited condylar resorption at the anchor region and bone apposition at all other condylar surfaces being the lateral pole the most frequent region (**Fig. 7**). An ongoing study further compared the 2 groups mentioned (MMA × MMA-Drep), now with a surface correspondent analysis based on spherical harmonics (SPHARM-PDM; opensource, available at: http://www.nitrc.org/projects/spharm-pdm)[59,60] that allows correspondent surface measurements among 2 or more 3D volumes from the same patient. In this study, maxillomandibular stability was also addressed and it was concluded that patients with TMJ disc displacement submitted to maxillomandibular advancement and articular disc repositioning have the

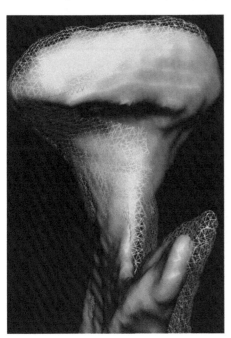

Fig. 5. Maxillomandibular advancement (MMA) group left condyle superimposition. Preoperatively (T1) solid 3-dimensional model in white and (T2) yellow in wiremesh overlay immediate postoperatively show condylar spatial change in upward, backward, and medial directions. (*From* Goncalves JR, Wolford LM, Cassano DS, et al. Temporomandibular joint condylar changes following maxillomandibular advancement and articular disc repositioning. J Oral Maxillofac Surg 2013;71(10):1759.e1–15; with permission.)

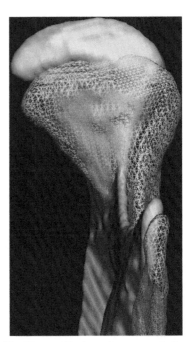

Fig. 6. Maxillomandibular advancement disc repositioning (MMA-Drep) group left condyle superimposition. Preoperatively (T1) solid 3-dimensional model in white and (T2) yellow in wiremesh overlay immediate postoperatively show condylar spatial change in downward, forward, and medial directions. (*From* Goncalves JR, Wolford LM, Cassano DS, et al. Temporomandibular joint condylar changes following maxillomandibular advancement and articular disc repositioning. J Oral Maxillofac Surg 2013;71(10):1759.e1–15; with permission.)

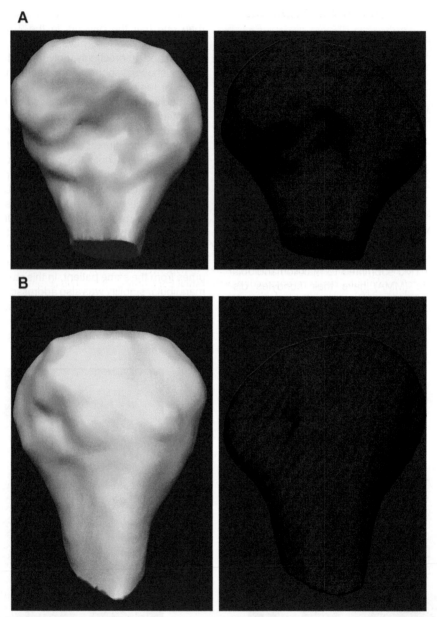

Fig. 7. (*A*) Maxillomandibular advancement disc repositioning (MMA-Drep) group left condyle anterior view. Immediately postoperative (T2) solid 3-dimensional (3D) model in yellow and (T3) 1-year follow-up in purple show condylar bone apposition in anterior, medial, and lateral surfaces. (*B*) MMA-Drep Group left condyle posterior view. Immediately postoperative (T2) solid 3D model in yellow and (T3) 1-year follow-up in purple show condylar bone apposition in posterior surface, and medial and lateral poles. Note bone resorption at the anchor region. (*Courtesy of* Larry M. Wolford, DMD, Dallas, TX.)

same stability as patients with normal TMJs submitted to maxillomandibular advancement only.

There are 3D quantitative analyses that have suggested that orthognathic surgery does not fix the TMJs and possibly will increase joint loading (observed even in patients with normal TMJs),[4] demonstrated by the significant reduction of TMJ space. This fact has been demonstrated before with plain radiographs,[61] cross-sectional computed tomography images,[62,63] and with 3D quantitative analysis,[4,64,65] showing that mandibular advancement promotes an upward, backward, and medial condyle displacement with likely change of the disc/condyle spatial relation. Individuals who received articular disc repositioning have their condyles moved in the opposite direction: Downward and forward to make room for the discs that preserved the overall condylar morphology.[4]

The relevance of 3D quantitative assessment with open-source software specifically designed for this purpose is the automatic algorithm used that dramatically decreases user interference and the possibility of unintentional bias.[59,66,67] This method also increases reliability because open source software can be freely evaluated over the Internet and the experiments can be replicated exactly the same way as initially presented in the literature, without the need for commercial software.

SURGICAL TECHNIQUE AND POSSIBLE PITFALLS

Annandale first described surgical repositioning of the displaced temporomandibular articular disc in 1887[68]; however, it was not until 1978 when Wilkes used arthrography to describe the anatomy, form, and function of the TMJ that disc repositioning became an accepted surgical technique.[69,70] Other surgeons, however, did not experience similar success, and this led to the development of modified techniques for disc repositioning surgery.[2,71–81] Some authors have proposed arthroscopic suturing techniques to reposition the disc.[82–86] Although various claims have been made, the reliability of an arthroscopic approach for predictably repositioning and stabilizing the disc in the TMJ has not been documented. The aim of this article was to evaluate our treatment outcomes with the use of the Mitek mini anchor in TMJ articular disc repositioning surgery.

Mitek Mini Anchor

Mitek anchors were originally developed for use in orthopedic surgery procedures such as rotator cuff repair, medial and lateral collateral ligament repair, bicep tendon reattachment, and other muscle, ligament, and tendon repair procedures.[2,87,88] Although available in various sizes, the Mitek mini anchor is the most adaptable Mitek anchor for TMJ disc stabilization. The successful use of the device for TMJ articular disc repositioning has been previously reported in the literature by Wolford and colleagues.[2,24,25,72] The United States Food and Drug Administration approves the use of the Mitek mini anchor specifically for use in the TMJ.

The Mitek mini anchor is cylindrical, measuring 1.8 mm in diameter and 5.0 mm in length. The body of the anchor is composed of titanium alloy (titanium 90%, aluminum 6%, vanadium 4%), and its arcs are composed of a nickel–titanium alloy (Nitinol), utilizing super elastic shape memory properties. An eyelet in the posterior aspect of the anchor allows placement of sutures that can function as artificial ligaments (**Fig. 8**).

Simultaneous surgical treatment would include repositioning the TMJ disc into a normal anatomic, functional position and stabilize it using the Mitek anchor (Mitek Surgical Products) technique[1–3,5,24–26,30] and then performing the indicated orthognathic surgery. The Mitek anchor technique uses a bone anchor that is placed into the lateral aspect of the posterior head of the condyle and the anchor will subsequently osseointegrate. Two 0-Ethibond sutures (Ethicon Inc., Somerville, NJ, USA) are attached to the anchor and are used as artificial ligaments to secure and stabilize the disc to the condylar head (**Fig. 9**).

High Success Rate with Disc Repositioning

Situations where the disc repositioning with the Mitek anchor has a high success rate:

1. Disc repositioning at the onset of displacement within 4 years of displacement provides the greatest predictability of outcome.
2. Adolescent internal condylar resorption patients who are treated within the first 4 years of disease onset.

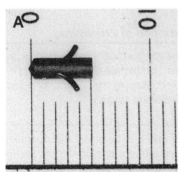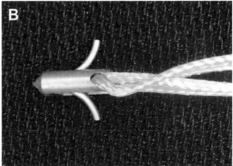

Fig. 8. (*A*) Body of the Mitek mini anchor is 1.8 × 5 mm and is composed of titanium alloy with wings of nickel titanium. (*B*) A doubled size 0 Ethibond suture has been passed through the eyelet of the Mitek mini anchor and these sutures function as artificial ligaments to stabilize the disc in the proper position.

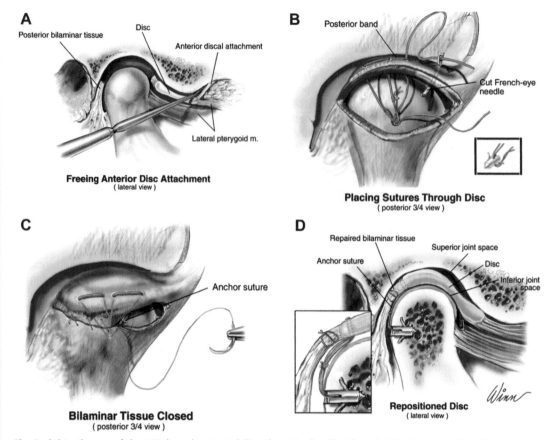

A

Posterior bilaminar tissue

Disc

Anterior discal attachment

Lateral pterygoid m.

Freeing Anterior Disc Attachment
(lateral view)

B

Posterior band

Cut French-eye needle

Placing Sutures Through Disc
(posterior 3/4 view)

C

Anchor suture

Bilaminar Tissue Closed
(posterior 3/4 view)

D

Repaired bilaminar tissue

Superior joint space

Anchor suture

Disc

Inferior joint space

Repositioned Disc
(lateral view)

Fig. 9. (*A*) In the use of the Mitek anchor to stabilize the articular disc, the joint first is exposed and the excessive bilaminar tissue excised. To mobilize the disc, the anterior attachment of the disc to the articular eminence is released so the disc can be positioned over the condyle passively. (*B, C*) The Mitek Mini Anchor (insert) has an eyelet that will support two 0-Ethibond sutures that can function as artificial ligaments. The anchor is inserted into the posterior head of the condyle lateral to the mid-sagittal plane and 5 to 8 mm below the top. One suture is placed in a mattress fashion through the medial aspect of the posterior part of the posterior band. The other suture is placed more lateral through the posterior band. (*D*) Cross-sectional sagittal view shows the Mitek anchor positioned in the condyle with the artificial ligaments attached to the disc to stabilize it to the condylar head. (*Courtesy of* Larry M. Wolford, DMD, Dallas, TX.)

3. No significant intracapsular inflammation, especially in the bilaminar tissues.
4. No history of connective tissue autoimmune diseases, such as rheumatoid arthritis, juvenile idiopathic arthritis, psoriatic arthritis, Sjögren syndrome, scleroderma, lupus, or ankylosing spondylitis.
5. Good remaining anatomy of the disc.
6. Reducing discs provide betters outcomes compared with nonreducing discs.
7. No other joint involvement.
8. No recurrent gastrointestinal, urinary, or respiratory tract problems.
9. No history of sexually transmitted diseases.

Successful surgical technique is the result of careful observation of details through a sequence of steps that have paramount importance. This section describes TMJ articular disc repositioning with all anatomic and surgical sequences that have proven to be effective and safe. Furthermore, it highlights possible mistakes that commonly affect outcomes.

Description of Procedure

A precise surgical intervention is paramount to obtain predictable outcomes; we present a detailed, step-by-step guide for a successful disc repositioning surgery.

Step 1

The patient is taken to the operating room and nasoendotracheal intubation is performed by the anesthesiologist. This is important, because it aids in the sterility of the field by allowing the surgeon to isolate the mouth of the patient using a tegaderm or ioband. It also helps in manipulating the patient's

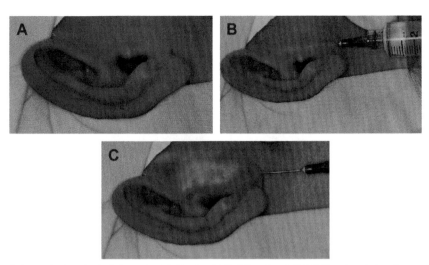

Fig. 10. (*A–C*) Preauricular site is injected with 5 mL of 1% lidocaine 1:100,000 epinephrine in a subcutaneous plane.

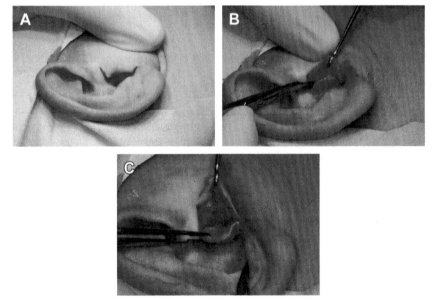

Fig. 11. (*A*) Modified endaural incision with #15 blade. (*B*) Sharp dissection with fine Iris scissors. (*C*) Tragal cartilage isolated 12 to 15 mm to the subcutaneous tissue.

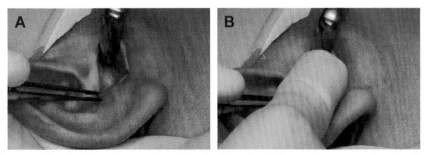

Fig. 12. (*A*) Long pickup holding the tragal cartilage backward and the small retractor showing the zygomatic area. (*B*) Digital manipulation to identify the zygomatic arch and to feel the condylar head.

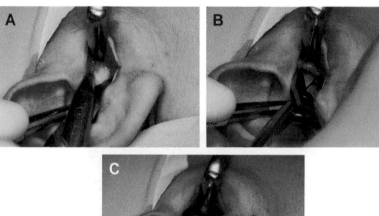

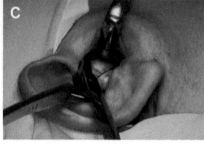

Fig. 13. (A) Sharp dissection with Dean scissors perpendicular to the arch 8 mm in front of the tragal cartilage. (B) Blunt dissection carried to the temporalis muscle fascia, below the fat tissue. (C) Blunt dissection is extended anteriorly to expose the articular eminence.

mouth while maintaining sterility and it permits the assessment of the occlusion during surgery.

Step 2
Bilateral preauricular sites are injected with 5 mL of 1% lidocaine 1:100,000 epinephrine in a subcutaneous plane (**Fig. 10**).

Possible Pitfalls: If you do not inject lidocaine, you will have more bleeding during the endaural incision and dissection of the subcutaneous plane.

Step 3
With a #15 blade, a modified short endaural incision is made with extension of 5 mm anterosuperiorly and 3 mm anteroinferiorly. Sharp dissection with fine Iris scissors is carried from tragal cartilage down approximately 12 to 15 mm to the subcutaneous tissue (**Fig. 11**). The preauricular approach is also preferred by some surgeons.

Possible Pitfalls: If you do not make the correct extension of endaural incision, you will not have a good surgical field to work in the TMJ; if you do not pay attention in the tragal cartilage during the sharp dissection, you can damage the cartilage, increasing the risk of perforating the external auditory meatus. The preauricular approach results in a more visible scar.

Step 4
Digital manipulation is done to identify the zygomatic arch and the condyle into the fossa when the mandible is moved laterally (**Fig. 12**).

Possible Pitfalls: If you do not do digital manipulation to identify the zygomatic arch you can incise in the wrong place, and potentially injure the frontal branch of cranial nerve VII or the external auditory canal.

Step 5
At this level, on top of the zygomatic arch, 8 mm in front of the tragal cartilage, blunt dissection is made with Dean scissors, perpendicular to the arch, carried to the temporal muscle fascia, below of the fat tissue. The dissection is extended anteriorly to expose the articular eminence (**Fig. 13**).

Possible Pitfalls: Visualizing the superficial layer of the deep temporal fascia is key in protecting the facial nerve.

Step 6
With a #9 periosteal elevator, the lateral rim of the glenoid fossa is demarcated (**Fig. 14**).

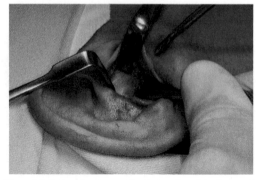

Fig. 14. Lateral rim of the glenoid fossa is demarcated.

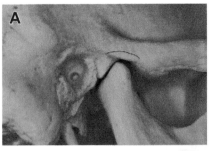
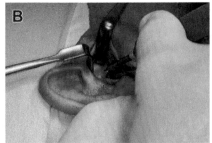
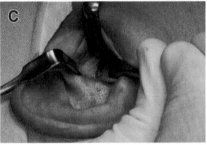

Fig. 15. (A) Extension of the C incision in the zygomatic arch. (B, C) Using Bovie electrocautery, a circular linear incision is performed on top of the arch, following the shape of the glenoid fossa.

Possible Pitfalls: This marking helps in delineating and identifying the condyle and protects the TMJ before the incision over the zygomatic arch.

Step 7
Using Bovie electrocautery, a curved linear incision is performed on top of the arch, following the shape of the glenoid fossa (**Fig. 15**).
Possible Pitfalls: The incision has to stay on bone on top of the arch to prevent inadvertent damage to the disc and fibrocartilage of the superior joint space.

Step 8
With a periosteal elevator, the fossa tissues are reflected inferiorly and laterally to expose inner capsule of the TMJ (**Fig. 16**).
Possible Pitfalls: If you do not reflect tissues to expose the inner capsule, you will have difficulty entering the superior joint space.

Step 9
Approximately 3 mL of 1% lidocaine 1:100,000 epinephrine is injected into the superior joint space to hydraulically displace the disc inferiorly. You can observe the mandible moving forward (**Fig. 17**).
Possible Pitfalls: This step hydraulically displaces the disc inferiorly and makes the access to the superior joint space safer.

Step 10
The lateral capsular attachments are incised superficially with a #15 blade 45° from inferior to superior aspect. The superior joint space is entered superficially with a freer elevator (**Fig. 18**).
Possible Pitfalls: The angulation of the blade is important in protecting the articular disc and the use of a freer elevator prevents scuffing and scratching of the fibrocartilage at the fossa, decreasing the risk of adhesions.

Step 11
Using Dean scissors, the lateral capsular attachments are cut along the margin of the glenoid fossa and articular eminence (**Fig. 19**).

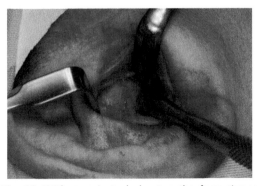

Fig. 16. With a periosteal elevator, the fossa tissues are reflected inferiorly and laterally to expose to the lateral capsule of the temporomandibular joint.

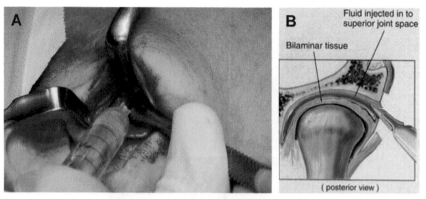

Fig. 17. (*A*) Lidocaine 1:100,000 epinephrine is injected into the superior joint space. (*B*) Anesthetic hydraulically displace the disc inferiorly to make an incision in the capsule securely. ([*B*] *Courtesy of* Larry M. Wolford, DMD, Dallas, TX.)

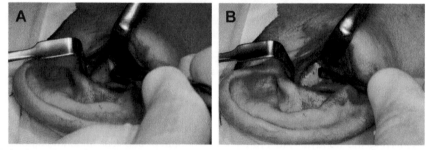

Fig. 18. (*A*) The lateral capsular attachments are incised with a #15 blade. (*B*) The superior joint space is entered with a freer elevator.

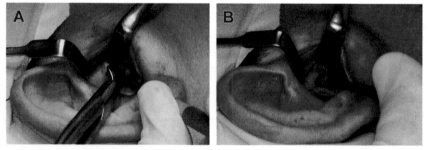

Fig. 19. (*A, B*) The lateral capsular attachments are dissect with Dean scissors countering the glenoid fossa beyond the articular eminence.

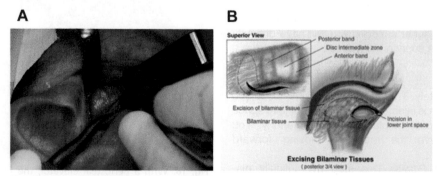

Fig. 20. (*A, B*) Using a #15 blade the lateral capsule is incised 10 mm below the lateral pole of the condyle from posterosuperior to inferoanterior aspect. ([*B*] *Courtesy of* Larry M. Wolford, DMD, Dallas, TX.)

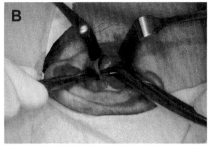

Fig. 21. (*A*) Using a #9 periosteal elevator, the condyle is dissected inferiorly. (*B*) Using the Dean scissors, the bilaminar tissue is cut around the posterior aspect of the condyle.

Possible Pitfalls: Failure to adequately dissect the capsular attachments at the glenoid fossa will cause limited visibility and greater difficulty in mobilizing the articular disc.

Step 12

Using a #15 blade, the lateral capsule is incised just above the lateral pole of the condyle from posterosuperior to inferoanterior (**Fig. 20**). The incision is made at this level to maintain and maximize soft tissue attachment and vascularity to the condyle.

Possible Pitfalls: Care must be taken to minimize damage to the fibrocartilage of the fossa and condylar head, as well as the disc, because injury to these structures can promote the formation of adhesions and degenerative changes postoperatively.

Step 13

Using a periosteal elevator, the condyle is retracted inferiorly to create a space to insert the Dean scissors and cut the bilaminar tissue around the posterior aspect of the condyle until the medial wall of the fossa is reached (**Fig. 21**).

Possible Pitfalls: If a piece of the retrodiscal tissue is not removed, there will not be adequate

space to reduce the articular disc and the condyle may be displaced forward. Also, access and visibility will be limited.

Step 14

In cases of anterior displacement, it is often necessary to free the disc anteriorly where the ligament attaches from the anterior band of the disc to the anterior slope of the articular eminence; sometimes, it is necessary to release the medial attachments as well.

Possible Pitfalls: The anterior release is critical to passively reposition the disc. Sometimes, a medial release is also necessary.

Step 15

Using a Mitek drill bit (2.1 mm diameter) with a built-in stop, a 2×10-mm hole is made in the posterior head of the condyle. The position of the anchor may vary slightly from case to case, but is generally positioned 8 to 10 mm below the superior aspect of the condyle, and just lateral to the midsagittal plane. It is not necessary to strip soft tissue from the posterior condyle for hole preparation, and generally the hole is drilled through the periosteum to maximize soft tissue attachment and blood supply to the condyle.

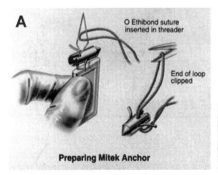

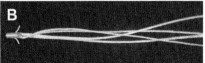

Fig. 22. (*A, B*) A doubled size 0 Ethibond suture has been passed through the eyelet of the Mitek mini anchor, and the loop is cut, thereby yielding 2 separate strands of suture material. ([A] *Courtesy of* Larry M. Wolford, DMD, Dallas, TX.)

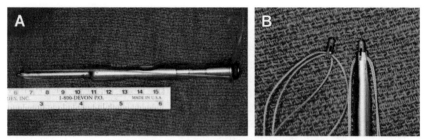

Fig. 23. (*A, B*) The anchor is then loaded onto an inserting device used to place the anchor in the condyle.

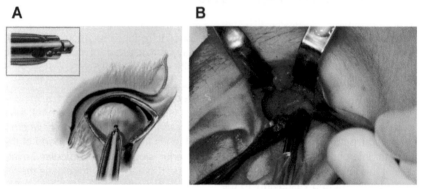

Fig. 24. (*A, B*) The 1.8-mm titanium Mitek anchor is then placed into the prepared hole. ([*A*] *Courtesy of* Larry M. Wolford, DMD, Dallas, TX.)

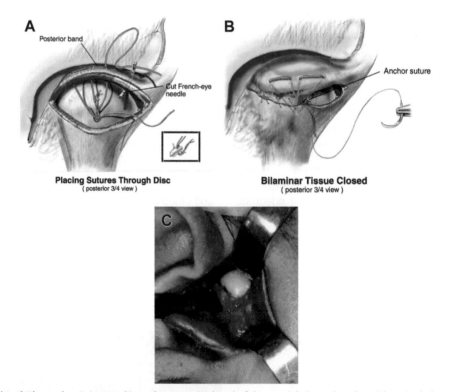

Fig. 25. (*A–C*) The anchor is inserted into the posterior head of the condyle lateral to the mid sagittal plane and 5 to 8 mm below the top. One suture is placed in a mattress fashion through the medial aspect of the posterior part of the posterior band. The other suture is placed more lateral through the posterior band. These sutures function as artificial ligaments to stabilize the disc in the proper position. ([*A, B*] *Courtesy of* Larry M. Wolford, DMD, Dallas, TX.)

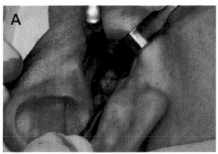

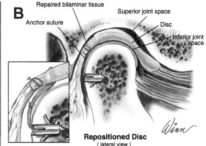

Fig. 26. (*A*) Disc is well-secured in new optimal position. (*B*) Cross-sectional sagittal view shows the Mitek anchor positioned in the condyle with the artificial ligaments attached to the disc to stabilize it to the condylar head. ([*B*] *Courtesy of* Larry M. Wolford, DMD, Dallas, TX.)

Possible Pitfalls: The position of the anchor can be modified to suit the type of reduction necessary.

Step 16

Before placing the implant, 1 size 0 polyester or other nonresorbable braided suture is doubled and threaded through the eyelet of the anchor (**Fig. 22**). The suture loop is then cut, thereby making 2 separate strands, and the anchor is placed into an inserting device (**Fig. 23**).

Possible Pitfalls: If you do not use a threader you will have difficulty to inserting the 0 Ethibond into the eyelet of the anchor.

Step 17

The 1.8-mm titanium Mitek anchor is then placed into the prepared hole using a special delivery device, and using hand pressure, the trigger is advanced, delivering the anchor below the cortical bone level into the softer medullary bone of the condyle (**Fig. 24**).

Possible Pitfalls: Failure to place the anchor into an inserting device with the permanent suture into the eyelet of the anchor will cause difficulty during the insertion of the anchor inside the hole and can break the wings.

Step 18

Using an 8-mm modified French-eye needle, the 2 sutures are then attached to the disc in a mattress or running fashion from the posteromedial to posterolateral aspect of the disc to reposition it in correct position on top of the condylar head (**Fig. 25**). The sutures are securely tightened and positioned with a double knot and 3 simple knots (**Fig. 26**). The condyle is manipulated in various directions noting the disc and condylar unit moved harmoniously and the disc well-secured in its new, optimal position.

Possible Pitfalls: The use of a double knot or a surgeon's knot is necessary to secure the suture as close as possible to the condylar head and stabilize the anchor.

Step 19

The surgical site is then profusely irrigated and the lateral capsule is sutured back into position.

Possible Pitfalls: If you do not irrigate the surgical site with saline solution, you will increase the risk of infection. If you do not suture the lateral capsule, you will not stabilize the disc laterally and it will take longer to heal the joint.

Step 20

A layered closure of the incision is completed with 4–0 Polydioxanone (PDS) for the deep tissue of temporomandibular fascia (**Fig. 27**) and to approximate the subcutaneous tissue of the endaural incision (**Fig. 28**). The skin is closed in a subcuticular fashion (**Fig. 29**).

CLINICAL CASE

A 19-year-old woman presented with bilateral TMJ anteriorly displaced articular discs (confirmed by MRI). Intermediate zone criteria is the location of the intermediate zone of the disk in relation to the condyle and the articular eminence. Using this criterion, we can observe articular disc displacement (**Fig. 30**). She had vertical excess

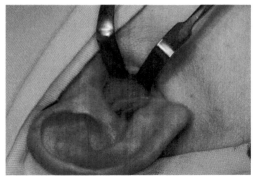

Fig. 27. A layered closure of the incision is completed with 4–0 PDS for the deep tissue of temporomandibular fascia.

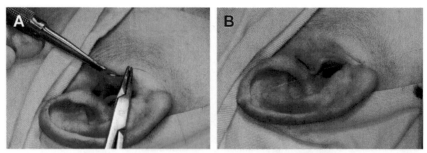

Fig. 28. (*A, B*) Approximation of the subcutaneous tissue of the endaural incision.

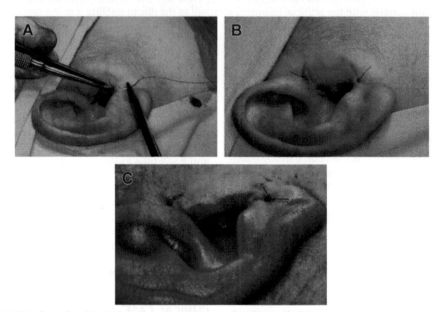

Fig. 29. (*A–C*) To close the skin, 5–0 Prolene is used in a subcuticular fashion.

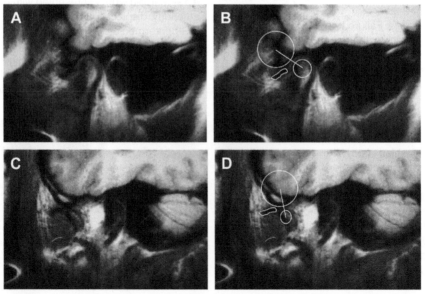

Fig. 30. (*A, B*) MRI of a temporomandibular joint showing a significantly anterior displaced articular disc using Intermediate Zone (IZ) criteria. (*C, D*) On opening, the disc remains anteriorly displaced and nonreducing with degenerative changes using IZ criteria. (*Courtesy of* Larry M. Wolford, DMD, Dallas, TX.)

of maxilla, lip incompetence, facial asymmetry, mandible retruded, high occlusal plane angle, and class II skeletal and occlusal dentofacial deformity (**Figs. 31** and **32**). She complained of moderate to severe TMJ pain, headaches, and myofascial pain, as well as clicking in the TMJs and difficulty eating. After orthodontic preparation, surgery was performed in a single operation, including bilateral TMJ disc repositioning with Mitek anchors, bilateral mandibular ramus sagittal split osteotomies and multiple maxillary osteotomies for maxillomandibular counterclockwise advancement at the pogonion. At 2 years postoperatively, the patient demonstrated good stability, esthetics, symmetry, smile, and occlusion with elimination of TMJ pain, headaches, myofascial pain, and TMJ noise, as well as improved jaw function and facial esthetics.

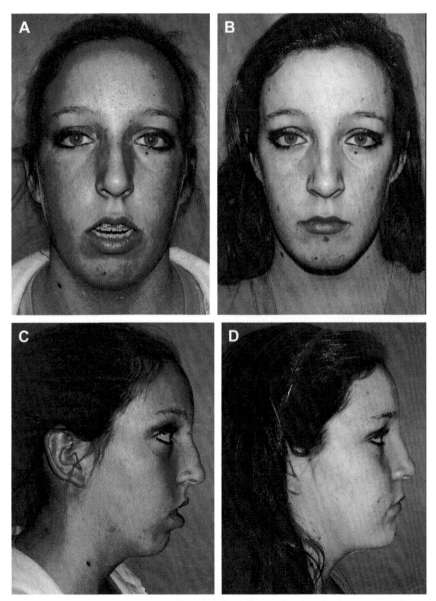

Fig. 31. (*A, C*) This 19-year-old woman presented with bilateral articular disc displacement and temporomandibular joint (TMJ) dysfunction. The mandible is significantly retruded, with a high occlusal plane angle and associated facial morphology. (*B, D*) The same patient 2 years after undergoing bilateral TMJ articular disc repositioning with Mitek mini anchors and simultaneous double jaw orthognathic surgery. (*Courtesy of* Larry M. Wolford, DMD, Dallas, TX.)

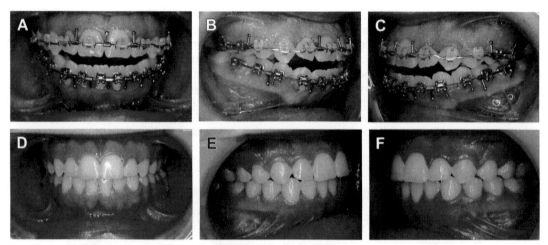

Fig. 32. (*A–C*) Preoperative occlusion demonstrating an anterior open bite and class II occlusal relationship. (*D–F*) The occlusion remained stable 2 years postoperatively. ([*B*] *Courtesy of* Larry M. Wolford, DMD, Dallas, TX.)

SUMMARY

Scientific evidence with regard to the effectiveness of TMJ disc repositioning remains scarce and needs further efforts to guide clinicians and patients among the clinical and surgical options to better treat TMJ internal derangement, mainly when associated with skeletal malocclusion that requires surgical interventions. Although scarce, we have reviewed several papers that showed outcomes after TMJ articular disc repositioning. These studies were undertaken with lateral cephalometric radiographs, tomograms, cone-beam computed tomography, MRIs, and visual analog scale assessments for reported pain and function. The lack of evidence that TMJ articular disc repositioning is an ineffective procedure points to a future when new TMJ biomarkers will support the technique effectiveness in more rigorously controlled studies.

Because this is a sensitive technique with a wide learning curve, many surgeons have practiced TMJ articular disc repositioning with a large range of outcomes. In this article, we have reviewed all the main steps for a successful surgery and the most frequent pitfalls that can compromise the procedure. Adequate training is important for achieving the best results possible.

REFERENCES

1. Wolford LM, Karras S, Mehra P. Concomitant temporomandibular joint and orthognathic surgery: a preliminary report. J Oral Maxillofac Surg 2002;60:356–62.
2. Mehra P, Wolford LM. The Mitek mini anchor for TMJ disc repositioning: surgical technique and results. Int J Oral Maxillofac Surg 2001;30(6):497–503.
3. Wolford LM, Cardenas L. Idiopathic condylar resorption: diagnosis, treatment protocol, and outcomes. Am J Orthod Dentofacial Orthop 1999; 116(6):667–77.
4. Goncalves JR, Wolford LM, Cassano DS, et al. Temporomandibular joint condylar changes following maxillomandibular advancement and articular disc repositioning. J Oral Maxillofac Surg 2013; 71(10):1759.e1–15.
5. Goncalves JR, Cassano DS, Wolford LM, et al. Postsurgical stability of counterclockwise maxillomandibular advancement surgery: affect of articular disc repositioning. J Oral Maxillofac Surg 2008;66(4):724–38.
6. US Agency for Healthcare Research and Quality. Evidence-based Practice Centers: evidence-based reports. Available at: http://www.ahrq.gov/research/findings/evidence-based-reports/index.html. Accessed March 7, 2014.
7. Institute for Scientific Information. ISI impact factor description. Available from: http://thomsonreuters.com/productsservices/science products/a-z/journal citation reports.
8. Pitak-Arnnop P. The 100 most cited articles in dentistry–some discussions. Clin Oral Investig 2014;18(2):683–4.
9. Sandhu A. The evidence base for oral and maxillofacial surgery: 10-year analysis of two journals. Br J Oral Maxillofac Surg 2012;50(1):45–8.
10. Harris AD, McGregor JC, Perencevich EN, et al. The use and interpretation of quasi-experimental studies in medical informatics. J Am Med Inform Assoc 2006;13(1):16–23.
11. Shaughnessy AF, Slawson DC, Bennett JH. Becoming an information master: a guidebook to the medical information jungle. J Fam Pract 1994; 39(5):489–99.

12. List T, Axelsson S. Management of TMD: evidence from systematic reviews and meta-analyses. J Oral Rehabil 2010;37(6):430–51.

13. Stavropoulos F, Dolwick MF. Simultaneous temporomandibular joint and orthognathic surgery: the case against. J Oral Maxillofac Surg 2003;61(10):1205–6.

14. Onizawa K, Schmelzeisen R, Vogt S. Alteration of temporomandibular joint symptoms after orthognathic surgery. J Oral Maxillofac Surg 1995;53(2):117–21.

15. Mercuri LG. Internal derangement outcomes reporting. J Oral Maxillofac Surg 2010;68(6):1455 [author reply: 1455–6].

16. Wolford LM, Reiche-Fischel O, Mehra P. Changes in temporomandibular joint dysfunction after orthognathic surgery. J Oral Maxillofac Surg 2003;61:655.

17. Karabouta I, Martis C. The TMJ dysfunction syndrome before and after sagittal split osteotomy of the rami. J Maxillofac Surg 1985;13:185.

18. Magnusson T, Ahlborg G, Finne K, et al. Changes in temporomandibular joint pain and dysfunction after surgical correction of dentofacial deformities. Int J Oral Maxillofac Surg 1984;15:707.

19. Upton G, Scott R, Hayward J. Major maxillomandibular malrelations and temporomandibular joint pain and dysfunction. J Prosthet Dent 1984;51:686.

20. Panula K, Somppi M, Finne K, et al. Effects of orthognathic surgery on temporomandibular joint dysfunction. Int J Oral Maxillofac Surg 2000;29:183.

21. Reiche-Fischel O, Wolford LM. Changes in TMJ dysfunction after orthognathic surgery. J Oral Maxillofac Surg 1996;54(Suppl 1):84.

22. Fuselier C, Wolford LM, Pitta M, et al. Condylar changes after orthognathic surgery with untreated TMJ internal derangement. J Oral Maxillofac Surg 1998;56(Suppl 1):61.

23. Wolford LM. Concomitant temporomandibular joint and orthognathic surgery. J Oral Maxillofac Surg 2003;61:1198.

24. Wolford LM, Cottrell DA, Karras SC. Mitek minianchor in maxillofacial surgery. In: Proceedings of SMST-94, the First International Conference on Shape Memory and Superelastic Technologies. Monterey (CA): MIAS; 1995. p. 477.

25. Wolford LM. Temporomandibular joint devices: treatment factors and outcomes. Oral Surg Oral Med Oral Pathol Oral Radiol Endod 1997;83:143.

26. Downie MJ, Wolford LM, Morales-Ryan CA. Outcome assessment following simultaneous orthognathic and TMJ surgery. J Oral Maxillofac Surg 2001;59(Suppl 1):51.

27. Cardenas L, Wolford LM, Gonçalves J. Mitek anchor in TMJ surgery: positional changes and condylar effects. J Oral Maxillofac Surg 1997;55(Suppl 1):14.

28. Fields T, Cardenas L, Wolford LM. The pull-out strengths of Mitek suture anchors from human cadaver mandibular condyles. J Oral Maxillofac Surg 1997;55:483.

29. Fields T, Franco PF, Wolford LM. The osseous integration of the Mitek mini anchors in the mandibular condyle. J Oral Maxillofac Surg 2001;59:1402.

30. Morales-Ryan CA, Garcia-Morales P, Wolford LM. Idiopathic condylar resorption: outcome assessment of TMJ disc repositioning and orthognathic surgery. J Oral Maxillofac Surg 2002;60(Suppl 1):53.

31. Wolford LM, Mehra P, Reiche-Fischel O, et al. Efficacy of high condylectomy for management of condylar hyperplasia. Am J Orthod Dentofacial Orthop 2002;121:136.

32. Garcia-Morales P, Mehra P, Wolford LM, et al. Efficacy of high condylectomy for management of condylar hyperplasia. J Oral Maxillofac Surg 2001; 59:106.

33. Wolford LM, Mehra P, Franco P. Use of conservative condylectomy for treatment of osteochondroma of the mandibular condyle. J Oral Maxillofac Surg 2002;60:262.

34. Wolford LM, Cottrell DA, Henry CH. Sternoclavicular grafts for temporomandibular joint reconstruction. J Oral Maxillofac Surg 1994;52:119.

35. Franco PF, Wolford LW, Talwar RM. Sternoclavicular grafts in congenital and developmental deformities. J Oral Maxillofac Surg 1997;55:104.

36. Wolford LM, Cottrell DA, Henry CH. Temporomandibular joint reconstruction of the complex patients with the Techmedica custom-made total joint prosthesis. J Oral Maxillofac Surg 1994;52:2.

37. Freitas RZ, Mehra P, Wolford LM. Autogenous versus alloplastic TMJ reconstruction in rheumatoid-induced TMJ disease. J Oral Maxillofac Surg 2002; 58:43.

38. Mehra P, Wolford LM. Custom-made TMJ reconstruction and simultaneous mandibular advancement in autoimmune/connective tissue diseases. J Oral Maxillofac Surg 2000;58:95.

39. Henry CH, Wolford LM. Treatment outcomes for TMJ reconstruction after Proplast-Teflon implant failures. J Oral Maxillofac Surg 1993;51:352.

40. Wolford LM, Karras SC. Autologous fat transplantation around a temporomandibular joint total joint prosthesis: preliminary treatment outcomes. J Oral Maxillofac Surg 1997;55:245.

41. Karras SC, Wolford LM, Cottrell DA. Concurrent osteochondroma of the mandibular condyle and ipsilateral cranial base resulting in temporomandibular joint ankylosis: report of a case and review of the literature. J Oral Maxillofac Surg 1996;54:640.

42. Wolford LM, Pitta MC, Reiche-Fischel O, et al. TMJ Concepts/Techmedica custom-made TMJ total joint prosthesis: 5-year follow-up. Int J Oral Maxillofac Surg 2003;32:268.

43. Nickerson JW, Boring G. Natural course of osteoarthrosis as it relates to internal derangement of the temporomandibular joint. Oral Maxillofac Surg Clin North Am 1989;1:27.

44. Cutbirth M, Sickels JEV, Thrash WJ. Condylar resorption after bicortical screw fixation of mandibular advancement. J Oral Maxillofac Surg 1998;56:178.

45. Hoppenreijs TJM, Stoelinga PJW, Grace KL, et al. CMG: long-term evaluation of patients with progressive condylar resorption following orthognathic surgery. Int J Oral Maxillofac Surg 1999;28:411.

46. Will LA, West RA. Factors influencing the stability of the sagittal split osteotomy for mandibular advancement. J Oral Maxillofac Surg 1989;47:813.

47. Hwang SJ, Haers PE, Seifert B, et al. Non-surgical risk factors for condylar resorption after orthognathic surgery. J Craniomaxillofac Surg 2004;32:103.

48. Schellhas KP, Piper MA, Omlie M. Facial skeleton remodeling due to temporomandibular joint degeneration. AJNR Am J Neuroradiol 1990;11:541.

49. Schellhas KP. Internal derangement of the temporomandibular joint: radiologic staging with clinical, surgical and pathologic correlation. Magn Reson Imaging 1989;7:495.

50. Kerstens HC, Tuinzing DB, Golding RP, et al. Condylar atrophy and osteoarthrosis after bimaxillary surgery. Oral Surg Oral Med Oral Pathol 1990; 69:274.

51. Moore KG, Cooris PJ, Stoelinga PJ. The contributing role of condylar resorption in orthognathic surgery: a retrospective study. J Oral Maxillofac Surg 1991; 49:448.

52. DeClercq CA, Neyt LF, Mommaerts MY, et al. Condylar resorption in orthognathic surgery: a retrospective study. Int J Adult Orthodon Orthognath Surg 1994;9:233.

53. Arnett GW, Tamborello JA. Progressive class II development: female idiopathic condylar resorption. Oral Maxillofac Surg Clin North Am 1990;2:699.

54. Crawford JG, Stoelinga PJ, Blijdrop PA, et al. Stability after reoperation for progressive condylar resorption after orthognathic surgery: report of seven cases. J Oral Maxillofac Surg 1994;52:460.

55. Bertram S, Moriggl A, Neunteufel N, et al. Lateral cephalometric analysis of mandibular morphology: discrimination among subjects with and without temporomandibular joint disk displacement and osteoarthrosis. J Oral Rehabil 2012;39:93–9.

56. Chemello PD, Wolford LM, Buschang MS. Occlusal plane alteration in orthognathic surgery, Part II: long-term stability of results. Am J Orthod Dentofacial Orthop 1994;106:434.

57. Satrom KD, Sinclair PM, Wolford LM. The stability of double jaw surgery: a comparison of rigid versus wire fixation. Am J Orthod 1991;6:550.

58. Cottrell DA, Sugimoto RM, Wolford LM, et al. Condylar changes after upward and forward rotation of the maxillomandibular complex. Am J Orthod Dentofacial Orthop 1997;111:156.

59. Cevidanes LHS, Hajati AK, Paniagua B, et al. Quantification of condylar resorption in temporomandibular joint osteoarthritis. Oral Surg Oral Med Oral Pathol Oral Radiol Endod 2010;110(1):110–7.

60. Paniagua B, Cevidanes L, Walker D, et al. Clinical application of SPHARM-PDM to quantify temporomandibular joint osteoarthritis. Comput Med Imaging Graph 2011;35(5):345–52.

61. Angle AD, Rebellato J, Sheats RD. Transverse displacement of the proximal segment after bilateral sagittal split osteotomy advancement and its effect on relapse. J Oral Maxillofac Surg 2007;65(1):50–9.

62. Harris MD, Van Sickels JE, Alder M. Factors influencing condylar position after the bilateral sagittal split osteotomy fixed with bicortical screws. J Oral Maxillofac Surg 1999;57(6):650–4 [discussion: 654–5].

63. Alder ME, Deahl ST, Matteson SR, et al. Short-term changes of condylar position after sagittal split osteotomy for mandibular advancement. Oral Surg Oral Med Oral Pathol Oral Radiol Endod 1999; 87(2):159–65.

64. Carvalho FD, Cevidanes LH, da Motta AT, et al. Three-dimensional assessment of mandibular advancement 1 year after surgery. Am J Orthod Dentofacial Orthop 2010;137(Suppl 4):S53.e1–12 [discussion: S53–5].

65. Motta AT, Cevidanes LH, Carvalho FA, et al. Three-dimensional regional displacements after mandibular advancement surgery: one year of follow-up. J Oral Maxillofac Surg 2011;69(5):1447–57.

66. Cevidanes LH, Bailey LJ, Tucker GR, et al. Superimposition of 3D cone-beam CT models of orthognathic surgery patients. Dentomaxillofac Radiol 2005;34(6):369–75.

67. Schilling J, Gomes LC, Benavides E, et al. Regional 3D superimposition to assess temporomandibular joint condylar morphology. Dentomaxillofac Radiol 2014;43(1):20130273.

68. Annandale T. On displacement of the interarticular cartilage of the lower jaw and its treatment by operation. Lancet 1887;1:411–2.

69. Wilkes CH. Arthrography of the temporomandibular joint in patients with TMJ pain dysfunction syndrome. Minn Med 1978;61:645.

70. Wilkes CH. Structural and functional alterations of the temporomandibular joint. Northwest Dent 1978; 57:287–90.

71. Anderson DM, Sinclair PM, McBride KM. A clinical evaluation of temporo- mandibular joint plication surgery. Am J Orthod Dentofacial Orthop 1991;100: 156–62.

72. Cottrell DA, Wolford LM. The Mitek mini anchor in maxillofacial surgery. J Oral Maxillofac Surg Educ Summ Outlines 1993;57(3):150.

73. Dolwick MF, Nitzan DW. The role of disc-repositioning surgery for internal derangements of the temporomandibular joint. Oral Maxillofac Surg Clin North Am 1994; 6:271–5.

74. Kerstens HC, Tuinzing DB, Van Der Kwast WA. Eminectomy and disco- plasty for correction of the displaced temporomandibular joint disc. J Oral Maxillofac Surg 1989;47:150–4.

75. McCarty WL, Farrar WB. Surgery for internal derangement's of the temporomandibular joint. J Prosthet Dent 1979;42:191–6.

76. Walker RV, Kalamchi S. A surgical technique for the management of internal derangement of the temporomandibular joint. J Oral Maxillofac Surg 1987;45:299–305.

77. Weinberg S, Cousens G. Meniscocondylar plication: a modified operation for surgical repositioning of the ectopic temporomandibular joint meniscus. Oral Surg Oral Med Oral Pathol 1987;63:393.

78. Santos GS, Nogueira LM, Sonoda CK, et al. Using endaural approach for temporomandibular joint access. J Craniofac Surg 2014;25(3):1142–3.

79. Ruíz CA, Guerrero JS. A new modified endaural approach for access to the temporomandibular joint. Br J Oral Maxillofac Surg 2001;39:371–3.

80. Dolwick MF, Kretzschmar DP. Morbidity associated with the preauricular and perimeatal approaches to the temporomandibular joint. J Oral Maxillofac Surg 1982;40:699–700.

81. Al-Kayat A, Bramley P. A modified pre-auricular approach to the temporomandibular joint and malar arch. Br J Oral Surg 1979;17:91–103.

82. Hoffman DC, Sansevere JJ. A new method of TMJ disc stabilization during open joint surgery. J Oral Maxillofac Surg Educ Summ Out- lines 1993;51(3):149.

83. Tarro AW. TMJ arthroscopic diagnosis and surgery: clinical experience with 152 cases over a 2 year period. Cranio 1991;9(2):108–19.

84. Yang CI, Cai XY, Chen MJ, et al. New arthroscopic disc repositioning and suturing technique for treating an anteriorly displaced disc of the temporomandibular joint: part I–technique introduction. Int J Oral Maxillofac Surg 2012;41(9):1058–63. http://dx.doi.org/10.1016/j.ijom.2012.05.025.

85. Zhang SY, Liu XM, Yang C, et al. New arthroscopic disc repositioning and suturing technique for treating internal derangement of the temporomandibular joint: part II–magnetic resonance imaging evaluation. J Oral Maxillofac Surg 2010;68(8):1813–7. http://dx.doi.org/10.1016/j.joms.2009.08.012.

86. Ingawalé S, Goswami T. Temporomandibular joint: disorders, treatments, and biomechanics. Ann Biomed Eng 2009;37(5):976–96. http://dx.doi.org/10.1007/s10439-009-9659-4.

87. Obrist J, Genelin F, Neureiter H. Bankart operation with the Mitek anchor system. Unfallchirugie 1991;17:208–13.

88. Pederson B, Tesoro D, Weetheimer SJ, et al. Mitek anchor system—a new technique for tenodesis and ligamentous repair of the foot and ankle. J Foot Surg 1991;30:48–52.

Complications of TMJ Surgery

David Hoffman, DDS[a], Leann Puig, DMD[b]

KEYWORDS

- TMJ surgery • TMJ surgical complications • TMJ surgical infections • Maxillary artery bleeds
- TMJ nerve damage

KEY POINTS

- The complications of temporomandibular joint (TMJ) surgery are a known event and, even in the best surgical hands and surgical intentions, complications can develop.
- There are no indications to suggest that a complication such as bleeding, infection, or failure of the prosthesis is necessarily the fault of the surgeon or the patient.
- For the most part, complications are rare and TMJ surgery can be done in a very successful manner.
- The advent of arthroscopic surgery has minimized untoward events and has been a major help to many surgical patients.
- Simplifying many of the arthroplasty procedures can be of benefit to patients and be performed in predictable and successful fashion with minimal complication rate.

Complications from temporomandibular joint (TMJ) surgery can be divided in true complications and untoward outcomes. The purpose of this article was to look at complications directly related to TMJ surgery and not dwell on the outcomes or the success of TMJ surgery. Needless to say, complications clearly affect surgical outcomes; however, there are many other factors that affect the success rate of TMJ surgery. The 3 main surgical procedures that could lead to complications are:

- Arthroscopic surgery
- Open arthroplasty; and
- Total joint reconstruction.

Although these 3 groups are general or broad categories, they each have their own specific surgical techniques and therefore their own potential complication rates. They are all done differently, and each one in successive order has an increasing rate of complications.

In general, complications can be divided into the following categories:

1. Anatomic
2. Neurovascular
3. Infectious
4. Autoimmune, and
5. Biomechanical.

Damage to adjacent anatomic structures can become a major concern when doing TMJ surgery of all kinds. Infections are a second important group of complications, and although rare (about 2% in all 3 categories), when they occur they have devastating effects on the patient. Infection rates can also be looked at as a comparison in what the overall infection rate is in other orthopedic joint-related procedures. There are so few publications on TMJ infections and the numbers are so low that, for any given group, the orthopedic literature has become the benchmark for comparisons. Hypersensitivity reactions

[a] Oral & Maxillofacial Surgery, Staten Island University Hospital, 256-C Mason Avenue, 3rd Floor, Staten Island, NY 10305, USA; [b] Kings County Hospital, Brooklyn, 451 Clarkson Ave, NY 11203, USA
E-mail address: swordfish1@me.com

Oral Maxillofacial Surg Clin N Am 27 (2015) 109–124
http://dx.doi.org/10.1016/j.coms.2014.09.008
1042-3699/15/$ – see front matter © 2015 Elsevier Inc. All rights reserved.

or hardware failures are rare, but also potentially incapacitating.

A basic understanding of the TMJ anatomy is inherent in understanding potential complications. The joint itself is surrounded by neurologic structures primarily derived from cranial nerves V and VII, and blood vessels branches of the internal maxillary and superficial temporal artery predominantly (**Figs. 1** and **2**). Additionally, the joint is intimately involved with the base of the skull, sharing the roof of the glenoid fossa with the middle cranial fossa, so that any damage to the bony structures of the joint has the potential to cause an intracranial hematoma or cerebrospinal fluid fistula. One of the problems associated with some of the vasculature surrounding the joint, in particular the maxillary artery, is that it is located medial to the joint and any damage to it during a surgical procedure runs the risk of having a bleed that is not approachable for routine tying off of the vessel. For most surgeons who have experienced a maxillary artery bleed, isolation and ligation is ideal; but, if not possible, packing and embolization should be considered. The close proximity of the ear potentiates damage to the external auditory canal, the tympanic membrane, and the middle ear. Additionally, the parotid gland is inferior but adjacent to the joint.

Certainly, the best approach to minimizing the complication rate of TMJ surgery is careful surgical planning, delicate technique, and

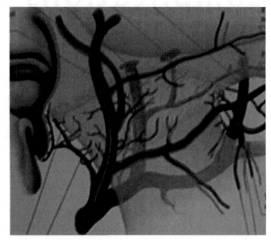

Fig. 2. Blood vessels in the field of the temporomandibular joint condyle. (*From* Quinn PD. Color atlas of temporomandibular joint surgery. Philadelphia: Mosby; 1998; with permission.)

preparedness to identify and treat a complication before it occurs or immediately upon its expression. With the advent of 3-dimensional modeling, computed tomography (CT) arteriograms, and MRI, the surgeon can anticipate many of the problems that might potentially occur and plan to avoid them, or treat them if they do occur. For example, when the CT arteriogram illustrates an artery directly in the field of an ankylosed joint, the use of interventional radiology either before or during surgery, can minimize or eliminate intraoperative bleeding with the use of selective embolization. This is just one of many examples of how the use of technology and imaging can help to plan and perform a safe TMJ surgery.

Another technology that lends itself to complex TMJ surgical procedures such as ankylosis is image-guided surgery. This technology, although developed either for intracranial surgery or ear, nose, and throat surgery, is directly applicable to TMJ surgery. In this instance, a surgical wand that allows the surgeon to identify their position on a computed axial tomography (CAT) during surgery can be very helpful. Currently, there are 3 companies that support this type of technology, each one having the maxillofacial component. They are Brain Lab, Stryker, and Medtronics (**Fig. 3**).

Another complication applicable to any type of TMJ surgical procedure is the effect of the TMJ on function and occlusion. Although arthroscopy has a minimal and temporary effect on mandibular occlusion, it does have significant effects on its function. The 2 other surgical procedures—arthroplasty and total joint reconstruction—directly

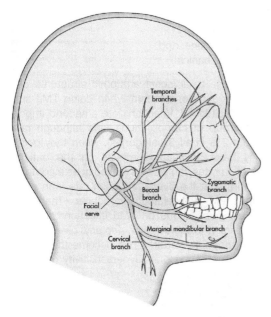

Fig. 1. Diagram of the facial nerve (VIIth cranial nerve) around the temporomandibular joint. (*From* Quinn PD. Color atlas of temporomandibular joint surgery. Philadelphia: Mosby; 1998; with permission.)

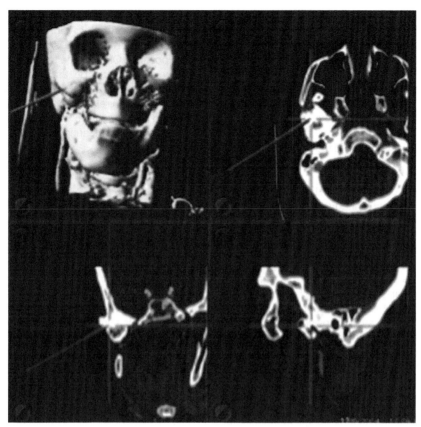

Fig. 3. Image-guided surgery in a case of temporomandibular joint ankylosis. Surgical wand shows the position of the wand in the bone.

affect occlusion because the joint becomes one of the stable structures in establishing a bite. Therefore, a surgical malocclusion as a result of TMJ surgery could easily be construed as a complication. For example, a malpositioned total joint replacement would be unforgiving if the bite were not exactly set right. Furthermore, failure to maintain the occlusion after ablative surgery of the TMJ can easily result in a malocclusion.

In some instances, surgical complications are directly related to the craniofacial structures and have similar comparisons to other skeletal joints. Occlusion and joint function are specific to the TMJ and cannot necessarily be compared with other orthopedic models. On the other hand, infections become similar to other orthopedic replacement systems and a comparison of the given TMJ surgical procedures can be extrapolated to see how they would fair against the orthopedic literature. Vallerand and Dolwick[1] reviewed TMJ surgical complications in 1990. At that time, TMJ arthroscopy had recently become popular, and alloplastic joint replacements were in a holding pattern owing to problems with proplast. Kieth[2]

published a similar review in 2003 with a substantial amount of data on arthroscopy, and a growing body of data on the latest generation of total joint replacement systems.

ARTHROSCOPIC SURGERY

Arthroscopic surgery is probably among the safest procedures performed by maxillofacial surgeons. In its simplest form, a 1.9 or smaller arthroscope is placed in the TMJ either through a posterior puncture or an anterior puncture or portal. Scopes as long as 2.3 have been used, and even working instruments as large as almost 3 mm can be utilized with or without the protective casing. Arthroscopy can be as simple as a single puncture in the TMJ with an outflow system created with an 18-gauge needle to a more complex procedure using multiport or triangulation techniques involving the use of 1 portal for the arthroscope and the second portal for instrumentation. Instrumentation can range from forceps to graspers, spinal needles to inject, shavers, electrocauteries, and lasers. In light of this multiport or triangular operative arthroscopic surgery, the complication potential of a broken instrument always exists. Instruments should be checked carefully before they are inserted, and if there is any question of work hardening or potential fractures, they should be changed for a newer version. If an instrument does break, the surgeon should be prepared to either retrieve it through the arthroscope or perform an open procedure at that time. Fortunately, broken instruments in the TMJ rarely occur, and there are virtually no reported instrument breaks in the literature.

The number 1 complication in terms of severity is damage to the ear by an inadvertent misplacement of the arthroscope. Routinely, the arthroscope is placed through a portal at approximately 10 mm anterior of the tragus along the tragal canthal line. Surgical placement of the trocar is the key to avoiding damage to the external or middle ear structures. The trocar for the posterior portal should always be angled anterior away from the ear. With the patient in a supine position and the head turn 90° and the side of face parallel to the floor, the potential of inadvertently placing the trocar or the scope into the ear canal is minimized (**Fig. 4**). Even though the markings of 10, 20, and 30 mm are good indicators of the position and contour of the glenoid fossa, it is important for the surgeon to take his finger and palpate the rim of the glenoid fossa to find the actual indentation and make a puncture wound along that line. To avoid complications of placement of the instrument inadvertently into the ear structures, the surgeon must first ensure that the scope is in the joint after placing the trocar in the joint itself. This is done by a combination of both feel, when the scope has free movement inside the joint space, and

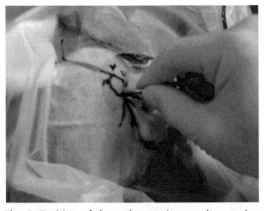

Fig. 4. Position of the arthroscopic cannula entering the posterior puncture site. Note that the scope is in the depression under the rim of the glenoid fossa, and is pointe forward.

visual sighting. If both these parameters are not met, the surgeon has to regroup and ensure that the cannula or arthroscope is inserted in the appropriate position. Once inside the joint, an inflow and outflow system can be established and further examination can occur. Several studies have been reported on related ear damage with arthroscopy and they vary from virtually none to minor or temporary issues; hearing was affected in fewer than 1% of cases.[3,4]

NERVE DAMAGE

The facial nerve could be considered the second most important structure at risk during arthroscopy of the TMJ. Understanding the anatomy of the facial nerve as it passes over the TMJ is key to all TMJ surgeries. Classical literature has described a safe zone approximately 0.8 to 1.8 mm in front of the tragus and approximately 10 mm inferior to the root of the glenoid fossa The concept of arthroscopic surgery with placement of a scope along the posterior portal at approximately 10 mm seems to be very safe and blunt dissection of a trocar has minimal chance of damaging the nerve. The second cannula, if we are using a multiport technique, is placed approximately 25 to 35 mm anterior to the tragus and usually is in front of the facial nerve. Accordingly, placement of the instruments into the TMJ has minimal potential to damage to the facial nerve. However, inadvertent bleeding, scarring, or aberrant moves can run the risk of facial nerve injury.

Cranial nerve V, particularly its third division, can also be damaged during arthroscopy. Patients report some numbness to their lip or teeth accordingly. This seems to be more the result of swelling, because the nerve itself is not in the surgical field. Fluid extravasation with into the surround tissues may cause a transient nerve injury to either cranial nerve V or VII.

Neuropraxia around the joint usually is related to temporary edema and is usually short lived. Should there be permanent nerve damage, it would potentially be to the frontal zygomatic branches and this can be treated appropriately with either the use of botulinum toxin on the contralateral side of the forehead or a gold weight into upper lid if it is permanent in nature. This author has had 2 patients with masseter nerve damage and secondary weakness. One of the patients went on to achieve full recovery, and the other had permanent dysfunction and atrophy of the muscle.

Arthroscopy also runs the risk of damaging the base of the skull by inadvertently putting the scope into a weak portion of the roof of the glenoid fossa.

Careful introduction of the trocar and appropriate siting of the joint space avoids this pitfall. Damage to medial structures is particularly uncommon if the surgeon knows the parameters of the joint itself. Most joints are within the 25 mm of width, and careful attention to the depth of the trocar can almost make this an unlikely possibility. The skin is of variable thickness, but McCain describes the medial wall at about 50 mm forms the skin.[4–6] The literature has not reported any significant damage to the middle cranial fossa, and certainly careful technique and staying with in the joint space are paramount.

Damage to joint structures is a potential complication. If the surgeon is just doing a simple lysis and lavage or injecting medications, the complication rate for the most part is negligible. The use of steroids inside the joint is somewhat controversial, and there has been some suggestion that a single unit of steroid injection may facilitate degenerative joint disease. On the other hand, steroids in the joints are commonly used in orthopedics for other associated joints and the literature does not substantiate that a 1-time use of a steroid in the joint is problematic. One can even suggest that the patient's joint is damaged to begin with and that the steroid is given for the purposes of improving joint function. For the most part, damage to related structures inside the joint such as the synovium, the disc, or the medial draping are minimal, and the joint has quite a bit of reparative effect. Most of the time, surgeons find damaged joints as a result of the disease process. The literature has no reported incidents of the surgeon doing permanent iatrogenic damage to a TMJ through manipulation or placement of an instrument into the disc or synovial tissue.

On certain occasions, the joint space is so obliterated that the joint cannot be well visualized and the surgeon is not sure the instruments are in the joint. In this instance, the discretion of the surgeon could be discontinuing the case or take instruments such as shavers or lasers and create a joint space. In doing so, the surgeon must be careful to always have the instrument in sight, and that they are comfortable with the performed procedure.

Potentially, when there is no joint space visible, the surgeon could become disoriented and easily slip into an area anterior to the joint such as sigmoid notch and hit the maxillary artery with a maxillary artery bleed (**Figs. 5** and **6**). This could be problematic. During arthroscopic surgery, on lysis and lavage, there can be on occasion bleeding that is more than just simple ooze. However, placing the patient into occlusion often stops any eventual bleeding, and it has not been reported that bleeding is a known risk of

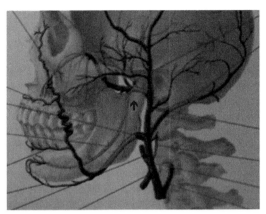

Fig. 5. Maxillary artery medial to the condyle (*arrow*). (*From* Quinn PD. Color atlas of temporomandibular joint surgery. Philadelphia: Mosby; 1998; with permission.)

arthroscopic surgery. Hemarthrosis can be a problem jeopardizing postoperative function. Bleeding from the puncture site can occur and this can easily be controlled with oversuturing the area. Misdiagnosis of a potential ankylosis could occur without the use of appropriate imaging, and an attempt to arthroscope the joint that has no true space could easily put the surgeon in a situation where the scope is misguided and some of the above complications could occur.

Patient selection is important for many reasons, some of which beyond the scope of this article. However, the heavier the patient is, the more difficult the procedure will be.

There has been a case report of an arteriovenous fistula and cardiac arrhythmias.[7–9]

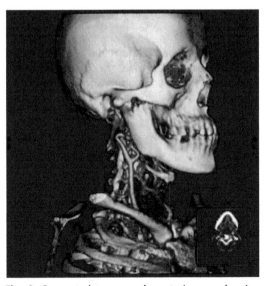

Fig. 6. Computed tomography arteriogram showing blood vessels around the ankylosis.

Overall, TMJ arthroscopic surgery can be considered a very safe and low-risk procedure. The incidence of nerve damage complications is almost negligible.[10] During a 10-year period, at one of the institutions of the author, we looked at the overall rate of infections in arthroscopic surgery, and it was approximately 1%. When further delineating the use, this was an operative arthroscopy where sutures were placed in a multiport technique. During this procedure, the few patients who have had infections were examined very carefully, and of the 6 patients who have had postoperative infections, 1 or 2 were stitch abscesses and the others were all immunodeficient patients. This is in line with the known incidence of infections in orthopedic literature, which is about 1%.[11–13] Obviously, careful selection of patients is paramount in any surgical procedure and the potential of infections in immunocompromised patients is always there.

Postoperative pain can occur in many patients and is beyond the scope of this discussion as a known complication. However, selection when dealing with chronic pain patients is important and should be taken into consideration before the decision to operate is made.

Distention of the joint can occur during an arthroscopic procedure. This is a result of constantly having more fluid flushed into the joint and not having an appropriate outflow. Surgeons who rely on a pump are more prone to having this problem. In addition, the surgeon who has an assistant pumping water through the inflow and outflow system and is not watching the appropriate outflow can also have this problem. Distension of the surrounding tissues can collapse the joint space and limit the ability to complete the operation. The swelling can be so severe that it can cause a shift medial to the joint and create a potential airway occlusion. Although this complication has been reported, it is not commonly seen and it is not among the known risks, other than that the surgeon should avoid distending the joint. Once the surrounding joint space is distended, the arthroscopic surgery is over and the surgeon has to stop the procedure with no benefit to the patient.[14,15]

TEMPOROMANDIBULAR JOINT ARTHROPLASTY

TMJ arthroplasties encompass surgical incisions into the TMJ through an external approach. The most common incision is the preauricular, although others have been discussed. Regardless of the diagnosis, the surgical procedure has a group of common potential complications, including damage to adjacent structures including nerves, vessels, the ear, parotid gland, base of the skull, and middle cranial fossa. In addition, infections and secondary issues such as ankylosis, functional disorders, and increase postoperative pain should be considered. Common surgical treatments for internal derangements, degenerative joint disease, tumors ankylosis, or part of total joint placement for the most part entail the same complication issues.

Nerve Injuries

Nerve injuries can occur to cranial nerves V and VII. The surgical approach stays within the safe zone and has been described elsewhere. Damage to the facial nerve is a known risk in this procedure and intuitively increases in the patient who has undergone previous operations. Damage can either be permanent or temporary, and can be the result of stretching to gain access to the joint or severing in the dissection. Nerve stimulators are helpful to avoid this problem.

Treatment of nerve injuries

In this instance, it is the same as from arthroscopy, and if weakness in the frontal branches is observed, cosmetic treatment of the injury can be done with either a forehead lift, or botulinum toxin to the adjacent side to give symmetry. An inability to close the eyelid is difficult to fix anatomically, but the use of a gold weight in the upper lid seems to resolve the problem.

Damage to the fifth mandibular division of cranial nerve V is not likely. However, patients do report having some numbness to that area, although it seems to be transient. It seems that it is either from swelling or retraction that has gone beyond that level of the capsule and causing some pressure on the mandibular nerve as it travels parallel to the joint and enters the inferior alveolar canal.[2,16]

Infections

Infections from arthroplasty of the joint are in the 1% to 2% range, as indicated by these authors and as compared with the orthopedic literature. Infections can be of 3 distinct routes in theory: Contamination during the operative procedure owing to some type of flora from the adjacent structures, for example, the external ear, or scalp; immunodeficient patients; and opportunistic infections. Patients with a localized infection may contaminate the wound and this may occur before surgery or postoperatively. For example, the patient in **Fig. 7** developed a secondary infection to an allergic reaction to tape and had a Staphylococcus infection surrounding the joint. Owing to the increased concentration of the

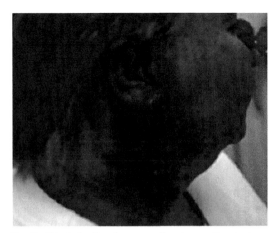

Fig. 7. Skin infection from an allergic reaction to tape in a total joint patient that spread to the joint itself.

bacterial flora in and around the joint, the joint became secondarily infected. These infections are known as acute infections and can often be treated with appropriate antibiotics and lavaging of the joint. Because there are no foreign bodies, in an arthroplasty per se, with the exception of a Mitek bone anchor or a suture, joints can often be treated with aggressive postoperative care. There have been reported instances where the patients themselves would seed the infection for some unforeseen psychological gain. These cases are difficult to treat and can have unlikely flora on culture. Drug addicts also have a propensity to infections in a joint and they often grow a serration-type infection. Indications of an occult joint infection start out with signs of pain, swelling, and inflammation around the joint. It may take several weeks before the joint opens up and starts to ooze. Certainly, arthroplasty patients who have an abnormal postoperative presentation with signs of swelling, lymphadenopathy, and edema should be considered for infection. This may include testing beyond the clinical examination, including bone scans and blood chemistry looking at C-reactive protein and sedimentation rates.

Surgical infections in general in joints can be divided into acute, subacute, and chronic infections. Acute infections lend themselves to aggressive wound care and antibiotics. Subacute infections are defined as one that occurs within the first year. Chronic infections often develop later and can be persistent. Chronic infections can come from a biofilm if an alloplastic material is used, although with no foreign body in the joint, a biofilm is an unlikely culprit. In either case, if there has been an autogenous grafting in the joint, then one must consider that the material that has been grafted is contaminated and may need to be removed. Chronic infections of the joint could lead to chronic osteomyelitis in the joint or spread the infection beyond the joint and into the adjacent structures, such as osteomyelitis of the base of skull and the glenoid fossa. Infection in the joint also may present through a fistula into the external auditory canal; the primary source may be the canal itself or the joint. Without foreign body, this circumstance is difficult to determine. With the foreign body, one would assume that the joint was the source of infection.

The use of Mitek bone anchors is the most common foreign body placed in the joint. There has been nothing in the literature to suggest that Mitek bone anchors have an higher incidence of infection fat grafting in the joint; other autogenous grafts bring along with them the potential site of contamination on the operating table or from the contamination of the donor site. When periumbilical fat is used, it should be carefully managed because it is proximal to the umbilicus, which is considered part of the dirty field and should be copiously given a sterile preparation.[2,12,13]

Damage to Adjacent Structures

Damage to adjacent structures of the joint can occur either through direct trauma during the time of surgery or secondary as a result of a bleed or infection. The ear is probably the most troublesome structure that could have severe effects if there is a hearing impairment that is related to the joint. Care should be taken so that the surgeon stays in front of the auditory canal and there is no bleeding or heavy instrumentation in that area that would potentially damage the middle ear or the ossicles per se.

The base of the skull again can be damaged if surgery extends too far medially. On either side of the joint, there is a capsule. Scar tissue and bony ankylosis can also penetrate the medial aspect and damage can occur there. Medial to the joint below the level of the condyle lies the maxillary artery, and this could be a significant vital structure that is discussed elsewhere.

Damage to Vessels

Bleeding and nerve damage often run hand in hand. In the attempt to stop bleeding with a cautery, the burn can propagate to a nearby nerve. Most bleeding in TMJ surgery occurs during the dissection and can be controlled with surgical technique. Damage to the maxillary artery is more ominous and is discussed under total joint replacements.

Frey Syndrome

Frey syndrome or gustatory sweating is a known complication of both parotid gland surgery and TMJ surgery. It is a mix up of the sympathetic and parasympathetic nerves around the face. Treatment includes the use of botulinum toxin, and or placement of a graft material under the skin in the effected area.

Diskectomy

Removal of the disk with or without a graft has become a standard procedure in TMJ surgery; the major complication is disease progression. This author presented a paper at an American Association of Oral and Maxillofacial Surgeons meeting on the outcome of diskectomy patients with or without fat grafts. Of note was the fact that at least 50% of patients went on to potentially require a total joint replacement.

Patients Undergoing Multiple Operations

One concern over arthroplasty patients is the need for serial operative procedures. This may be owing to disease progression or ectopic bone formation. Whether this scenario is a complication is debatable. The surgeon must consider in the surgical algorithm at least a stopgap measure to avoid multiple procedures and having their patients become chronically ill pain patients.

Alloplastic Implant

Historically, there have been several types of disk implants or substitutes, including Teflon/proplast implants and silicone sheeting. The problem with these materials is that they tend to break apart and cause foreign body cell reactions. Metal fossa implants were used for a time and avoided this problem, but have not been widely accepted and may not be available currently. All insertable materials run the risk of infections, instability, and host response problems.[17,18]

TMJ surgery is a technique-sensitive procedure. Attention to detail, preoperative planning, a patient expectations should all be part of the decision-making process. Intraoperative problems are real and can occur, even in the best of hands. Thinking ahead and surgical preparation become key factors.

TOTAL JOINT REPLACEMENTS

Of the 3 surgical procedures discussed herein, total joint replacements are probably the most complex and demanding. Whether the surgeon is using a custom-made or stock joint, the surgical procedures are for the most part the same and the complications are nearly identical. It is not the intent of this paper to compare different prostheses. Because total joint replacements add the element of a foreign body into the equation, surgical sterility becomes paramount. Replacement of a total joint requires 2 surgical incisions. The first incision is identical to the arthroplasty incision and incorporates a preauricular incision in front of the ear. The second incision has some variation, but is either a retromandibular or submandibular incision; either one has its proximity to the facial nerve and related vasculature, facial artery, and vein. The incisions for this procedure are well-described in these clinics as well as other surgical approaches to the facial skeleton. It is probably important that both incisions are made with careful attention to cranial nerve VII and that either a nerve stimulator or a nerve locator be used.

It is important that surgeons spend a reasonable amount of time in planning the surgical procedure when it comes to total joint replacements. Usually, detailed computed axial tomography scans are obtained and a surgical plan is developed well before the time in the operating room. Particularly in the case of ankylosis patients, there are many procedures that could be done preoperatively to delineate the extent of the ankylosis and the vascularity surrounding the ankylosis. The use of CT, especially in conjunction with arteriograms, can clearly define the surgical anatomy as well as the abnormal surgical structures.

Nerve Damage

As described in the discussion on an arthroplasty, cranial nerve VII lies directly over the surgical field of entry. In this instance, not only does the preauricular incision involve part of the facial nerve, but so does the retromandibular or submandibular approach. Damage to any one of these branches can result in either a true severing of the nerve or purely a stretching of the nerve. In a case of nerve stretching, nerve function generally returns, whereas if there is inadvertent severing of the nerve, it is unlikely that function will return to normal. Unlike a TMJ arthroplasty, it is possible to damage isolated branches of the facial nerve in the retromandibular or submandibular incision while leaving the main trunk alone. The preauricular incision alternatively can have either the frontal or zygomatic branch damage and/or potentially damage in severe cases the entire trunk of the facial nerve, including all 5 branches involved. It is unlikely for complete facial nerve paralysis to occur, but in theory it is possible. Again, careful surgical technique and either a nerve stimulator or a nerve locator will help to avoid this problem.

It is important to instruct the anesthesiologist not use muscle relaxants if possible so that this testing can be done.[16]

Potentially, a nerve can be damaged through the use of electrocautery. In this instance, in an attempt to stop bleeding, a nerve injury can occur where the radiation of the electrical charge spreads in a circular fashion around the point. The use of a Colorado tip or bipolar cautery minimizes this problem. In addition, when bleeding occurs, especially at the root of the incision of the preauricular approach, it may be safer to try to correct the problem with the use of local anesthetic and oversew the area with an absorbable suture in lieu of trying to cauterize the minor bleed that could potentially spread to a nerve injury.

In general, complications related to TMJ or total joint replacements can be classified as immediate intraoperative complications or postoperative complications. Bleeding is be an intraoperative complication, as is nerve damage. Often, the attempt to stop a continuous bleed or ooze with the use of a cautery leads to nerve injury.

Damage to cranial nerve V is possible in both the placement of the joint with the screws leading into the inferior alveolar canal, or exceeding the medial aspect of the joint and entering into the base of the skull. Cranial nerve V can be damaged, because its foramen lies medial to the medial draping of the glenoid fossa. In this instance, the damage may be permanent or transient. In this author's series of approximately 250 joint replacements, inferior alveolar nerve damage has been minimal, and it if occurs, it is most likely the result of the an unavoidable screw placed into the nerve canal as a result of abnormal or compromised mandibular anatomy. In the case of big counterclockwise rotations were the mandible is repositioned anteriorly, traction to the inferior alveolar nerve occur, causing temporary or potentially permanent damage to the nerve.

Custom and stock joints are designed so that the screw fixation should lie posterior to the inferior alveolar canal and that minimal damage would occur as a result of fixation of the condylar component.

Bleeding Issues

Intraoperative bleeding in total joint replacements can occur from some of the major vessels located in the surgical field, including the maxillary artery, temporal artery, masseteric artery, and facial artery. In addition, the associated veins can also be injured. Furthermore, because there is muscle stripping and cutting, especially of the masseter and both pterygoid muscles, there can be a significant amount of oozing of that musculature. Inadvertent damage to the masseteric artery can occur when the area underlying the sigmoid notch is not protected in an attempt to remove sufficient bone to place the joint, during ankylosis, or in attempts to remove the coronoid process. Knowledge of the vascular anatomy and adherence to good surgical technique of isolating the soft tissue away from the bone can minimize intraoperative bleeding. Several surgeons favor the use of a Piezo saw when they get close to the adjacent soft tissue next to bone and find this as another form of safety to minimize bleeding.

The most clinically important vessel that could be damaged in TMJ surgery is the maxillary artery, which runs behind the neck of the condyle and at the level just above the sigmoid notch (see **Fig. 5**). In most instances, this area can be protected with the use of instrumentation that is posterior and medial to the bony cuts of the condyle. Should the maxillary artery bleed, it poses a significant intraoperative threat because of the lack of accessibility to tie it off, especially in ankylosis. There are discussions in the literature that suggest that tying off the branch of the maxillary artery as it comes off the external carotid will not suffice because there will be retro-flow and the bleed will continue. However, surgeons who have been in this situation have reported that either tying off the visible artery or tying off the branch can help in stopping the bleeding. Careful preoperative planning in cases of ankylosis can allow the surgeon to embolize the artery 1 or 2 days before surgery. An alternative to that procedure can be exposure of the branches of the external carotid during the surgery and immediate embolization, if a bleed occurs, can be undertaken (**Figs. 8** and **9**).

Adjunctive therapies to stop bleeding should always be available such as thrombin-soaked Surgicel or the use of some of the fibrin products. Often packing in the area and allowing a sufficient amount of time stops most oozing or minor joint bleeds.

Damage to Adjacent Structures

Intraoperative damage to adjacent structures is always a concern as an intraoperative complication. Most relevant structures related to joint replacement TMJ surgery are the 3 areas surrounding the condylar component, including the external and internal structures of the ear, the anatomic areas medial to the joint (specifically the base of the skull), and damage to the superior aspect of the glenoid fossa into the intracranial space. All these potential areas of damage require

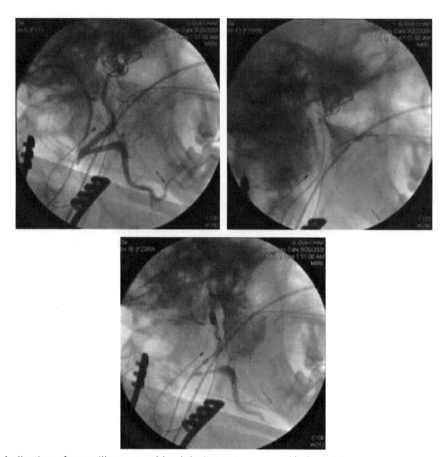

Fig. 8. Embolization of a maxillary artery bleed during temporomandibular joint surgery.

careful surgical dissection to minimize the potential hazard. Careful presurgical workup with computed axial tomography can identify areas that would be of concern in situations such as tumors or ankylosis. Again, the use of image-guided surgery and careful dissection can help to

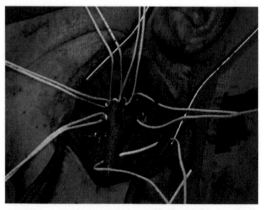

Fig. 9. Branches of the external carotid artery and the maxillary artery exposed in case of a maxillary artery bleed.

minimize this problem. The literature does not report any significant complications to the base of the skull, although in an ankylosis case there is potential to go beyond the medial envelope of the joint. Certainly, in an attempt to remove sufficient tissue for placement of prosthesis, the surgeon can enter the base of the skull and damage some of the structures located in that area, because their foramens are just medial (see **Fig. 2**).

Damage to the ear can happen if the surgeon is misguided or the ankylosis extends into the ear canal. In addition, aggressive use of instrumentation such as a chisel and a hammer can cause trauma to the related areas. The surgeon should have some type of anatomic guide when approaching ankylosis that extends adjacent to the ear canal. Damage to the ear canal itself can occur during the surgery, but again this is a rarely described event.

Perforation of the roof of the glenoid fossa will lead into the intracranial exposure the parietal lobe of the brain. In this event, if the dura is intact, it is probably not going to be a considerable problem. Should there be a cerebrospinal fluid leak or perforation that seems sufficiently large, it needs to be addressed with both a neurosurgical consultation and the potential for sealing off the space. A bone graft, dural patch, or use of the prosthesis itself may suffice as a safeguard. Potentially, a bone graft can be placed and the surgery can be aborted and returned at a later date. One concern is that a foreign body, such as prosthesis, becomes infected; it could lead to an intracranial infection. However, it is not uncommon to use a foreign body to seal the bony structure of the cranial cavity during routine neurosurgical procedures, and the TMJ could be considered as any other intracranial approach. A neurosurgical consultation would be required. The literature does not discuss this problem, but this author has seen a few clinical cases and presentations by others on this topic. This complication is always a concern in the event that the roof of the glenoid fossa is violated.

Malposition of the Prosthesis

Malpositioning of the prosthesis can occur in several different clinical manifestations. The dental occlusion must be set appropriately before the condylar and fossa components are set. It is advisable to double check this surgical step in the operating room, because a mistake will lead to redoing the surgery. Many times, attempts are made to reposition the mandible during surgery, and there is a significant amount of pulling and an inability to release some of the scarring from previous surgical endeavors. Passive stable occlusion should be obtained. The surgeon should always have some system of checking the occlusion once the patient is taken out of intermaxillary fixation during the surgical procedure before all the screws are placed. A second possibility is that the condyle is poorly situated, and even though the occlusion is stable as soon as the intermaxillary fixation is released, the condyles returns back to an unfavorable spot. Again, surgical technique requires that the condyle be seated appropriately during fixation of the components. The

fossa itself has to be positioned appropriately, and if it is not secured into good bone stock, the potential for the fossa to slip postoperatively can occur (**Fig. 10**).

Additionally, postoperative dislocations can occur. These can occur inadvertently during the time of surgery, upon extubation, or in the immediate postoperative period when the patient may be suffering from severe nausea or vomiting and puts abnormal stretch on the joint. It can occur in the postoperative period during the healing phase as well, but is not a common event any time after the first few weeks postoperative. The most common time for dislocations to occur is when both the medial and lateral pterygoid muscles are stripped so that there are no constraining muscles (**Fig. 11**). It is helpful for the surgeon to check the condyle at the time of fixation of the components, after fixation, and before closing the incisions, confirming that the condyles are visible and in the most posterosuperior position. Last but not least, the surgeon should check the mobility of the condyle, and if it easily dislocates while they are visualizing the joint, then the patient should be considered a candidate for some type of fixation with interarch wiring or elastics.

Dislocation of the condyle is easily detectable owing to malocclusion and can be addressed either with an attempt at repositioning the condyle with sedation and then placement in a short period of intermaxillary fixation or, in the worst case scenario, the incision sites have to be opened and the condyle has to be manipulated into its proper position.

INFECTIONS OF THE TEMPOROMANDIBULAR JOINT

The most ominous of all problems of a total joint replacement are postoperative infections. Infections can be divided into acute, subacute, or chronic. In the acute phase, it is conceivable to treat the patient with antibiotics and/or open the joint, wash it out, and reseal it. In the chronic phase, it is almost imperative that the components

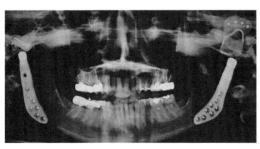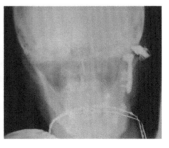

Fig. 10. Displaced fossa on the left joint.

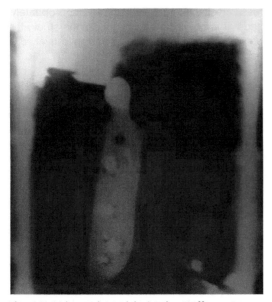

Fig. 11. Dislocated condyle in the Hoffman Pappas joint.

be removed, especially the fossa. The probability that there is a biofilm is likely. The subacute phase is somewhat less clear, and can have a mixed response. This author has treated several total joint infections by removing the fossa in the acute phase and then aggressively trying to sterilize the condylar component intraoperatively. The fact that it is smooth and can be washed especially with a sterilizing agent such as Betadine has seemingly worked in many patients. However, clinical examination and appropriate imaging should be able to determine if the infection has spread along the ramus area. CT to see a collection of purulent material or a bone scan to see if anything lights up other than in the joint space alone helps to make the diagnosis. If in doubt, the surgeon needs to remove both components and place some type of temporary spacer in the joint. This author has treated infections with methyl methacrylate mixed with tobramycin in removal of both joint components and in many instances just the fossa alone. There is an higher incidence of infections after secondary surgeries on total joints and placement of a new fat graft. Therefore, this author has abandoned the placement of fat grafts as a secondary procedure for this purpose. As a primary procedure, there has not been any indication that there is any further incidence of infection.[19–22]

In a study done at Staten Island University Hospital and presented in an abstract at the American Association of Oral and Maxillofacial Surgeons meeting, our infection rate was approximately

2% to 3%, which is even lower than the published percentage unit in the orthopedic literature, which is anywhere from 3% to 5%. The questions around infections often required the decision to remove either part or the entire prosthesis. In either case, the use of a 6-week course of intravenous antibiotics and an infectious disease consultation are important. The literature on biofilms in joint replacements has been established and it seems to be the significant cause of infection[23]; other causes are immunosuppressed patients and intravenous drug usage. The use of prophylactic antibiotics for dental procedures is debatable, but owing to the proximity of the condyle to any type of dental infection, it would be prudent to take the same precautions that orthopedics does in having no obvious dental or skin infections in the area before placement and to treat them aggressively if an infection occurs.

Replacement of the total join or fossa component can be performed when the patent is deemed to be infection free. Following the sedimentation rate, white blood cell count, and the C-reactive protein levels are all helpful indicators.

This author has had 2 patients with a fistula between the external auditory canal and the joint space with secondary infections. Both required removal of the fossa, and one the entire joint. The etiology is unclear, but both have been treated with revisions.

LOOSENING OF PROSTHESIS

The joints are generally very secure. Most total joint systems involve at least 6 to 8 screws. There has been some debate in the biomedical engineering as to the total number of screws needed to secure the condylar component to the ramus. It seems that fewer than 5 screws would suffice, and some form of microlocking helps to avoid micromovement, which can lead to screw failure. An attempt to have the ramus component stay as close as possible to the existing bone is seemingly important. In the use of stock joint, we would require re-contouring of the bone to get a flat surface against a flat surface. Custom joints can avoid this problem, but at the same time, if they do not get an exact fit, there can be an irregular surface against an irregular surface. In any respect, it seems that there have been no indications in the literature that a small gap in the interface is of any significance as long as the joint has what is termed as 3-point stabilization and has no wobbling per se. The fossa runs the risk of being displaced postoperatively when screws can loosen and bone stock is not strong enough to hold the joint in place. Displacement of the fossa runs hand in hand with screw loosening and it is difficult to determine the cause. The cause for the displacements or screw loosening should be identified. Infections, trauma, or misplacement all should be considered. Screws can loosen especially when the bone is thin and there is some micromovement associated. The concept again is that a custom joint would have a better fit and a non-custom joint would have at least 3-point stabilization in trying to maintain a flat surface against the flat surface. In any respect, the patient should be followed on routinely with appropriate imaging. Because the polyethylene is often not visible on imaging, surgeons who have less experience with total joint replacements can be fooled into thinking that there is an abnormal position owing to a shadow or space between the condylar component and the metal fossa.

In the use of the Biomet joint with no metal-backed fossa, screw fixation is directly into the polyethylene. A theoretic problem associated with polyethylene would be that there is micro-movement and migration of particles along the screw fixation of the polyethylene head without metal backing. This has been shown to occur in the hip literature with propagation of a screw in the polyethylene. This has not been a known problem with the Biomet joint, and it seems that the data available now, which are starting to become long term, show that these joints are not more prone to a dislodgement in any other joint than a metal-backed fossa.

In the same vein of discussion, the use of a highly polished metal condyle against a polyethylene fossa has a potential problem of wear debris, although this has not been shown to occur.

In addition to displacement of a prosthetic joint, the possibility of a component fracture exists. Chromium cobalt, when used as a condylar stem, can fatigue and fracture. Fractured components are rare and the current group of joints approved by the US Food and Drug Administration

have only isolated cases that some manufacturers have shared (**Fig. 12**).

Allergy to Materials

Reaction to foreign bodies, especially nickel or titanium, can occur. Patients who are known to be allergic to metals can be tested for metal allergy both by an allergist and also by getting some of the metal that these joints are made of from the company to give them a skin test. The area of metal allergy seems to be controversial. However, a patient with a known history of sensitivity to metals may not be a candidate for a joint replacement.

Recurrent Bone Formation

Recurrent ankylosis is always a concern when the patients have had previous ankylosis whether it is fibrous, fibro-osseous, or bony ankylosis. The general surgical rule is to try and create as large gap as possible so that if bone does form, it will have trouble connecting from the mandible to the base of the skull. The use of fat grafts has seemingly minimized this event, as well as the use of very wide resections. There have been no controlled studies suggesting that fat grafts are mandatory, but several leading surgeons in this field routinely use fat grafts; however, others do not. It does seem prudent that, if one is concerned with an ankylosis, patients have wide resection of bone to minimize the ability of the bone to reapproximate itself. Additionally, reducing the bone to levels of clean periosteum may very well help and avoid a fibro-osseous union.

The use of postoperative low-dose radiation and medications such as indomethacin and Didrinal can help with this problem.

In addition to considerations that minimize recurrent ankylosing, the ability to get good range of motion is important. In this instance, removal of the coronoid process may be helpful in improving

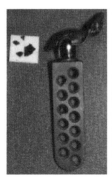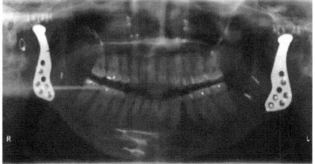

Fig. 12. Fracture of the condyle (*right*) and the fossa on (*left*).

postoperative range of motion. The use of post-operative physical therapy, especially with the patient continuing with it themselves over the long run, would be seemingly helpful.

Should ankylosis recur, it sometimes can be approached with a rearthroplasty, but in many instances the joint has to be removed because the bone has grown medial to the joint and could not be visualized. Many times the patient will form bone completely around the joint itself encapsulating the entire condyle in casing of bone.

Postoperative Pain

Postoperative pain can be considered a potential complication. It is not uncommon for a patient who has had bilateral joints to complain that 1 side feels perfectly well and the other side is painful. It is unclear exactly what the mechanism of pain is. Intuitively, one would think that the more surgical procedures the patient has had leading up to surgery, the higher index of suspicion of postoperative chronic pain may exist. However, the discussion of pain related to TMJ surgery is beyond the scope of this discussion. It would be fair to say that pain, as a postoperative problem, is a real factor and should be addressed with the patient both preoperatively as well as treated postoperatively with appropriate pain management.

One source of postoperative pain, especially at the 1-year mark, may be scarring inside the joint with tissue growing in the interface of the condyle and the fossa. If this is the case, it is difficult to tell clinically that this is occurring, other than that the patient was doing fine and then begins to have pain on motion of the joint. This can be remedied relatively easily, with a simple arthroplasty and removal of scar tissue. It is unclear as to why any tissue that slowly evolves as the interface between the movable parts would be a problem; however, it is easy to understand that a tissue that has been squeezed on a persistent basis could become painful.

Range of Motion

Poor range of motion after surgery can be another postoperative problem. Most patients have lost their pterygoid muscular function and therefore cannot translate or go side to side, although rarely a patient can. However, rotation movement should allow the patient to open at least 30 mm, and in many cases reportedly upwards of 40 mm. Aggressive physical therapy after surgery can be helpful. Some surgeons prefer to send their patients for several months to physical therapist, whereas others feel that the use of home physical therapy with a device such as a TheraBite may

allow the patient to do this on a more regular basis. Two of the main objectives related to surgery in total joint replacement include reduction of pain and improvement of movement. It is inherent to provide some type of therapy to improve the range of motion that has been obtained from the surgical procedure. It seems that patients tend to form a fibrous scarring around the joint and this needs to be reduced with postoperative physical therapy. From time to time, the patient may have joint reoperated on to reduce some of the scarring.

There are other postoperative complications related to TMJ surgery, but are general surgical problems associated with any type of facial surgery. Patients who have an allergy to the postoperative dressing can often develop a skin reaction and in case of a total joint replacement, owing to the high concentration of bacteria adjacent to the joint, can develop a joint infection. Wound care varies from surgeon to surgeon from some biological dressings. Overall, it does not seem that the surgical dressing plays a significant role in postoperative infection. Unfavorable scarring in some of the areas would be more related to surgical technique than the procedure itself. In general, the surgical scars created by the TMJ surgeon are usually minimal and are not any more specific than any other surgical procedure of the face.

In summary, for complications related to TMJ infections, it is clear that, in going from arthroscopy to arthroplasty to total joint replacements, the infections and complications become more involved and more troublesome. Overall, surgeons can separate arthroscopy and arthroplasty from total joint replacements with regard to complications. The latter group has to be monitored for issues related to the prosthesis itself on long-term basis.

Overall, the prostheses used today, which are highly polished metal (either titanium and chrome-cobalt or combinations of the 2 against a polyethylene surface), seem to be the standard. There have been joints using metal-on-metal and there have been some discussion of the materials' interface. However, there seem to be no hard data suggesting that a metal-on-metal joint in the TMJ would be a problem. On the other hand, the orthopedic industry has subsequently stopped using metal-on-metal joints. A discussion on choice of materials is beyond the scope of this article of complications TMJ surgical complications. However, there are concerns along the lines of prosthetic joints in terms of fatiguing of the joint with subsequent fractures of the prosthesis. Originally in the pure chromium-cobalt joints made by Christensen, Inc, there was fracturing of the condylar component. Fracturing of the condylar component now in any of the joint seems to be a rare event. Certainly, it is not advisable for any surgeon to bend or try to reconfigure these joints because this maneuver may cause fatigue in the metal and make it subject to a fracture. However, breaking of the prosthesis at this junction does not seem to be a reported problem. Furthermore, wearing out of the polyethylene has not been reported, and does not seem to be problematic. In summary, with regard to problems associated with wear debris, joint fracture or choice of the metals, the 2 or 3 joints that are made today seem to be safe. With regard to the longevity of these joints, they have all been established for greater than 10 years. However, there are no indications that they should not last a lifetime of a patient, although the data are yet to be collected. Retrieval of a joint for any reason can sometimes be a problem if the screws are covered in bone, stripped, or metals have integrated with the bone. This type of surgery can be very demanding.

Total joint replacements in a growing individual have relative contraindications, although there are cases where they may be indicated if no other alternatives exist. Again, this is not necessarily a complication, but potentially a problem if joint replacement is needed in a growing patient and then needs to be replaced again at a later date.

Overall, the complications of TMJ surgery are known and, even in the best surgical hands, complications can develop. There are no indications to suggest that a complication such as bleeding, infection, or failure of the prosthesis is necessarily the fault of the surgeon or the patient. In many patients, these are complex surgical procedures and placed in a very difficult anatomic location. For the most part, complications are rare and TMJ surgery can be done in a very successful manner. The advent of arthroscopic surgery has minimized untoward events and has been a major help to many surgical patients. Furthermore, simplifying many of the arthroplasty procedures can be of benefit to patients and be performed in predictable and successful fashion with minimal complication rate. With regard to total joint replacements, as more time passes and despite their potential complications, they have clearly become a predictable procedure that has minimal complications and a well-trained surgeon can perform in a very satisfying manner for both patient and doctor. Clearly, as generations of surgeons place prosthetic joints, the confidence level will build and they will hopefully find their place in treating the patients in a similar fashion for surgical placement of hips and knees.

REFERENCES

1. Vallerand WP, Dolwick MF. Complications of TMJ surgery. Oral Maxillofac Surg Clin North Am 1990; 3:481.
2. Kieth DA. Complications of temporomandibular joint surgery. Oral Maxillofac Surg Clin North Am 2003; 15:187.
3. Van Sickels JE, Nishioka GJ, Hegewald MD, et al. Middle ear injury resulting from temporomandibular joint arthroscopy. J Oral Maxillofac Surg 1987;45:962.
4. Westesson PL, Erickson L, Liedberg L. The risk of damage to facial nerve, superficial temporal vessels, discs, and articular surfaces during arthroscopic examination of the temporomandibular joint. Oral Surg Oral Med Oral Pathol 1986;62:124.
5. McCain JP. Complication of TMJ arthroscopy. J Oral Maxillofac Surg 1998;46:256.
6. Sugisaki M, Ikai A, Tanabe H. Dangerous angles and depth for cranial fossa injury during arthroscopy of the temporomandibular joint. J Oral Maxillofac Surg 1995;53:803.
7. Sacho RH, Kryshtalskyj B, Krings T. Arteriovenous fistula of the middle meningeal artery- A rare complication after arthroscopic temporomandibular joint surgery readily amenable to endovascular treatment. J Oral Maxillofac Surg 2014;72:1258.
8. Martín-Granizo R, Caniego JL, de Pedro M, et al. Arteriovenous fistula after temporomandibular joint arthroscopy successfully treated with embolization. Int J Oral Maxillofac Surg 2004;33:301–3.
9. Roberts RS, Best JA, Shapiro RD. Trigeminocardiac reflex during temporomandibular joint arthroscopy: report of a case. J Oral Maxillofac Surg 1999;57:854.
10. González-García R, Rodríguez-Campo FJ, Escorial-Hernández V, et al. Complications of temporomandibular joint arthroscopy: a retrospective analytic study of 670 arthroscopic procedures. J Oral Maxillofac Surg 2006;64:11.
11. Chossegros C, Cheynet F, Conrath J. Infratemporal space infection after temporomandibular arthroscopy: an unusual complication. J Oral Maxillofac Surg 1995;53:949.
12. Norden C, Gillespie WJ, Nade S. Infections in bones and joints. Boston: Blackwell Scientific Publications; 1994. p. 291–319.
13. Krueger K, Hoffman D, Stracher M, et al. Abstract presentation: "Infection of the temporomandibular joint after surgery", American Association of Oral and Maxillofacial Surgeons 1996 Annual Meeting. The Fountainbleau, Miami, Florida, September 20, 1996.
14. Tsuyama M, Kondoh T, Seto K, et al. Complications of temporomandibular joint arthroscopy: a retrospective analysis of 301 lysis and lavage procedures performed using the triangulation technique. J Oral Maxillofac Surg 2000;58:500.

15. Carter JB, Testa L. Complications of TMJ arthroscopy: a review of 2225 cases. Review of the 1988 Annual Scientific Sessions Abstract. J Oral Maxillofac Surg 1988;46:M14.

16. Gokkulakrishnan S, Singh S, Sharma A, et al. Facial nerve injury following surgery for temporomandibular joint ankylosis: a prospective clinical study. Indian J Dent Res 2013;24:521.

17. US Food and Drug Administration. Serious problems with proplast coated TMJ Implant. Rockville (MD): Department of Health and Human Services; 1990.

18. Kearans GJ, Perrott DH, Kaban LB. A protocol for the management of failed alloplastic temporomandibular joint disc implants. J Oral Maxillofac Surg 1995;53:1240–7.

19. Sidebottom AJ, Speculand B, Hensher R. Foreign body response around total prosthetic metal-on-metal replacements of the temporomandibular joint in the UK. Br J Oral Maxillofac Surg 2008; 46:288–92.

20. Mercuri LG, Psutka D. Perioperative, postoperative, and prophylactic use of antibiotics in alloplastic total joint temporomandibular joint replacement surgery: a survey and preliminary guidelines. J Oral Maxillofac Surg 2011;69:2106.

21. Sidebottom AJ, Gruber E. One-year prospective outcome analysis and complicationsfollowing total replacement of the temporomandibular joint with the TMJ Concepts system. Br J Oral Maxillofac Surg 2013;51:620–4.

22. Lidgren L, Knutson K, Stefánsdóttir A. Infection of prosthetic joints. Best Pract Res Clin Rheumatol 2003;17:209.

23. Mercuri L. Microbial biofilms: a potential source for alloplastic device failure. J Oral Maxillofac Surg 2006;64:1303–9.

Temporomandibular Joint Dislocation

Aaron Liddell, DMD, MD[a], Daniel E. Perez, DDS[b],*

KEYWORDS

- Temporomandibular joint • Dislocation • Luxation • Hypermobility • Eminectomy • Subluxation

KEY POINTS

- Temporomandibular joint (TMJ) dislocation is uncommon and presents most times as an acute process that can be solved with conservative therapies.
- Chronic TMJ dislocation usually requires surgical intervention.
- Medications and specific syndromes can cause recurrent dislocation.
- Subluxation refers to the condition were the joint is partially displaced without complete loss of articulating function and is usually self-reduced by the patient.
- It is extremely hard, if not impossible, to reduce a joint back to its functional anatomic position after prolonged (>6 mo) dislocation.

Dislocation of the temporomandibular joint is one of many pathophysiologic joint conditions that the oral and maxillofacial surgeon is challenged with managing. Although not particularly common, managing a dislocated joint will inevitably be the challenge of most surgeons or physicians, whether in private or academic practice. Accordingly, this article will address the pathophysiology associated with dislocation, in addition to treatment strategies (both historical and current practice techniques) aimed at managing acute, chronic, and recurrent dislocation.

DEFINITION

Temporomandibular joint (TMJ) dislocation involves a non self-limiting displacement of the condyle, outside of its functional positions within the glenoid fossa and posterior slope of the articular eminence (**Fig. 1**).[1] Although the most common condylar dislocation is anterior to the articular eminence, onto the preglenoid plane, there have also been reports of medial, lateral, posterior, and intracranial dislocations.[2–5] Anterior and anteromedial are the most common dislocations observed.

Subluxation refers to a condition in which the joint is transiently displaced without complete loss of the articulating function, and is usually self-reduced by the patient.

CLASSIFICATION

Despite a variety of classification schemes, the most common divides dislocation into 3 categories: acute, chronic, and chronic recurrent, as described by Adekeye and colleagues[6] and Rowe and Killey (**Fig. 2**).[7]

Acute dislocations may be associated with any number of etiologies, including prolonged mouth opening during a lengthy dental procedure, vomiting, yawning, and singing. There have also been reports of acute dislocation secondary to epileptic seizures, acute facial trauma, and direct laryngoscopy. Frequent dislocation may also be seen in patients with connective tissue disease, such as Ehlers-Danlos syndrome (EDS) or muscular dystonias (**Box 1**).

Acute dislocations are typically isolated events, which, when managed appropriately, usually have no long-term sequelae. Acute dislocations may

[a] Former Chief Resident, Oral & Maxillofacial Surgery, University of Texas HSC San Antonio, 7703 Floyd Curl Drive, MC 7908, San Antonio, TX 78229-3900, USA; [b] Oral & Maxillofacial Surgery, University of Texas HSC San Antonio, 7703 Floyd Curl Drive, MC 7908, San Antonio, TX 78229-3900, USA
* Corresponding author.
E-mail address: perezd5@uthscsa.edu

Oral Maxillofacial Surg Clin N Am 27 (2015) 125–136
http://dx.doi.org/10.1016/j.coms.2014.09.009
1042-3699/15/$ – see front matter © 2015 Elsevier Inc. All rights reserved.

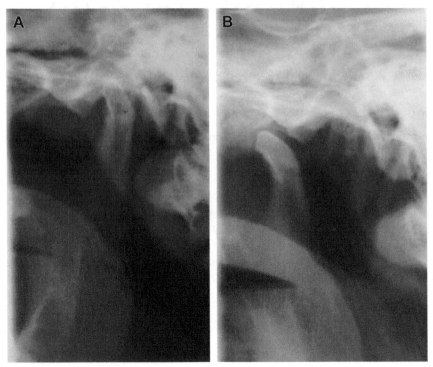

Fig. 1. (*A*) TMJ showing normal position within the glenoid fossa. (*B*) TMJ dislocated anterior to the eminence outside of the glenoid fossa. (*From* Güven O. Management of chronic recurrent temporomandibular joint dislocations: a retrospective study. J Craniomaxillofac Surg 2009;37(1):27; with permission.)

predispose an individual to progressing to the spectrum of chronic dislocations.

Chronic dislocations include acute dislocations that are not self-limiting and progress without treatment, in addition to chronic recurrent dislocations, wherein individuals experience multiple, recurrent dislocations as a result of everyday activities. Chronic recurrent dislocations can create significant interference in a patient's everyday life, and can become both physically and emotionally distressing.

ANATOMY

The glenoid fossa houses the mandibular condyle, and is essentially a depression in the temporal bone of the skull base. In many ways, this articular fossa can be considered a functionally developed structure. In children, the glenoid fossa is nearly flat, with an underdeveloped eminence. With functional loading, apposition anteriorly and resorption in the fossa base creates the contour and morphology of the adult temporomandibular articulation.[8]

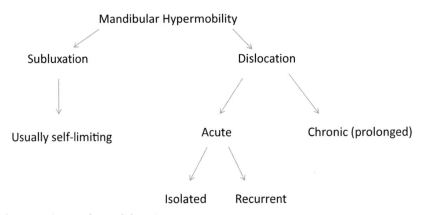

Fig. 2. Classification scheme of TMJ dislocations.

Bony apposition creates the articular eminence, wherein condylar translation occurs. The anterior slope of the articular eminence, the preglenoid plane, arises from the squamous temporal bone and gently rounds its way to the posterior slope of the articular eminence, where the bulk of mandibular load occurs. This gently rounded transition between the preglenoid plane and articular eminence serves to minimize condylar dislocation, inasmuch as at extremes of mandibular opening, the condylar head translates onto the proximal slope of the preglenoid plane.[9]

The TMJ capsule, which inserts circumferentially around the condylar neck, has skull-base condensations at the squamous temporal bone, articular eminence, preglenoid plane, and glenoid fossa.

The thickened lateral capsular condensations make up the temporomandibular ligament (TML). Although there is some controversy as to the exact ligamentous/capsular relationship, it suffices to say that the TML is a broad, fan-shaped bilayered tissue band that typically has a superficial, broad plane, and a thinner, deep plane.[10] The fibers of the TML have reproducibly defined directional orientation, including horizontal, vertical, and oblique bands, which flow from the articular tubercle of the zygoma to the lateral pole and posterior neck of the condyle. This dense capsulo-ligamentous apparatus functionally restricts extremes of mandibular movement, including tendencies for anterior, vertical, and postero-medial condylar dislocation.

PATHOGENESIS

The coordination of mandibular movement is very complex, and outside of the scope of this review. Suffice it to say, the myofascial sling can be compartmentalized into functional groups, including elevators (masseter, temporalis, medial pterygoid), retruders (temporalis, digastric), protruders (lateral pterygoid), and depressors (digastric, mylohoid, geniohyoid). Depending on origin/insertion and orientation, any of the previously mentioned muscles may contribute to functionally opposing movements, underscoring the beauty and complexity of mandibular motion. In addition, at rest and during function, the aforementioned myofascial apparatus serves to stabilize and orient the condylo-fossa articulation.

The pathogenesis of TMJ dislocation is multifactorial, attributed to capsular weakness, ligamentous laxity, atypical eminence size (morphology or projection), myospasm, trauma, or aberrancy in masticatory movements. Recurrent dislocation may contribute to ligamentous laxity and capsular weakness, and internal derangement, thus predisposing to arthritic joint degeneration and chronic recurrent dislocation.

It is generally accepted that initial dislocation is caused by lack of muscular coordination during initiation of jaw closure.[11] This may include a lack of relaxation of the protractors with concomitant firing of the elevators, causing myospastic contraction. This spasm causes feedback loops that perpetuate spastic contraction, thus prohibiting self-reduction/relocation, as the condylar head is intruded into the soft tissues of the infratemporal fossa. If one has a predilection for joint laxity (EDS or chronic recurrent joint dislocations) or muscle spasms (Duchenne Muscular Dystrophy [DMD], psychotropic dystonia, or epilepsy), it is not uncommon for chronic dislocation to be a persistent problem.

ACUTE DISLOCATIONS

When looking at various treatment modalities, one must consider the nature of the dislocation. Acute dislocations are typically addressed in a nonsurgical fashion. Conventional nonoperative methods have been described by multiple authors.[7,12,13] The typical maneuver is described as bimanual intraoral traction, placing the thumbs at the retromolar pad/external oblique ridge and pressing inferiorly and then posteriorly, manipulating the condylar head over the preglenoid plane, seating it back in the articular fossa. This maneuver is typically done asking the patient to open the mouth so that the elevators of the mandible are relaxed.

In some instances, this may be accomplished utilizing local anesthesia for auriculotemporal nerve blocks (**Fig. 3**). Litler has advocated for intra-articular anesthetic distribution into the empty glenoid fossa, aimed at minimizing myospasm prior to digital manipulation. In some cases, the acute myospasm is significant enough that general anesthetics, occasionally including intravenous paralytics, are required.

In addition to conventional digital intraoral reduction, as described previously, there are less known techniques that have been described. Ardehali and colleagues[14] described an external method wherein 1 hand creates anterior traction at the mandibular angle with fingers along the ascending ramus using the thumb at the malar eminence as a fulcrum while the other thumb places posterior directed pressure antero-superior to the displaced

coronoid process, with fingers creating traction at the mastoid process. This technique is said to minimize bite risk to the practitioner.

Awang[15] described initiating a gag reflex for reduction of the acutely dislocated condylar head. In this procedure, a mouth mirror is used to stimulate a gag by soft palate/pharyngeal contact. As impulses are carried to the central nervous system (CNS), there is stimulation of depressors/protruders, and reflex inhibition of the associated antagonists (elevators), enabling the mandible to relocate into the fossa.

Regardless of the employed technique, once the condylar head has been reduced, a period of functional restriction is advocated. Muscle relaxants may also be prescribed. In many instances, however, a tendency toward redislocation requires use of a chin strap/face-lift bandage for vertical

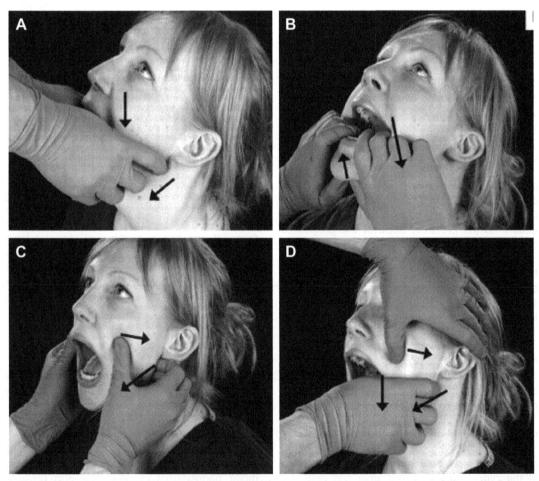

Fig. 3. Maneuver to reduce an acutely dislocated TMJ. (*A*) Downward and anterior traction is followed by (*B*) superior repositioning. (*C*) Pulling anteriorly while asking the patient to open (note how the zygoma is used for stabilization). (*D*) Unilateral maneuver pushing down and forward while using the other hand to stabilize while pushing back at the same time. (*From* Oliphant R, Key B, Dawson C, et al. Bilateral temporomandibular joint dislocation following pulmonary function testing: a case report and review of closed reduction techniques. Emerg Med J 2008;25(7):435–6; with permission.)

traction or even frank intermaxillary fixation for 7 days.[16] Injection of the lateral pterygoid muscle with botulinum toxin, as will be described later, has also been advocated as a conservative post-reduction treatment, aimed at decreasing the force of translation of the muscle, therefore decreasing the risk of continued dislocation.

CHRONIC DISLOCATIONS

Often, acute dislocations are self-limiting, without any adverse long-term sequelae or recurrent problems. With that in mind, however, acute dislocations may lead to a predilection toward chronic dislocation, or chronic recurrent dislocation. Regardless of the subtype, chronic dislocation can be managed via surgical or nonsurgical treatment modalities. Nonsurgical/minimally invasive therapy typically includes autologous blood transfer, sclerotherapy, botulinum toxin injection, or a combination thereof. Surgical/invasive interventions are aimed at anatomic modification of the eminence, condyle or musculo-capsular tissues. Managing the malocclusion without operating in the TMJ is also possible, utilizing conventional intraoral osteotomies like a sagittal split osteotomy or vertical ramus osteotomy. A brief discussion of the aforementioned procedures will ensue below.

MINIMALLY INVASIVE/MYOFASCIAL
Autologous Blood Injection/Sclerotherapy

Autologous blood injection (ABI) was initially described by Brachmann in 1964; he reported successful management of 60 patients with chronic dislocation. Since that article, scattered case reports have intermittently appeared in the literature.[17–20] Intra-articular blood injections are aimed at initiating an intra- and peri-capsular inflammatory response, perpetuated by transferred platelets and damaged nonplasma blood constituents. This inflammation creates fibrosis and adhesions, as is seen in the post-traumatic hemarthrosis model. Fibrosis and cicatricial maturation cause a physiologic decrease in compliance to the periarticular soft tissues, culminating in a decrease in range of motion (ROM).[18]

ABI has been described using a variety of techniques; however, the global methodology and end points are similar. The procedure can be unilateral or bilateral, depending on joint laxity and clinical symptoms. ABI may be completed with local anesthetic alone, intravenous sedation, or general anesthesia. Previously elaborated steps of arthrocentesis are followed, placing 2 needles into the superior joint space (**Fig. 4**).[1] The space is gently lavaged with normal saline or lactated ringers.

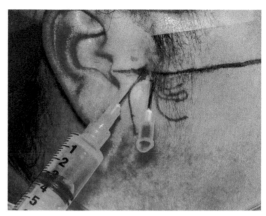

Fig. 4. Typical approach for arthrocentesis or injection into the TMJ.

The outflow needle is removed, and whole blood is then drawn from the patient and deposited into the superior joint space and infiltrated into the extracapsular tissue. The remaining needle is removed, and patients are given specific instructions to minimize jaw function for 2 weeks postoperatively.[18,21] At 2 weeks, patients can resume restricted function. Depending on clinical improvement, repeat injections can be completed. Variations of this technique have been described, wherein injections are completed multiple times a week over 2 to 3 weeks, followed by a period of intermaxillary fixation.[22]

Not unlike ABI, intracapsular deposition of sclerosing agents exerts effects by inducing an inflammatory response, which is followed by secondary localized fibrosis, resulting in joint hypomobility. Various sclerosing agents have been described, including cyclophosphamide, alcohol, tetracycline, ethanolamine oleate, Iodine, and OK-432.[23]

Given the conservative nature of this treatment, there are few risks, and the potential for prolonged neurosensory or neuromotor deficits, as is occasionally seen with open intervention, are minimal. That being said, despite the seemingly benign nature of the treatment, there are those who feel that exposure of the articular cartilage to blood/slcerosants may cause chondrocyte degeneration and lead to degenerative joint changes.[18] Because of the risk of intra-articular injection, there are proponents of arthroscopic guidance for the deposition of sclerosents.

Botulinum Toxin

Therapeutic use of botulinum toxin type A in the head and neck region has significantly increased over the past decade. Botulinum toxin type A induces a dose-related weakness of skeletal muscle by inhibition of acetylcholine release at the neuromuscular junction. When used in the treatment of dystonia or other neurogenic disorders, repeat injections at 3- to 6-month intervals are required for maximal therapeutic efficacy.[24]

In the context of chronic recurrent TMJ dislocation, there are many reports of the use of botulinum toxin type A, both as a primary therapy, and as an adjunct to other reductive techniques.[24–27] It is often employed in patients who may not be candidates for surgery, based on age, medical comorbidities, and other factors.

Most frequently, the targeted muscle is the lateral pterygoid, which is often implicated in myospasm associated with dislocation. That being said, it may also be infiltrated into any of the masticatory musculature. Computed tomography (CT) imaging can be completed preoperatively, so as to create accurate measurements from the skin surface to muscle belly. Fu and colleagues[24] described accessing the lateral pterygoid percutaneously through the sigmoid notch, inferior to the zygomatic arch. Twenty-five to 50 units of botulinum toxin type A are deposited directly into the muscle belly, aspirating prior to injection to avoid inadvertent intravascular injection.[24] In addition to percutaneous injection, botulinum toxin type A may also be injected transorally into the lateral pterygoid under continuous electromyography (EMG) control/guidance.[27] In many instances, a single injection may be sufficient.[24,26,28]

Adverse effects of injection include hemorrhage and intravascular injection. Additionally, there is risk of toxin-induced transient velopharyngeal insufficiency, dysarthria, and dysphagia.[26,28] Fortunately these events are unlikely, and symptoms typically subside between 2 and 4 weeks.

Proliferation Treatment

Proliferation treatment, also referred to as prolotherapy has been used since the 1930s in the management of temporomandibular dysfunction.[29] Prolotherapy, or regenerative injection therapy, is described as the infiltration of a nonpharmacologic solution into pericapsular, tendinous tissues, with aims of initiating a mixed inflammatory process.[29,30] This inflammatory process is thought to initiate localized fibrous proliferation, causing an increase in tissue robustness, which increases joint stability and bolsters joint laxity. Historically, various solutions have been used, including dextrose, psyllium seed oil, and various combinations of dextrose, glycerin, and phenol.[31–33]

The technique for prolotherapy is not unlike that described previously for ABI (see **Fig. 4**). After the patient is prepared and draped, an auriculotemporal nerve block is completed. 2 mL of 10% to 50%

dextrose may then be infiltrated into the superior joint space (as described for arthrocentesis), retrodiscal tissues, periarticular tissues, or a combination thereof.[29] Upon completion of the procedure, patients are put on a soft diet and jaw rest for 2 weeks. Patients are then followed, with repeat injections as needed in the event of recurrent dislocation. When using prolotherapy, the literature would suggest that although patients may only require a single series of injections, often, patients require 3 to 5 injections for optimal therapeutic effect.[29–31]

Temporalis Scarification/Lateral Pterygoid Myotomy

In the context of recalcitrant chronic recurrent or protracted dislocation of the TMJ, surgery is often indicated. Alteration of the juxta-articular musculature has been described as one of many surgical options, aimed specifically at alteration of the implicated spastic muscle units. Ultimately, it is likely the formation of intramuscular scar tissue that facilitates hypomobility of the mandible.

Lateral pterygoid myotomy has been described as being performed transorally and percutaneously, using a preauricular incision.[34] The transoral approach is completed with the patient under general anesthesia. The patient is opened maximally, and local anesthesia is infiltrated along the medial and lateral upper mandibular ramus. A vertical incision is then created, extending from the coronoid process, along the ascending ramus to the distal of the most posterior tooth. Soft tissues are elevated from the medial mandible, followed by blunt/scissor dissection to visualize the lateral pterygoid. The lateral pterygoid is then detached from the condyle/anterior capsule.[34] The wound is closed, and the patients are placed into maxillomandibular fixation (MMF) for 7 days.

Briefly, not unlike lateral pterygoid myotomy, temporalis scarification is a treatment modality aimed at creating cicatricial restriction of dynamic muscular function, so as to reduce condylar translation.

Arthroscopy

Arthroscopy is yet another treatment modality, occasionally employed in the management of TMJ dislocation.[35] An in-depth discussion of arthroscopy, including surgical approach/landmarks and technique is beyond the scope of this article. That being said, the aim of arthroscopy, in this context, is to facilitate posterior capsulorrhaphy and contracture, using either laser (Hol:YAG) or electrothermal devices.[35] Not unlike external capsulorrhaphy, the aim of this technique is to create cicatricial contracture and scarification of the retrodiscal synovial tissue and oblique pro-tuberance.[35] This procedure has been described using laser/cautery alone, or adding a retrodiscal sclerosing agent (sodium tetradecyl sulfate) under arthroscopic guidance.[35,36]

OPEN SURGICAL TREATMENT
Eminectomy

Initially described by Myrhaug in 1951, eminectomy is completed with aims of reducing the vertical height of the articular eminence, such that in the event of condylar hypermobility and dislocation, the condyle will slip posteriorly back into the fossa without significant anatomic restriction.[37]

The procedure is typically completed using a standard endaural or preauricular incision, with anterior/temporal extension. Dissection is carried to the superficial layer of the deep temporal fascia. This fascia is incised, with anterior release as needed (extending obliquely antero-superiorly at a 45° angle so as to minimize trauma to the temporal branch of the facial nerve).[38,39] At this point, the periosteum is incised on the zygomatic arch, and dissection is carried anteriorly, to the level of the articular eminence. The eminence is then reduced to its medial margin with burs, osteotomes, or a combination thereof (**Fig. 5**).[39] The lateral tubercle of the eminence may be left in place as a guide plane, or removed.[39] The decision as to whether this is a unilateral or bilateral procedure depends on the underlying joint aberrancy.

Patients are encouraged to comply with a soft diet for the first week postoperatively. Gentle physical therapy then ensues, to ensure maintenance of functional opening. Risks of this procedure include intracranial violation and damage to local neuromotor bundles.

Dautrey's Procedure

Because eminectomies alone can turn a dislocation into a subluxation, techniques aimed at creating a mechanical interference to condylar translation have been described extensively in the literature (**Fig. 6**). In 1933, Mayer described segmental dislocation of the zygomatic arch to act as a physiologic obstruction to condylar hypermobility.[40] 10 years later, LeClerc and Girard described a similar procedure, wherein a vertical osteotomy was created in the zygomatic arch, inserting the osteotomized segment to impede the path of the hypermobile condyle.[41,42] Modifying the paradigm yet again, in 1967 Gosserez and Dautrey described a similar procedure, similarly aimed at greenstick fracture of the zygomatic arch, with fossa inset.[43] Despite the variations, all of the procedures share a similar end point.

The technique is described as follows. A preauricular incision is created, with a slight anterior temporal extension. Dissection ensues to the superficial layer of the deep temporal fascia. This fascia is incised through, proximally, near the root of the zygoma. The TMJ capsule is not violated. An osteotomy is then created in the zygomatic arch, anterior to the eminence, extending from posterior–superior to anterior inferior, in an oblique fashion. Gentle pressure is exerted proximally on the osteotomized arch, to create a greenstick fracture, anteriorly. The osteotomized proximal arch is then mobilized medially or laterally and inset under the articular eminence. Once inset, the segment may be held in place by a mini plate, or simply left passively.[44–47] Once the procedure has been completed, patients are placed on a soft diet, with restriction of function over 2 to 3 weeks, followed by ROM treatment.[44]

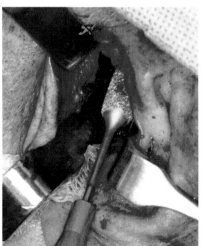
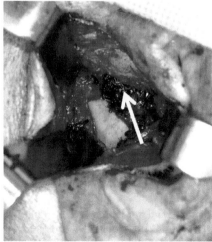

Fig. 5. TMJ eminectomy. Note (*white arrow*) how the eminence is completely flat after ostectomy.

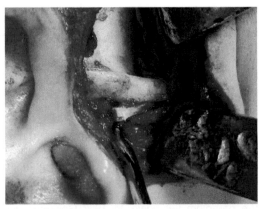

Fig. 6. Oblique osteotomy of the eminence and wedge formed bone graft inserted tightly into the osteotomy site. (*From* Güven O. Management of chronic recurrent temporomandibular joint dislocations: a retrospective study. J Craniomaxillofac Surg 2009;37(1):25; with permission.)

Complications of Dautrey's procedure include localized neurosensory and neuromotor aberrancies. Additionally, there is risk of complete fracture of the zygomatic arch, which requires rigid stabilization. Occasionally, grafting of the surgical site is indicated, in the event that the osteotomized segment is not robust enough to prohibit movement.

Other Blocking Procedures

Not unlike Dautrey's procedure, blocking procedures are aimed at interfering with translation by increasing the overall mass of the articular eminence, so as to act as a physical stop to prevent excessive translation of the condylar head. There have been a variety of techniques described, all with the common end point of creating a physiologic stop. This can be accomplished using a titanium miniplate, interpositional bone graft, or blocks of hydroxyapatite.[48,49]

Glenotemporal osteotomy with autogenous grafting can be completed using various graft donor sites; however, the most frequently described techniques typically use iliac crest or cranium.[48–51] In this technique, the joint is accessed as previously described, with subperiosteal dissection to the articular eminence. A sagittal saw or fissure bur is used to create a horizontal osteotomy along the eminence, which is subsequently downfractured, maintaining intact periosteum.[48,49] Once the eminence has been downfractured, the harvested bone is then shaped and inset as an interpositional graft between the zygomatic arch and downfractured eminence (see **Fig. 6**). Depending on the stability of the inset graft, wires, screws, or mini-plates may be used to secure the graft.[49]

Mini-plates have also been described in the context of physiologic blocking procedures. There are many clinical permutations; however, the end point is the same. The approach to the TMJ is completed as heretofore described. Once the articular eminence has been visualized, an L plate is placed, with the short arm fixed laterally to the eminence with 2 6 mm screws and the long arm

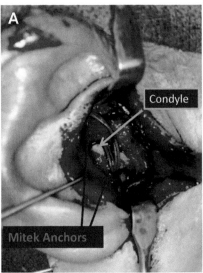
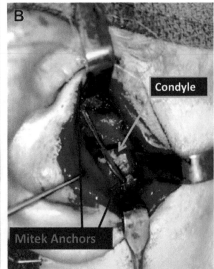

Fig. 7. Preventing forward translation. (*A*) The Mitek anchors have been placed in the lateral pole of the condyle and the posterior root of the zygomatic arch. The #2 Ethibond sutures are seen secured to the Mitek anchors. Note the laxity of the sutures. (*B*) The condyle is protracted forward to the extent the ligaments will allow, preventing subluxation.

being contoured and placed along the eminence, inferiorly, to act as a mechanical obstruction.[52] Careful attention is given so as to remain extracapsular during the procedure.

Proponents of mini-plate placement advocate the procedure based on its reversibility and relatively less invasive nature.[52] That being said, there is risk for plate fracture, in addition to a lager reduction in maximum interincisal opening.[52–54] In the event of plate fracture, a second surgery must be undertaken, to remove the hardware, and a decision must be made as to whether additional treatment might be undertaken.

Wolford's Procedure

This relatively simple procedure uses 2 Mitek mini-bone anchors (Mitek Products Incorporated, Westwood, Massachusetts) with osseointegration potential. A #2 Ethibond suture (Ethicon,

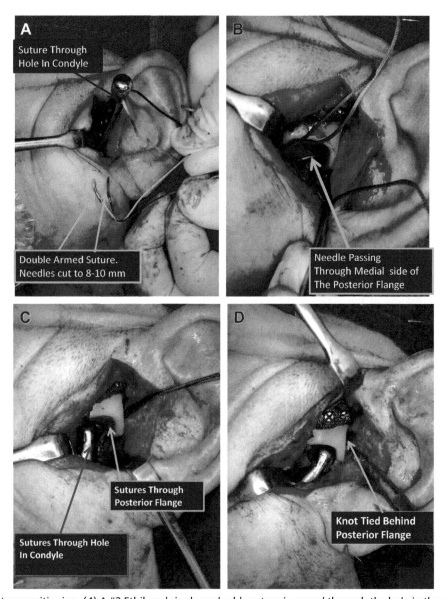

Fig. 8. Suture positioning. (*A*) A #2 Ethibond single or double suture is passed through the hole in the prosthesis. A suture with double-armed needles makes the procedure easier. The needles are cut to about 8 to 10 mm length. (*B*) The needle on the medial side of the prosthesis (*arrow*) is passed through the medial side of the posterior flange and pulled through the posterior wall of the flange. (*C*) The needle on the lateral side of the prosthesis (*arrow*) is passed through the lateral aspect of the posterior flange and pulled through the posterior wall of the flange. (*D*) The sutures are tied on the back wall of the posterior flange.

Incorporated, Somerville, New Jersey) is looped through the threading device and pulled through the eyes of both Mitek anchors. The looped end is cut, so now there are 2 separate artificial ligaments through the eye of each Mitek anchor. An endaural or preauricular incision is used for access to the TMJ and dissection completed exposing the zygomatic arch and lateral capsule. If the articular disc is in proper position, then neither joint space needs to be entered. The lateral pole of the condyle is exposed, and 1 anchor is placed in the lateral pole of the condyle. The other anchor is placed in the very posterior root of the zygomatic arch. The 2 sutures are then adjusted for the amount of mobility desired and tied. If the patient has chronic forward posturing of the mandible, then the 2 artificial ligaments can be tightened to keep the condyle seated in the postero-superior aspect of the fossa, preventing forward translation (Fig. 7). If the procedure is used to prevent dislocation anterior to the articular eminence, then the artificial ligaments can be left slack to provide translation but limit forward movement so the condyle cannot translate beyond the articular eminence. This will allow relatively normal movement of the condyle including excursive movements. No eminectomy is needed with this procedure. If the articular disc is dislocated, then a third anchor can be used to reposition the disc into a normal relationship.[55]

Potential risks with these techniques include rupture or breakage of the sutures or failure of the Mitek anchors. Wolford and colleagues[55] reported good success in 5 cases treated with this technique.

This same tethering philosophy can be applied to patients with total joint prostheses that can become displaced. For the TMJ concepts total joint prosthesis, dislocation or subluxation can occur, although rare. In cases of large tumor resection, in which the muscles of mastication are reflected or partially removed, there is a risk of condylar displacement and dislocation related to the lack of vertical support. When it is anticipated that this could be a problem before surgery, the manufacturer can place a hole through the condylar neck of the prosthesis. If it is a dislocation or subluxation problem that develops after surgery, then a secondary surgery can be performed and a hole drilled through the neck of the prosthesis with carbide burs. In either case, 1 or 2 #2 Ethibond sutures can be placed through the hole in the condylar neck and the sutures passed through the posterior flange (polyethylene) of the fossa component in a mattress fashion and tied securing the condylar component into the fossa (Fig. 8).[56]

Box 2
Summary of treatment

- Minimally Invasive/Myofascial
  - Autologous Blood injection
  - Sclerotherapy
  - Botulinum toxin
  - Proliferation treatment
  - Arthroscopy (+/− sclerotherapy)
  - Temporalis scarification
  - Lateral pterygoid myotomy
- Open/surgical
  - Eminectomy
  - Glenotemporal osteotomy
    - As described by LeClerc and later modified ay Gosserez and Dautrey
  - Blocking procedures
    - Titanium mini-plate
    - Interpositional autologous grafting
    - Alloplastic/allograft block inset
  - Artificial ligament/anchors
    - As described by Wolford
  - Alloplastic joint replacement
  - Sagittal Split/Vertical Ramus Osteotomy

In cases of chronic dislocation where the joint has been out of the fossa for more than 6 months, an intraoral vertical ramus osteotomy (IVRO) or sagital split osteotomy (SSO) may be considered to correct the occlusion if the patient is asymptomatic. Sometimes a total joint prosthesis (TJP) is indicated if the patient has significant functional problems and pain. It is extremely hard if not impossible to reduce a joint back to its normal position after more than 6 to 12 months of dislocation.

In summary, there are myriad etiologies that can create acute or chronic TMJ dislocations. Accordingly, it is up to the astute practitioner to create a patient-centered treatment algorithm when deciding on which treatment modality to employ (Box 2). As important as symptom palliation is, the underlying cause of dislocation should be analyzed, and thoughtful consideration should be given to etiology, so long-term resolution may be attained.

REFERENCES

1. Nitzan D. Temporomandibular joint "open lock" versus condylar dislocation: signs and symptoms,

imaging, treatment, and pathogenesis. J Oral Maxillofac Surg 2002;60:506–11.

2. Rattan V. Superolateral dislocation of the mandibular condyle: Report of 2 cases and review of the literature. J Oral Maxillofac Surg 2002;60:1366–9.

3. Akers JO, Narang R, DeChamplain R. Posterior dislocation of the mandibular condyle into the external Ear Canal. J Oral Maxillofac Surg 1982; 40(6):369–70.

4. Li Z, Shang Z, Wu Z. An unusual type of superolateral dislocation of mandibular condyle: discussion of the causative mechanisms and clinical characteristics. J Oral Maxillofac Surg 2009;67:431–5.

5. Imai T, Machizawa M, Kobayashi M. Anterior dislocation of the intact mandibular condyle caused by fracture of the articular eminence: an unusual fracture of the temporomandibular joint apparatus. J Oral Maxillofac Surg 2011;69:1046–51.

6. Adekeye EO, Shamia RI, Cove P. Inverted L-shaped ramus osteotomy for prolonged bilateral dislocation of the temporomandibular joint. Oral Surg Oral Med Oral Pathol 1976;41:568–77.

7. Rowe NL, Killey HC. Fractures of the facial skeleton. 2nd edition. Edinburgh: E & S Livingstone; 1970. p. 23–34.

8. Atherton GJ, Peckitt NS. Bilateral dislocation of the temporomandibular joints in a 2-year-old child: report of a case. J Oral Maxillofac Surg 1997;55:646–7.

9. Laskin DM, Green CS, Hylander WL. TMDs. An evidence-based approach to diagnosis and treatment. Chicago (IL): Quintessence; 2006. p. 219–28.

10. Du Brul EL. Evolution of the temporomandibular joint. In: Sarnat BG, editor. The temporomandibular joint. Springfield (IL): Charles C Thomas; 1964. p. 3–27.

11. Merrill RG. Mandibular dislocation. In: Keith DA, editor. Surgery of the temporomandibular joint. London: Blackwell Publications; 1988. p. 135–68.

12. Fordyce GL. Long-standing bilateral dislocation of the jaw. Br J Oral Surg 1965;2:222–5.

13. Howe AG, Kent JN, Farrell CD. Implant of articular eminence for recurrent dislocation of TMJ. J Oral Surg 1978;36:523–6.

14. Ardehali MM, Kouhi A, Meighani A, et al. Temporomandibular joint dislocation reduction technique: a new external method vs. the traditional. Ann Plast Surg 2009;63(2):176–8.

15. Awang MN. A new approach to the reduction of acute dislocation of the temporomandibular joint: a report of three cases. Br J Oral Maxillofac Surg 1987;25:244–9.

16. Pinto AS, McVeigh KP, Bainton KP. The use of autologous blood and adjunctive 'face lift' bandage in the management of recurrent TMJ dislocation. Br J Oral Maxillofac Surg 2009;47:323–4.

17. Brachmann F. Autologous blood injection for recurrent hypermobility of the temporomandibular joint. Dtsch Zahnarztl Z 1964;15:97–102.

18. Machon V, Abramowicz S, Paska J, et al. Autologous blood injection for the treatment of chronic recurrent temporomandibular joint dislocation. J Oral Maxillofac Surg 2009;67:114–9.

19. Daif ET. Autologous blood injection as a new treatment modality for chronic recurrent temporomandibular joint dislocation. Oral Surg Oral Med Oral Pathol Oral Radiol Endod 2010;109:31–6.

20. Kato T, Shimoyama T, Nasu D, et al. Autologous blood injection into the articular cavity for the treatment of recurrent temporomandibular joint dislocation: a case report. J Oral Sci 2007;49: 237–9.

21. Hegab AF. Treatment of chronic recurrent dislocation of the temporomandibular joint with injection of autologous blood alone, intermaxillary fixation alone, or both together: a prospective, randomized, controlled clinical trial. Br J Oral Maxillofac Surg 2013;51:813–7.

22. Schulz S. Evaluation of periarticular autotransfusion for therapy of recurrent dislocation of the temporomandibular joint. Dtsch Stomatol 1973;23:94–8 [in German].

23. Matsushita K, Abe T, Fujiwara T. OK-432 (Picibanil) sclerotherapy for recurrent dislocation of the temporomandibular joint in elderly edentulous patients: case reports. Br J Oral Maxillofac Surg 2007;45: 511–3.

24. Fu K, Chen HM, Sun ZP, et al. Long term efficacy of botulinum toxin type A for the treatment of habitual dislocation of the temporomandibular joint. Br J Oral Maxillofac Surg 2010;48:281–4.

25. Aquilina P, Vickers R, McKellar G. Reduction of a chronic bilateral temporomandibular joint dislocation with intermaxillary fixation and botulinum toxin A. Br J Oral Maxillofac Surg 2004;42:272–3.

26. Moore AP, Wood GD. Medical treatment of recurrent temporomandibular joint dislocation using botulinum toxin A. Br Dent J 1997;183:415–7.

27. Martinez-Perez D, Ruiz-Espiga PG. Recurrent temporomandibular joint dislocation treated with botulinum toxin: report of 3 cases. J Oral Maxillofac Surg 2004;62:244–6.

28. Zigeler CM, Haag C, Muhling J. Treatment of recurrent temporomandibular joint dislocation with intramuscular botulinum toxin injection. Clin Oral Investig 2003;7:52–5.

29. Zhou H, Hu K, Ding Y. Modified dextrose prolotherapy for recurrent temporomandibular joint dislocation. Br J Oral Maxillofac Surg 2014;52:62–6.

30. Refai H, Altahhan O, Elsharkawy R. The efficacy of dextrose prolotherapy for temporomandibular joint hypermobility: a preliminary prospective, randomized, double-blind, placebo-controlled clinical trial. J Oral Maxillofac Surg 2001;69:2962–70.

31. Schultz LW. A treatment of subluxation of the temporomandibular joint. JAMA 1937;109:1032.

32. Hauser R, Hauser M, Blakemore K. Dextrose prolotherapy and pain of chronic TMJ dysfunction. Practical Pain Management 2007;49–55.

33. Klein RT, Bjorn CE, DeLong B, et al. A randomized double blind trial of dextrose-glycerine-phenol injections for chronic lower back pain. J Spinal Disord 1993;6(1):23–33.

34. Sindet-Pedersen S. Intraoral myotomy of the lateral pterygoid muscle for treatment of recurrent dislocation of the mandibular condyle. J Oral Maxillofac Surg 1968;46:445–9.

35. Torres DE, McCain JP. Arthroscopic electrothermal capsulorrhaphy for the treatment of recurrent temporomandibular joint dislocation. Int J Oral Maxillofac Surg 2012;41(6):681–9.

36. McCain JP, Hossameldin RH, Glickman AG. Preliminary Clinical Experience and Outcome of the TMJ Arthroscopic Chemical Contracture Procedure in TMJ dislocation patients. J Oral Maxillofac Surg 2014;72(9):e16–7.

37. Myrhaug H. A new method of operation for habitual dislocation of the mandible; review of former methods of treatment. Acta Odontol Scand 1951;9: 247–60.

38. Al-Kayat A, Bramley P. A modified pre-auricular approach to the temporomandibular joint and malar arch. Br J Oral Surg 1979;17:91–103.

39. Williamson RA, McNamara D, McAuliffe W. True eminectomy for internal derangement of the temporomandibular joint. Br J Oral Maxillofac Surg 2000; 38:554–60.

40. Mayer L. Recurrent dislocation of the Jaw. J Bone Surg 1933;15:889–96.

41. Leclerc GC, Girard C. Un nouveau procédé de dutée dans le traitement chirurgical de la luxation recidivante de la machoire inferieur. Mem Acad Chir 1943;69:457–659.

42. Undt G, Kermer C, Piehslinger E, et al. Treatment of recurrent mandibular dislocation, Part 1; LeClerc blocking procedure. Int J Oral Maxillofac Surg 1997;26:92–7.

43. Gosserez M, Dautrey J. Osteoplastic bearing for treatment of temporomandibular luxation. Transaction of Second Congress of the International Association of Oral Surgeons, Copenhagen, Munksgaard. Int J Oral Surg 1967;IV:261.

44. Gadre KD, Kaul D, Ramanojam S, et al. Dautrey's procedure in treatment of recurrent dislocation of the mandible. J Oral Maxillofac Surg 2010;68: 2021–4.

45. Lawler MG. Recurrent dislocation of the mandible: treatment of ten cases by the Dautrey procedure. Br J Oral Surg 1982;20:14.

46. Kobayashi H, Uamazaki T, Okudera H. Correction of recurrent dislocation of the mandible in elderly patients by the Dautrey procedure. Br J Oral Maxillofac Surg 2000;38:54.

47. Izuka T, Hidaka Y, Murakami K, et al. Chronic recurrent anterior luxation of the mandible. Int J Oral Maxillofac Surg 1988;17:170.

48. Fernandez-Sanroman J. Surgical treatment of recurrent mandibular dislocation by augmentation of the articular eminence with cranial bone. J Oral Maxillofac Surg 1997;55(4):333–8.

49. Medra A, Mahrous A. Glenotemporal osteotomy and bone grafting in the management of chronic recurrent dislocation and hypermobility of the temporomandibular joint. Br J Oral Maxillofac Surg 2008; 46:119–22.

50. Costas Lopez A, Monje Gil F, Fernandez Sanroman J, et al. Glenotemporal osteotomy as a definitive treatment for recurrent dislocation of the jaw. J Craniomaxillofac Surg 1996;24:178–83.

51. Gray AR, Barker GR. Idiopathic blepharospasm-oromandibular dystonia syndrome (Meige's syndrome) presenting as chronic temporomandibular joint dislocation. Br J Oral Maxillofac Surg 1991;29:97–9.

52. Vasconcelos BC, Porto G. Treatment of chronic mandibular dislocations: a comparison between eminectomy and miniplates. J Oral Maxillofac Surg 2009;67:2599–604.

53. Kuttenberger JJ, Hardt N. Long-term results following miniplate eminoplasty for the treatment of recurrent dislocation and habitual luxation of the temporomandibular joint. Int J Oral Maxillofac Surg 2003;32:474.

54. Puelacher WC, Waldhart E. Miniplate eminoplasty. A new surgical treatment for TMJ dislocation. J Craniomaxillofac Surg 1993;21:176.

55. Wolford LM, Pitta MC, Mehra P. Mitek anchors for treatment of chronic mandibular dislocation. Oral Surg Oral Med Oral Pathol Oral Radiol Endod 2001;92(5):495–8.

56. Rodrigues DB, Wolford LM, Malaquias P, et al. Concomitant treatment of mandibular ameloblastoma and bilateral tempomandibular joint osteoarthritis with bone graft and total joint prostheses. J Oral Maxillofac Surg 2014. http://dx.doi.org/10.1016/j.joms.2014.06.461.

Surgical Management of Congenital Deformities with Temporomandibular Joint Malformation

Larry M. Wolford, DMD*, Daniel E. Perez, DDS

KEYWORDS

- Hemifacial microsomia (HFM) • Treacher Collins syndrome (TCS) • TMJ reconstruction
- Autogenous tissue grafts • Patient-fitted total joint prostheses • Periarticular fat grafts
- Orthognathic surgery • Counterclockwise rotation

KEY POINTS

- Hemifacial microsomia (HFM) is the second most common facial birth defect and can present with an ipsilateral hypoplasia of the soft tissues and temporomandibular joint (TMJ) or absent TMJ, ramus, and body of the mandible and decreased airway.
- Although autogenous tissues or distraction techniques have been advocated for TMJ and mandibular reconstruction, a patient-fitted total joint prosthesis can provide the best skeletal and occlusal stability as well as the best functional and esthetic outcomes.
- Treacher Collins syndrome (TCS) presents with bilateral hypoplasia of the facial soft tissues and bone structures, including hypoplasia or aplasia of the TMJs, retrusion of the jaws, and significantly decreased oropharyngeal airway.
- Autogenous tissues have been used to reconstruct the major facial and TMJ deformities associated with TCS with compromised success, but patient-fitted total joint prostheses are highly predictable to secure a stable functional and esthetic outcome as well as correct the airway.
- Patients with HFM and TCS benefit functionally and esthetically from counterclockwise rotation of the maxillomandibular complex.
- Virtual surgical planning can be used in the surgical preparation to improve quality of treatment outcome.

Surgical correction of congenital deformities in which the temporomandibular joints (TMJs) are affected and cause dentofacial malformations can be difficult to manage. Two deformities are particularly challenging: hemifacial microsomia (HFM) and Treacher Collins syndrome (TCS). These deformities commonly have hypoplastic or absent TMJ structures requiring TMJ reconstruction in conjunction with orthognathic surgery to provide stable and predictable functional and esthetic outcomes. HFM and TCS are similar and

can be confused, but the latter shows a well-defined pattern of inheritance and is usually symmetric.

The 2 primary methods to reconstruct the TMJs involve the use of autogenous tissues (ie, rib or sternoclavicular grafts [SCGs]) versus alloplastic total joint prosthetic devices. Understanding the nature of the deformities; the timing of the reconstruction; the surgical treatment options, including TMJ reconstruction and orthognathic surgery; and the predictability and stability of these options

Departments of Oral and Maxillofacial Surgery and Orthodontics Texas, A&M University Health Science Center Baylor College of Dentistry, Baylor University Medical Center, 3409 Worth St. Suite 400, Dallas, TX 75246, USA
* Corresponding author.
E-mail address: lwolford@drlarrywolford.com

Oral Maxillofacial Surg Clin N Am 27 (2015) 137–154
http://dx.doi.org/10.1016/j.coms.2014.09.010
1042-3699/15/$ – see front matter © 2015 Elsevier Inc. All rights reserved.

enables surgeons to apply this knowledge to these and similar deformities. This article concentrates on the more involved and complex cases with absent TMJs that are not amendable to conventional orthognathic surgery repair.

HEMIFACIAL MICROSOMIA

HFM is a specific condition of unilateral incomplete or hypoplastic development of the facial soft tissues and skeleton. HFM is the second most common facial birth defect after cleft lip and palate, with an estimated occurrence rate of 1 in 5600 live births.[1] It is also known as Goldenhar syndrome, oculoauriculovertebral spectrum, otomandibular dysostosis, lateral facial dysplasia, and branchial arch syndrome. HFM occurs sporadically in most cases and can be considered as a nonspecific symptom complex that is etiologically and pathogenetically heterogeneous. Extreme variability of expression is characteristic of this disorder.[2]

Clinical and Imaging Features

HFM features include some or all of the following characteristics: (1) unilateral hypoplasia or absence of the mandibular condyle, ramus, and body;

(2) retruded chin deviated toward the ipsilateral side; (3) facial morphology with high occlusal plane angle; (4) hypoplasia of the ipsilateral maxilla, zygomatico-orbital complex, and temporal bone; (5) ipsilateral soft tissue deficiency affecting muscles, nerves, subcutaneous and glandular tissues, as well as skin; (6) decreased ipsilateral facial height; (7) class II skeletal and occlusal relationship; (8) premature occlusal contact on the ipsilateral side; (9) transverse cant in the occlusal plane and skeletal structures; (10) ipsilateral hypoeruption of the teeth and partial anodontia; (11) eye, ear, and vertebral anomalies; and (12) decreased oropharyngeal airway and sleep apnea in cases with significant penetration (**Figs. 1** and **2**). Facial deformity and asymmetry usually worsen with growth. The contralateral TMJ articular disc may become anteriorly displaced, induced by the abnormal condylar rotation caused by the mandibular asymmetry and the functional overload on that joint. Typical TMJ symptoms may accompany the condition, such as TMJ pain, headaches, myofascial pain, and ear symptoms.

Classification

There are several proposed classifications that identify the severity of this syndrome, but this

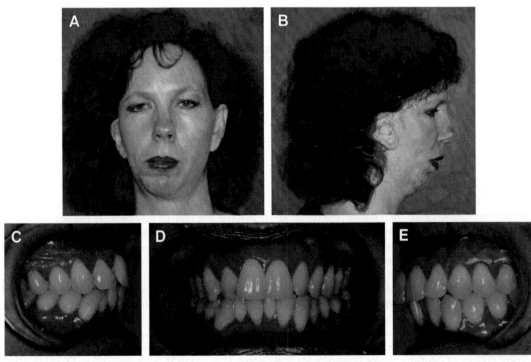

Fig. 1. (*A, B*) Patient with HFM with right side affected. Facial asymmetry with vertically shorter ipsilateral side and chin shifted to the right. In profile, the retruded maxilla and mandible are evident. (*C–E*) The occlusion has a transverse cant, being vertically higher on the ipsilateral side and can be class I or commonly class II with or without an anterior open bite.

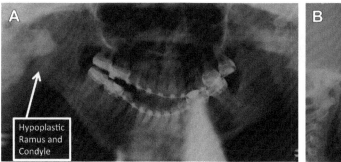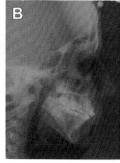

Hypoplastic Ramus and Condyle

Fig. 2. (A) These representative radiographs of HFM show a panogram with a hypoplastic ramus and TMJ. It is common for mandibular teeth to be congenitally missing. (B) The vertical asymmetry at the occlusion and inferior border of the mandible is evident. The high occlusal plane angle is noted as well as the decreased oropharyngeal airway.

article uses the classification system proposed by Pruzansky in 1969 and later modified by Mulliken and Kaban in 1987.[3,4] This system assigns patients with HFM to one of 3 categories based on size and function of the TMJ. Type I is a small mandible with normal TMJ morphology. Type IIa is a ramus with abnormal size and shape but with the glenoid maintaining its position, whereas type IIb is a ramus and TMJ with abnormal size, shape, and function that is displaced outside the plane of the contralateral side. Type III describes an absent condyle, ramus, and TMJ. This classification system may be the most useful to surgeons in the preoperative evaluation because of its simplicity and inclusion of TMJ anatomy and function.

The lateral cephalometric radiograph can be used to analyze the anteroposterior (AP) and vertical hard and soft tissue dimensions as well as to quantify left to right side vertical discrepancies by measuring between the double images of the occlusal plane and inferior borders of the mandible (see **Fig. 2**B).

Superimposing bilateral tracings of cephalometric tomograms that include the TMJ as well as the mandibular body and posterior teeth allows quantification of the asymmetry involving the condyles, rami, and bodies of the mandible. The use of three-dimensional (3D) computed tomography (CT) scans and virtual surgical planning (VSP) is advocated to obtain more consistent and predictable results. MRI evaluation shows the deformed or absent TMJ of the ipsilateral side, whereas the contralateral TMJ may show a displaced disc.

TREACHER COLLINS SYNDROME

TCS is a specific condition of bilateral incomplete, or hypoplastic development of, the facial soft tissues and skeleton from the first and second

pharyngeal arch. TCS is an autosomal dominant inheritance (although 60% represent new mutations), with an estimated occurrence rate of 1 per 50,000 live births. It is also known as mandibulofacial dysostosis and Franceschetti-Zwahlen-Klein syndrome.

Clinical and Imaging Features

TCS features include some or all of the following characteristics: (1) mandibular hypoplasia with vertical deficiency of the rami and significant gonial notching; (2) bilateral severe hypoplasia or aplasia of the mandibular condyles, articular eminences, and coronoid processes; (3) significantly retruded chin; (4) facial morphology with high occlusal plane and mandibular plane angles; (5) class II occlusion with anterior open bite; (6) posterior vertical maxillary hypoplasia; (7) hypoplastic zygomatico-orbital complex and temple bones; (8) downward-sloping palpebral fissures and absence of the medial lower eyelashes; (9) malformed pinnae; (10) decreased oropharyngeal airway; and (11) condyle covered with hyaline cartilage rather than fibrocartilage (**Figs. 3** and **4**).

The facial deformity usually worsens with growth. Sleep apnea is a common finding in TCS. Lateral cephalometric radiographs can be used to analyze the AP and vertical hard and soft tissue dimensions (see **Fig. 4**B). Cone beam imaging, CT scans, 3D imaging, and modeling can aid in diagnosis and treatment planning for these cases.

AGE OF SURGICAL INTERVENTION

The patient's age can affect the treatment protocol. For instance, patients with HFM or TCS who are less than 12 years of age and who have severe hypoplasia and malformation or absence of the TMJ may benefit from a growth center transplant,

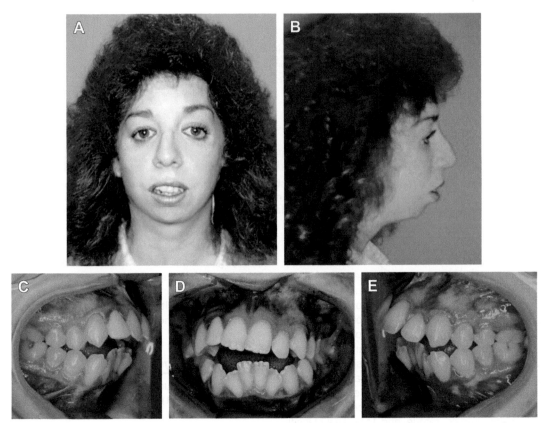

Fig. 3. (*A, B*) Patient with TCS with typical facial presentation. The mandible is significantly retruded and the facial morphology with high occlusal plane is characteristic. The zygomatico-orbital complexes are hypoplastic and the lateral palpebral ligaments are inferiorly positioned with associated palpebral deformities. (*C–E*) The occlusion can be class I or commonly class II with or without an anterior open bite.

using a rib graft[5,6] or sternoclavicular graft (SCG).[7] Rib grafts are unpredictable relative to growth and stability and often significantly overgrow, creating dentofacial deformities.[5,8] SCGs tend to have better growth potential, similar to normal TMJ growth, and better stability than a rib graft.[9] With either graft system there is a possibility that the grafts will not grow or will overgrow, resorb, or fracture during the initial healing phase.

Another option for early intervention is the use of distraction osteogenesis.[10,11] This technique has shown mixed results in the literature because it

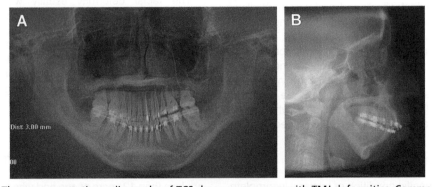

Fig. 4. (*A*) These representative radiographs of TCS show a panogram with TMJ deformities. Commonly there is gonial notching and a short ramus height. (*B*) The lateral cephalogram shows the typical high occlusal plane angle, retruded mandible, vertically hypoplastic posterior maxilla, and decreased oropharyngeal airway.

usually requires multiple operations to place and remove the distractors, and this can lead to difficulty in controlling the vector of growth. Lengthening of the ramus under the pressure of the pterygomasseteric sling is difficult to accomplish and may significantly overload the already hypoplastic TMJs causing further degenerative changes. Orthognathic surgery is usually necessary following completion of growth to maximize the functional and esthetic results. Other treatment methods include hard and soft tissue grafting techniques.

Improving the predictability of results and limiting correction of the jaw and TMJ deformities to 1 major operation can best be achieved by waiting until growth is complete, provided that the patient is functionally and psychologically stable. Girls usually have most of their facial growth (98%) complete by the age of 15 to 16 years, and boys by the age of 17 to 18 years.[12] Because asymmetric growth is a component of HFM and some required orthognathic surgical procedures may have further adverse effects on subsequent facial growth, performing orthognathic surgery during the growing years may result in the need for additional surgery at a later time to correct the asymmetry, AP discrepancy, and malocclusion that may develop during the completion of growth.

There are definite indications for early surgery, such as requirement for growth center transplant (ie, rib or SCGs) to correct masticatory dysfunction, airway obstruction, sleep apnea, and psychological factors. Wolford and colleagues[13,14] have published on maxillary and mandibular orthognathic surgery and the effects on growth, with age consideration guidelines for surgical intervention as well as age consideration and surgical treatment protocols for the common TMJ pathologic conditions.[15]

Patients with TCS can receive definitive treatment earlier than patients with HFM for TMJ reconstruction using patient-fitted total joint prostheses and orthognathic surgery because of its bilateral nature. Patients with HFM have one side of the mandible with a normally growing condyle that rarely requires TMJ reconstruction; hence the requirement to wait until growth of that condyle is complete to achieve predictable treatment outcomes. Patients with TCS have bilateral TMJ malformation and hypoplastic growth. Therefore, both TMJs require reconstruction in conjunction with orthognathic surgery and can be performed at the age of 13 to 14 years in girls and 15 to 16 years of age in boys, with subsequent growth occurring in a vertical direction with a down and backward rotation of the maxillomandibular complex as the residual vertical maxillary and mandibular alveolar growth is completed. The occlusion should stay together.

Autogenous Tissue Grafts

There are several different sources for autogenous bone grafts that can be used to replace the condyles in HFM and TCS. These sources include (1) costochondral grafts, (2) SCGs, (3) iliac crest grafts, (4) vascularized grafts (fibula, ileum, metatarsal, or scapula), (5) posterior border of the mandible (only applicable in cases in which significant ramus is available; ie, types I and II). For growth center transplants, costochondral grafts or SCGs may provide growth potential. An SCG grows more like a mandibular condyle, whereas a costochondral graft grows more like the rib that it is.

Advantages of using autogenous bone grafts are (1) native bone is readily available, (2) growth potential (rib, SCG), (3) vascularized grafts are available (fibula, metatarsal), and (4) articular disc is attached to the graft (SCG).

Disadvantages of autogenous bone grafts are (1) they require graft harvest, significantly increasing the operating time; (2) donor site morbidity; (3) grafts are subject to physiologic loading with subsequent bone resorption; (4) grafts can bend, warp, and fracture; (5) significant dentocraniofacial deformities cannot be corrected predictably; (6) unpredictable growth; (7) difficult to control occlusion; (8) risk of ankylosis caused by the immobilization period needed for healing; and (9) possible vascular compromise at the recipient site.

Indications for condylar replacement using autogenous bone grafts include (1) absent TMJ condyle, (2) zero to 1 previous TMJ surgeries (for free grafts), (3) good vascular bed (for free grafts), (4) both hard and soft tissues are required (vascularized fibula graft), (5) growth center transplant indicated (rib or SCG), (6) custom-fitted total joint prostheses are unavailable, (7) patient preference, (8) allergy to all metals in total joint prosthesis, and (9) requires minimal repositioning of the dentoskeletal structures.

Contraindications for free bone grafts include (1) multiply operated TMJ (2 or more previous procedures); (2) connective tissue autoimmune disease or inflammatory disease present in the TMJs; (3) previously failed TMJ allografts or autogenous grafts; (4) conditions causing decreased vascularization, prolonged healing, and so forth; (5) presence of polyarthropathies; and (6) concomitant TMJ and orthognathic surgery are indicated, requiring significant movement of the dentoskeletal structures.

COSTOCHONDRAL GRAFTS (RIB)

Rib grafts have been the most popular and published technique to reconstruct the TMJ with autogenous bone graft. It is easy to harvest and stabilize to the ramus. The costochondral junction fits well into the glenoid fossa. It does have growth potential but it is unpredictable. It can have no growth, or commonly shows significant overgrowth. The elasticity and flexibility of the rib, often with thin cortex, presents a structure that when stressed or loaded excessively can bend, warp, resorb, or fracture, resulting in positional shifting of the mandible and occlusion.

STERNOCLAVICULAR GRAFTS

SCGs overall may function better than costochondral grafts for autogenous reconstruction of the TMJ because SCG has a thick cortex, lots of medullary bone, and an articular disc attached to the condylar head. The upper half of the clavicle is harvested along with the articular disc attached to the upper head of the clavicle, providing a more normally functioning condyle. For patients with HFM and TCS, it usually fits best by placement on the medial side of the ramus or along the posterior border of the mandible. The primary complication of concern is the risk of postsurgical clavicle fracture, because the donor site is significantly weakened and may take a minimum of 6 months to regain significant strength.

VERTICAL RAMUS OSTEOTOMY

Vertical ramus osteotomy with superior repositioning of the proximal segment has significant limitations as to the amount of forward movement that can be achieved, particularly in patients with HFM and TCS who often require large advancements. The vertical height of the rami in these patients is generally much shorter than normal, thus significantly limiting the application of this technique.

FIBULA AND METATARSAL VASCULARIZED GRAFTS

Vascularized fibula and metatarsal grafts have not been documented consistently for use in patients with HFM and TSC. However, the fibula graft could be a viable autogenous alternative. A vascularized fibula or metatarsal graft could be used in reconstructing these HFM and TCS cases in which there is vascular compromise from previous surgeries. The advantages of a vascularized graft are (1) native tissue, (2) vascularized graft increasing survival rates, and (3) can harvest extensive bone and soft tissue if indicated (fibula). Disadvantages for vascularized grafts are (1) unsightly scar (fibula), (2) foot deformity (metatarsal), (3) subject to physiologic loading and adaptations, (4) unpredictable outcomes for correcting significant dentofacial/craniofacial deformities, (5) may require 2 surgical teams, and (6) significantly longer surgery.

DISTRACTION OSTEOGENESIS

Distraction osteogenesis has become popular recently, particularly in treating patients with HFM. Distraction osteogenesis requires placing a distraction device, performing an osteotomy, then distraction of the segments to produce new bone, increasing ramus length and protracting the mandible forward. Advantages of this technique are (1) native bone is used, (2) no bone harvest is required, and (3) it can be a pedicled graft.

Disadvantages of distraction osteogenesis are (1) requires at least 2 operations, the first to place the device and the second to remove it; (2) difficult to control the vector of distraction; (3) significant facial scaring with extraoral placement of distraction devices; (4) significant fibrosis around mandible because of the 2 surgeries, making subsequent reconstruction surgery more difficult and potentially compromising jaw function; (5) cannot correct a significant dentocraniofacial deformity concomitantly; (6) narrow mediolateral width of the neocondyle; (7) significantly longer treatment time; (8) subject to physiologic loading and adaptations; (9) likely to require additional orthognathic surgery procedures to achieve optimal outcomes; and (10) patient compliance is important.

PATIENT-FITTED TOTAL TEMPOROMANDIBULAR JOINT PROSTHESIS

Developed originally in 1989 by Techmedica Inc (Camarillo, CA) and since 1997 manufactured by TMJ Concepts, Inc (Ventura, CA), the patient-fitted TMJ total joint prosthesis is manufactured to meet patients' specific anatomic requirements for TMJ reconstruction and mandibular advancement. CT scan data are acquired presurgery and a 3D plastic model of the patient's jaws, TMJs, and cranial base structures is produced (Fig. 5). These devices have been extensively evaluated through clinical studies.[16–22]

The TMJ Concepts total joint prosthesis has the following advantages: (1) patient-fitted device that can be used to correct major dentofacial/craniofacial deformities; (2) the ramus component has a titanium alloy shaft and a chromium cobalt alloy condylar head; (3) the patient-fitted fossa is made of a titanium shell covered with a titanium mesh with ultra-high molecular weight polyethylene

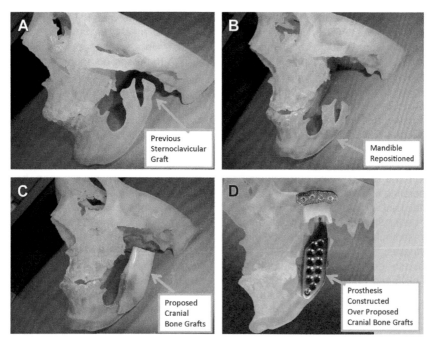

Fig. 5. Case 1. (*A*) CT scan data are acquired presurgery and a 3D plastic model of the patient's jaws, TMJs, and cranial base structures is produced. (*B*) The mandible is then reposition and the model is fixed in the new position with quick-cure acrylic. (*C*) The left ramus is simultaneously reconstructed with cranial bone grafts (pink wax-up area). This model is sent to TMJ Concepts for manufacturing of the prosthesis. (*D*) The prosthesis is manufactured over the wax-up, which represents the cranial bone grafts for simultaneous placement with the total joint prosthesis.

(UHMWPE) as the articulating surface; (4) it is metal on polyethylene articulation; (5) there is a defined posterior stop of the fossa component, which is a key component for stability in correcting significant dentofacial/craniofacial deformities; (6) osseointegration of the fossa and ramus components occurs; (7) orthognathic surgery can be done at the same operation; (8) surgeon has input for design; (9) prosthesis works in poorly vascularized recipient bed; and (10) 3D stereolithic model constructed for surgical planning and manufacturing of the patient-fitted prosthesis.

Disadvantages include (1) requires presurgical stereolithic model preparation time or virtual planning, (2) takes 6 to 8 weeks for manufacture of the device, (3) alloplastic materials with no growth potential, and (4) possible allergic reaction to materials in patients with multiple hypersensitivities.

PERIARTICULAR FAT GRAFTS

With any of the autogenous tissue grafts or the alloplastic joint replacement, the placement of fat grafts around the articulating areas of the new joint significantly improves the treatment outcomes for the following reasons: (1) the fat grafts eliminate dead space around the articulating areas, (2) prevents blood clots from forming around the grafts or total joint prostheses, (3) inhibits bone growth

and fibrosis, (4) decreases pain, and (5) increases joint function.

Wolford and colleagues[23–25] have reported a technique in which fat grafts harvested from the abdomen or buttock were packed around the articulating components of the total joint prosthesis. This technique significantly decreased the postoperative incidence of peri-implant fibrosis and heterotopic/reactive bone formation. Patients with fat grafts did better clinically with less pain and increased jaw function compared with similar patients reconstructed without fat grafts. Before the use of fat grafts, approximately 35% of patients with total joint prostheses required additional surgery to remove heterotopic/reactive bone and dense fibrosis that developed around the prostheses. Using the fat grafts has reduced reoperation to less than 2% for heterotrophic bone and fibrosis. Wolford and colleagues[23–25] also described the use of fat grafts to replace the deficient soft tissues on the ipsilateral side of the face in patients with HFM.[26]

COMPARATIVE STUDIES: AUTOGENOUS BONE GRAFTS VERSUS ALLOPLASTIC TOTAL TEMPOROMANDIBULAR JOINT PROSTHESIS

There have been comparison studies of autogenous tissues versus total joint prostheses. Henry and Wolford[27] in 1993 presented a comparative study of 107 patients exposed to Proplast Teflon implants (Vitek, Inc, Houston, TX). Various autogenous tissue grafts were used to reconstruct the TMJs (eg, ribs, SCG, conchal cartilage, dermal, temporal muscle/fascia grafts) with extremely high failure rates (only 8%–31% success). The Techmedica total joint prosthesis had an 86% success rate. Freitas and colleagues[28] compared costochondral grafts, SCGs, and total joint prostheses. The patients with total joint prostheses had better objective and subjective outcomes compared with the patients with autogenous tissues. The operating time was significantly reduced with the total joint prostheses, and there was significantly better skeletal and occlusal stability with maxillomandibular advancements with the total joint prostheses.

McPhillips and colleagues[29] compared outcomes for ankylosed patients using costochondral grafts, SCGs, and total joint prostheses. The costochondral grafts had no fat placed around the periarticulating area and these cases reankylosed. For the SCGs, two-thirds of the patients had fat grafts placed around the articulating area of the joint and this resulted in no recurrence of ankylosis. A third of the SCGs did not have fat placed around them and they reankylosed. In the total joint prostheses cases, all patients had fat placed around the articulating area. There was no reankylosis or mandibular relapse, but there was significant improvement of jaw function.

Saeed and colleagues[30] did a comparative study of costochondral grafts versus to total joint prostheses. There was a significantly greater rate of reoperation following costochondral grafts (55% of the patients required reoperation) compared with the 6 patients (12%) who received total joint prostheses. The patients with total joint prostheses had better objective and subjective outcomes. The investigators recommended total joint prostheses in cases of ankylosis, multiply operated joints, or previous alloplastic failure.

SURGICAL MANAGEMENT OF PATIENTS WITH HEMIFACIAL MICROSOMIA AND TREACHER COLLINS SYNDROME

The most consistently predictable treatment outcomes functionally and esthetically for the patients with HFM (type IIB and III) as well as TCS are achieved by reconstructing the TMJs and advancing the maxillomandibular complex in a counterclockwise direction on the affected sides, with a patient-fitted (custom-made) total joint prosthesis and orthognathic surgery.[31–37] The TMJ Concepts system is the prosthesis of choice

because of the material selection, patient-fitted design to meet the patient's specific anatomic requirements, presence of a defined posterior stop in the fossa component, and osseointegration of the fossa and mandibular components. For patients with HFM, a contralateral mandibular ramus sagittal split osteotomy is performed to aid in repositioning the mandible, and the indicated maxillary osteotomies are completed as well as any other adjunctive procedures (eg, turbinectomies, nasoseptoplasty, genioplasty, rhinoplasty). All procedures can be done at 1 operation, or separated into 2 or more operations if the surgeon prefers. Additional secondary reconstruction procedures to correct residual bony and soft tissue deficiencies may be necessary in more complex HFM and TCS cases using bone grafts, synthetic bone, alloplastic implants, and so forth to build up the residual deformed skeletal structures as well as soft tissue reconstruction to fill out the soft tissue defects using fat grafts,[26] tissue flaps, free vascularized grafts, and so on.

TRADITIONAL PRESURGICAL PLANNING

Traditional presurgical preparation requires the surgeon to reposition the mandible on the 3D model to its predetermined new position based on the clinical evaluation, dental model analysis, and the prediction tracing. The mandible is usually repositioned downward and forward, advancing in a counterclockwise direction decreasing the mandibular occlusal plane angle, and transversely leveling. The mandible is fixed in its new position with quick-cure acrylic (see **Fig. 3**). Recontouring of the ramus and base of skull is completed if indicated. The model is sent to TMJ Concepts, and the patient-fitted total joint prosthesis is manufactured, consisting of a mandibular/condylar component and a fossa component. The TMJ Concepts prosthesis delivers appropriate functional and esthetic results with excellent stability.[16–22] The technique of using the total joint prosthesis for TMJ reconstruction and simultaneous mandibular advancement with counterclockwise rotation of the maxillomandibular complex was developed by Wolford[22] in 1990 and was first used for HFM in 1997.

Before surgery, dental models mounted on an anatomic articulator are used to replicate the mandibular repositioning performed on the 3D plastic model for construction of the intermediate surgical stabilizing occlusal splint necessary for precise positioning of the mandible at surgery. The maxilla is sectioned if required and placed into the best occlusal fit. If the maxilla is segmentalized, then a palatal splint is constructed for surgical stabilization.

VIRTUAL SURGICAL PLANNING

VSP is currently available to aid in performing the preliminary surgery by reproducing the repositioning of the mandible and maxilla on a computer model and incorporating the repositioned jaw structures into the 3D model, eliminating the need for the mandibular repositioning on the 3D model by the surgeon as well as eliminating the requirement for articulator-mounted dental model surgery.[38] The VSP model is used for manufacturing the prostheses. Two weeks before surgery, final dental models are prepared, which usually requires 1 mandibular dental model and 2 maxillary models if the maxilla is to be segmentalized (one sectioned and used to establish the surgical occlusion and an uncut model). These models are sent to the VSP company for incorporation into the computer model and construction of the surgical splints. See chapter 9 for specific details in VSP.

SURGICAL SEQUENCING

The surgical sequencing used by the authors for treating patients with HFM is outlined in **Box 1**. Because HFM cases usually benefit from counterclockwise rotation of the maxillomandibular complex to get the best functional and esthetic outcomes,[31–37] repositioning the mandible first with the total joint prosthesis and contralateral sagittal split osteotomy (before the maxillary osteotomies are performed) simplifies the model surgery and splint construction, and improves the accuracy of the patient's surgery and outcome compared with the traditional orthognathic surgical sequencing of performing the maxillary osteotomies first.[36] Performing the counterclockwise rotation of the mandible first creates posterior open bites, being greater on the ipsilateral side as the transverse cant of the mandibular occlusal plane is also corrected. If segmentalization of the maxilla is required to optimize the occlusion, a palatal splint is indicated to stabilize the upper arch and allow maximum interdigitation of the occlusion as the maxilla is stabilized.[28]

The surgical sequencing for patients with TCS is outlined in **Box 2**. These patients benefit from counterclockwise rotation of the maxillomandibular complex to maximize the functional and esthetic outcomes as well as open the oropharyngeal airway to a normal dimension, correcting the sleep apnea issues that commonly accompany this syndrome.

Box 1
Surgical sequencing for HFM

1. Contralateral disc repositioning if displaced (Mitek anchor technique)
2. Mobilize ipsilateral mandible (through preauricular or endaural and submandibular incisions)
3. Contralateral mandibular ramus sagittal split osteotomy
4. Mandibular counterclockwise rotation, intermediate splint, MMF
5. Rigid fixation to contralateral mandibular ramus osteotomy, close incision
6. Ipsilateral placement of TMJ Concepts total joint prosthesis
7. Pack fat graft around articulation area of prosthesis (harvest fat from abdomen or buttock)
8. Close extraoral incisions
9. Maxillary osteotomies and mobilization, placement of palatal stabilizing splint if indicated
10. Intranasal procedures if indicated (eg, turbinectomies, nasoseptoplasty)
11. MMF, maxillary stabilization with bone plates and bone or synthetic bone grafting
12. Remove MMF, place light elastics
13. Other indicated procedures (eg, genioplasty, rhinoplasty, facial augmentation)

Abbreviation: MMF, maxillomandibular fixation.

Patients with HFM, and particularly TCS, commonly have sleep apnea issues as a result of the retruded mandible, decreased oropharyngeal airway, and/or nasal airway obstruction. Counterclockwise rotation of the maxillomandibular complex with advancement of the mandible is highly effective and predictable in opening the oropharyngeal airway. In conjunction with correcting any nasal airway obstruction (eg, turbinectomies, nasoseptoplasty) these patients have significant improvement in the airway and elimination of sleep apnea after surgery.[39–41]

SURGICAL PROTOCOL

The surgical procedures are done under general anesthesia with nasoendotracheal intubation. The HFM surgical sequencing is outlined in **Box 1**. For patients with HFM with contralateral TMJ disc displacement, an endaural incision is made and the disc repositioned and stabilized

Box 2
Surgical sequencing for TCS

1. Bilateral mandibular condylectomy and co-ronoidectomy (via endaural or preauricular incisions)

2. Detach masseteric and medial pterygoid muscles (via submandibular incisions)

3. Mobilize mandible with counterclockwise rotation

4. Placement of intermediate splint, MMF

5. Bilateral placement of TMJ Concepts total joint prosthesis

7. Pack fat graft around articulation area of the prostheses (harvest fat from abdomen or buttock)

8. Close extraoral incisions

9. Maxillary osteotomies and mobilization, placement of palatal stabilizing splint if indicated

10. Intranasal procedures if indicated (eg, tur-binectomies, nasoseptoplasty)

11. MMF, maxillary stabilization with bone plates and autogenous bone or synthetic bone grafting

12. Remove MMF, place light elastics

13. Other indicated procedures (eg, genio-plasty, rhinoplasty, facial augmentation)

The soft tissues surrounding the mandible (skin and muscles) are usually not a problem because they can stretch to accommodate large advancements. Any bony modifications to the temporal bone or ramus/body of the mandible are completed as determined from the 3D model surgery work-up.

The oral cavity is entered and a contralateral mandibular ramus sagittal split osteotomy is completed using the Wolford modified technique.[26,44] The mandible is mobilized and a pre-fabricated intermediate occlusal splint is placed to position the mandible into its final predetermined position. Maxillomandibular fixation (MMF) is applied and the contralateral mandibular sagittal split osteotomy is stabilized with a bone plate and screws, the incision closed, and mouth resealed with a Tegaderm dressing. The surgeons change gloves. The fossa component of the patient-fitted TMJ Concepts prosthesis is placed through the endaural/preauricular incision and secured to the temporal bone with 4 to 5 screws of 2-mm diameter and 4-mm length. The mandibular component is inserted through the submandibular incision, and the condyle seated into the fossa component against the posterior flange and secured to the ramus/body with 8 to 9 bicortical screws of 2-mm diameter. Fat is harvested from the abdomen through a suprapubic or umbilicus incision, or from the buttock, and packed around the fossa/condyle articulating area to prevent heterotrophic bone and scar tissue formation.[23–25] The incisions are closed.

The MMF and the occlusal splint are removed. Through a maxillary vestibular incision, the maxillary osteotomies are completed. The maxilla is downfractured, mobilized, and segmented when indicated between the cuspids and lateral incisors, and down the midline of the palate. The maxillary palatal splint is secured in place.[37] Intranasal procedures such as turbinectomies and/or nasal septoplasty are performed if indicated to eliminate preexisting nasal airway obstruction. The new occlusion is established and secured with MMF. Four bone plates and screws are used to stabilize the maxilla with at least 2 screws above and 2 screws below the osteotomy site for each plate. Autogenous bone or porous block hydroxyapatite (Inter-pore 200, Interpore Inc, Irvine, CA) grafts are placed into the osseous gaps in the lateral maxillary walls. An alar base cinch suture is placed to redefine nasal width, and the incision closed in a V-Y fashion.[46] Adjunctive procedures such as genioplasty and rhinoplasty are then completed. MMF is removed and light elastics applied to guide the occlusion and decrease stress on the muscles of mastication.

with the Mitek Mini Anchor (Mitek Products Inc, Westwood, MA) technique.[42,43] The ipsilateral side is approached via an endaural or preauricular incision. The zygomatic arch may be absent as well as the glenoid fossa, therefore the dissection is carried down to the temporal bone anterior to the internal meatus and extended medially beneath the cranial base to develop a foundation to place the patient-fitted fossa component.

An ipsilateral submandibular incision is made, exposing the hypoplastic ramus, and the hypoplastic pterygomasseteric sling is reflected off the mandible. A subperiosteal tunnel is created over the ramus to connect to the base of the temporal bone. The hypoplastic temporalis muscle, if present, is reflected from the remnant of the coronoid process. The ipsilateral mandible is then mobilized so it can be repositioned downward and advanced to its new position; this is a critical aspect for the success of the surgery. If the mandible is not completely stripped of all its attachments and fully mobilized, an adequate position of the mandible will not be achieved.

Case 1

This 15-year-old girl was born with left-sided Goldenhar HFM, Kaban type III, left transverse facial cleft, and cleft palate (**Figs. 6A–C and 7A–C**). She had several previous surgeries, including repair of a left transverse facial cleft at 5 months and cleft palate repair at 1 year. An SCG and cranial bone grafts for reconstruction of the left ramus and TMJ joint were performed at age 6 years. Although the graft took, it did not grow. Presurgery maximum incisal opening (MIO) was 33 mm; right excursion, 1 mm; left excursion, 5 mm; facial pain/headache, 0; TMJ

pain, 0; jaw function, 1; diet, 1; and disability, 0. AP chin deficiency was 20 mm (**Fig. 8A**), mandibular dental midline was 7 mm, and chin midline was 14 mm to the left. Presurgical orthodontics aligned and leveled the arches. At age 15 years, she was surgically treated with (1) left TMJ reconstruction and mandibular advancement counterclockwise with TMJ Concepts patient-fitted total joint prosthesis (see **Fig. 5**), (2) simultaneous reconstruction of the left ramus with cranial bone grafts (see **Fig. 5C**), (3) left TMJ fat graft harvested from the abdomen, (4) right mandibular ramus sagittal split osteotomy, (5) multiple maxillary osteotomies, and (6) nasal turbinectomies

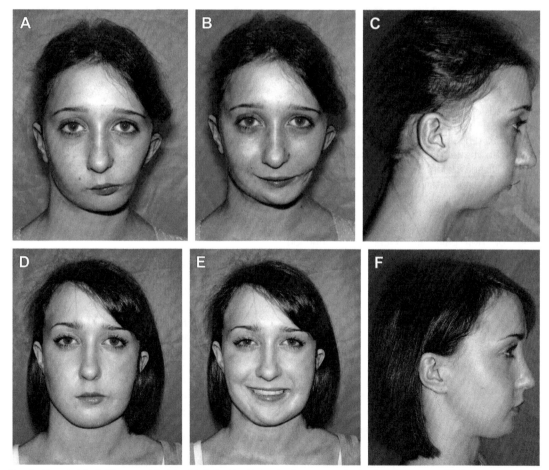

Fig. 6. Case 1: (A–C) 15-year-old girl with left-sided HFM (Kaban type III). She has (1) repaired left transverse facial cleft, (2) maxillomandibular hypoplasia and asymmetry, (3) absence of left TMJ with previously placed SCG that failed to grow, and (4) nasal airway obstruction secondary to hypertrophied turbinates. The patient underwent surgery for (1) left mandibular ramus reconstruction with cranial bone grafts, (2) left TMJ reconstruction and left mandibular advancement in a counterclockwise rotation with TMJ Concepts total joint prosthesis (pogonion advanced 18 mm), (3) right mandibular ramus osteotomy, (4) left TMJ fat graft, (5) multiple maxillary osteotomies for counterclockwise advancement, and (6) bilateral partial inferior turbinectomies. Second stage surgery included (1) osseous augmentation genioplasty (9 mm), (2) left facial augmentation with a fat graft, and (3) repositioning of the left ear. (D–F) The patient is seen 4 years after surgery with improved jaw function and facial esthetics.

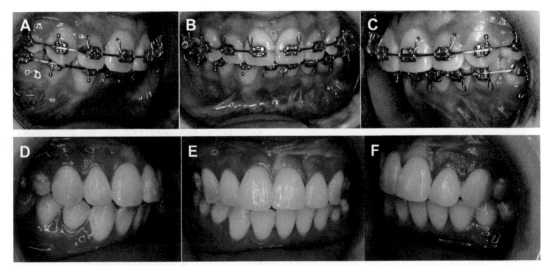

Fig. 7. Case 1. (*A–C*) Before surgery, this patient had a class II end-on occlusion and transverse cant of the occlusal plane. (*D–F*) At 4 years after surgery the patient has a stable class I occlusion.

(see **Fig. 8**B). A secondary surgical stage was performed at age 16 years that included (1) osseous AP augmentation genioplasty (9 mm), (2) vertical repositioning of the left ear, and (3) fat graft to the left side of the face to augment the soft tissue defect (**Fig. 9**).[37] The patient is seen at 4 years after surgery (see **Figs. 6**D–F and **7**D–F) with improved facial balance and function; MIO was 35 mm; right lateral excursion, 1 mm; left excursion, 3 mm; no facial pain/headaches or TMJ pain; and facial nerve function was unchanged compared with presurgery.

Case 2

This 30-year-old woman was born with TCS (**Figs. 10**A–C and **11**A–C). She had been in orthodontic treatment of 16 months with 4 first bicuspid extractions before initial surgical consultation. She had moderate TMJ pain and headaches, and MIO of 33 mm with right excursion of 1.5 mm and left excursion of 3.5 mm. She had an oropharyngeal airway of 2 mm (normal 11 mm) and sleep apnea. Her diagnosis was (1) TCS; (2) bilateral TMJ condylar deformation, arthritis, and articular disc dislocation; (3) mandibular AP and posterior

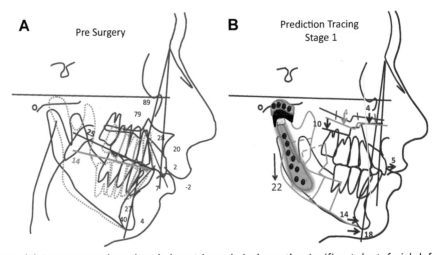

Fig. 8. Case 1. (*A*) Pretreatment lateral cephalometric analysis shows the significant dentofacial deformity with maxillary and mandibular hypoplasia as well as vertical asymmetry. The numbers refer to Wolford's cephalometric analysis.[31,32] (*B*) The prediction tracing shows the surgical treatment plan for stage 1 surgery. The numbers represent the surgical movements in millimeters. Arrows indicate direction of movement.

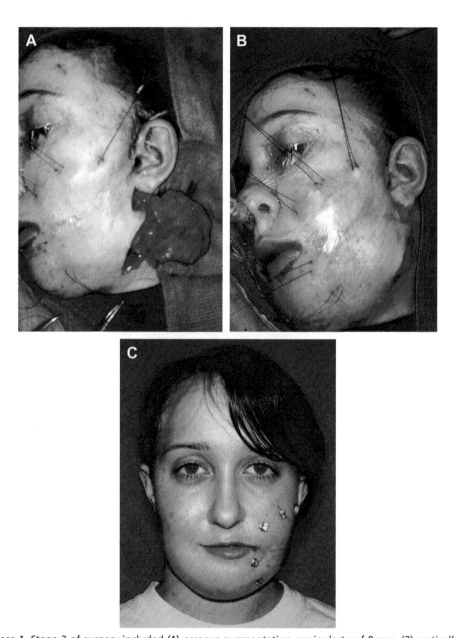

Fig. 9. Case 1. Stage 2 of surgery included (1) osseous augmentation genioplasty of 9 mm, (2) vertically repositioning the left ear, and (3) left facial augmentation with fat graft harvested from the abdomen. (*A*) The dissection for the recipient site is created with a facelift approach. Sutures are placed at the margins of the dissection in a mattress fashion through the fat graft to aide in delivery and for postsurgical stabilization. (*B*) The graft is positioned by pulling the sutures. The sutures are tied over cotton bolsters. (*C*) The patient is seen 1 week after surgery.

vertical hypoplasia; (4) maxillary posterior vertical hypoplasia; (5) high occlusal plane angle; (6) AP microgenia; (7) class II end-on occlusion; (8) absent zygomatic arches; and (9) sleep apnea (see **Figs. 10**A–C and **11**A–C; **Fig. 12**A). Treatment consisted of (1) bilateral TMJ reconstruction and mandibular advancement with counterclockwise rotation with TMJ Concepts total joint prostheses (pogonion advanced 25 mm before chin augmentation), (2) multiple maxillary osteotomies for counterclockwise rotation, (3) bilateral TMJ fat grafts (harvested from abdomen), (4) bilateral coronoidotomies, (5) bony genioplasty to advance the chin 10 mm (pogonion advanced a total of 35 mm) (see **Fig. 12**B), and (6) postsurgical orthodontics to finish and retain the occlusion.[45] The

150

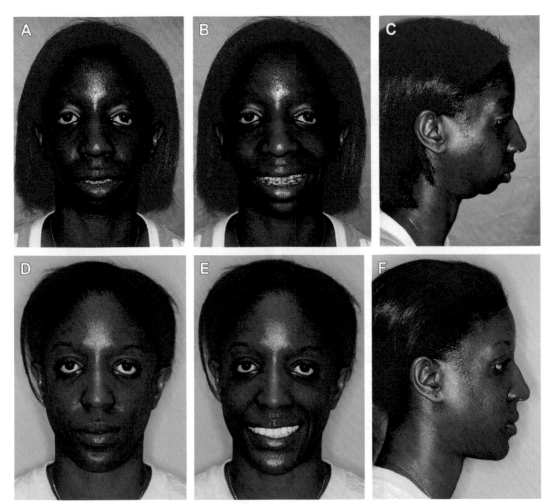

Fig. 10. Case 2. (*A–C*) A 30-year-old woman with TCS before treatment. Diagnosis included (1) TCS, (2) severely retruded mandible, (3) posterior maxillary vertical hypoplasia, (4) AP microgenia, (5) class II end-on occlusion (after 16 months of orthodontics with 4 first bicuspid extractions), and (6) severely decreased oropharyngeal airway. Surgery performed in a single stage included (1) bilateral TMJ reconstruction and mandibular advancement in a counterclockwise rotation (pogonion advanced 25 mm), (2) multiple maxillary osteotomies for counterclockwise rotation, (3) bilateral coronoidotomies, (4) bilateral TMJ fat grafts (harvested from the abdomen), (5) osseous augmentation genioplasty of 10 mm (pogonion advanced a total of 35 mm). (*D–F*) The patient is seen 4 years after surgery, showing improved function and occlusion, establishment of good facial balance, as well as elimination of pain and sleep apnea.

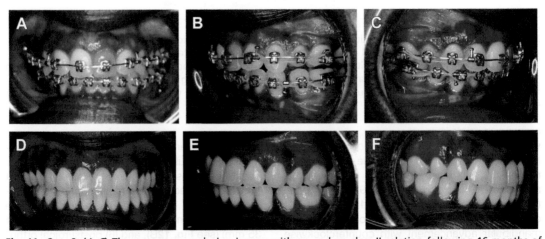

Fig. 11. Case 2. (*A–C*) The presurgery occlusion is seen with an end-on class II relation following 16 months of orthodontics that included 4 first bicuspid extractions. (*D–F*) The patient is seen 4 years after surgery with a class I stable occlusion.

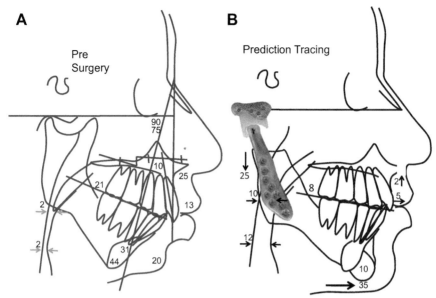

Fig. 12. Case 2. (*A*) Cephalometric analysis shows the severe jaw deformity with high occlusal plane angle of 21° (normal 8°) facial morphology and severely decreased oropharyngeal airway. Numbers refer to angular and linear measurements using Wolford's cephalometric analysis.[31,32] (*B*) The surgical plan includes counterclockwise rotation of the mandible with TMJ Concepts total joint prostheses, maxillary counterclockwise rotation, and a genioplasty, with pogonion projected to advance 35 mm. Numbers with arrows represent surgical change in millimeters.

patient is seen 4 years after surgery with good stability, function, and esthetics (see **Figs. 10**D–F and **11**D–F). MIO is 41 mm and excursions are 1 mm to the right and 2 mm to the left. She has no pain or headaches and normal facial nerve function. She has not proceeded with the second stage of surgery for orbital bony and soft tissue reconstruction because of financial reasons.

SURGICAL OUTCOME EXPECTATIONS

Kaban and colleagues[4] advocated early treatment of patients with type I, IIa HMF, and for some patients with type IIb HMF with mandibular osteotomies. The costochondral graft has been popular for reconstruction of the ipsilateral TMJ in young patients with type IIb and III HFM because of the growth center at the costochondral junction and for reconstruction of the glenoid fossa.[8–11] However, other investigators have shown that rib graft growth is unpredictable with either no growth or significant overgrowth, creating a deformity that required additional surgery.[5,6]

Wolford and colleagues[9] used the SCG to reconstruct the absent TMJ and to lengthen the mandible on the affected side. The upper half of the clavicle and associated portion of the articular disc were harvested. The mandible was advanced as predetermined and the graft was secured against the medial side of the residual ramus/

body secured with bone screws and the condylar head seated against the base of the skull. This grafting system provided a better normal growth potential and stability compared with a rib graft. Placing the graft on the medial side of the ramus and against the skull base eliminated the need for the bony reconstruction of the glenoid fossa. Wolford and colleagues[9] recommended the use of the SCG after the age of 6 years, because the clavicle is too small at an earlier age to provide adequate bone for grafting the mandible as well as enough integrity to support the remaining clavicle during the healing phase.

Wolford and colleagues[47] evaluated 6 patients with HFM treated with the surgical protocol. Average age at surgery was 23.5 years (range, 14–39 years) and average follow-up was 6 years 2 months (range, 1–11.4 years). For all subjective parameters, including facial pain and headaches, TMJ pain, jaw function, diet, and disability, all patients improved or remained the same. No patients were worse in any of the subjective parameters after surgery. Incisal opening average at T1 was 36.3 mm and at T3 was 39.2 mm. Excursive movements decreased moderately. One patient had a presurgery ankylosed ipsilateral TMJ as a result of failed previous rib grafts for TMJ reconstructive surgeries. Although he significantly improved in all parameters, including total elimination of pain, he retained limitations in jaw function, diet, and disability. For all patients, the mean surgical changes showed that the forward horizontal movement of anterior nasal spine was 1.3 mm; upper incisor tip advanced 7.4 mm; lower incisor tip, 8.9 mm; point B, 14.8 mm; pogonion, 18.6 mm; and menton, 17.5 mm. The occlusal plane angle decreased by a mean of 12.3°. Postsurgical stability analysis showed that point A, posterior nasal spine, and upper incisor tip had moved approximately 1 mm posteriorly at long-term follow-up. All mandibular anatomic points remained stable, as did the occlusal plane angle, with virtually no change at 6 years after surgery.

The longevity of the TMJ Concepts total joint prosthesis is unknown. Mercuri and colleagues[20] in 1995 reported a multicenter study on 215 patients with multiply operated TMJs (363 joints) reconstructed with the TMJ Concepts prosthesis. The results at 2 years after surgery showed statistically significant favorable changes in many subjective and objective evaluations. In 2003, Wolford and colleagues[19] published a 5-year follow-up study on 36 patients with 65 TMJs reconstructed with the Techmedica/TMJ Concepts total joint prosthesis. The overall success rate for long-term occlusal and skeletal stability after reconstruction was 90%, and pain reduction was recorded in 89% of patients. These study data contributed significantly to US Food and Drug Administration approval of the TMJ Concepts total joint prosthesis.[48]

In 2009, we published a series of articles[16–18] on the use of TMJ Concepts total joint prostheses and simultaneous counterclockwise rotation of the maxillomandibular complex to correct severe TMJ disorder or failed previous TMJ surgeries and coexisting dentofacial deformities. All patients were operated by the senior author (LMW). There were 47 women with an average follow-up of 40.6 months. Part I of the series[16] evaluated postsurgery skeletal and occlusal stability. The mandible was advanced an average of 18 mm at pogonion and the occlusal plane was decreased an average of 15°. At longest follow-up, the skeletal and occlusal structures remained stable with no statistically significant changes.

In part III of the series[18] the same patient group was evaluated for long-term pain and jaw function results. Many of the patients (22 of 47) had multiple previous failed TMJ surgeries. Facial pain/headache decreased 2.8 points, representing an improvement percentage (IP) of 43%. TMJ pain decreased 3.2 points, IP 52%; jaw function improved 2.3 points, IP 37%; diet improved 2.2 points, IP 39%; and disability decreased 2.1 points, IP 47%. Patients with 0 to 1 previous TMJ surgeries had a 73% reduction in pain, 37% increase in jaw function, and 61% decrease

in disability. The fewer previous TMJ surgeries, the better the surgical outcome. These results are consistent with our HFM study[47] in which all patients improved or remained the same in all subjective parameters: facial pain/headaches decreased 2.3 points, IP 100%; TMJ pain 1.7 points, IP 100%; jaw function improved 2.3 points, IP 48%; diet improved 2.3 points, IP 53%; and disability improved 1.6 points, IP 70%. In our HFM study, 4 of the 6 patients had previous ipsilateral TMJ reconstruction with rib grafts or SCGs, and only patient #3, who had 6 previous surgeries with repeated ankylosis of the rib grafts, had increased subjective results for jaw function, diet, and disability, but who was significantly improved compared with the presurgery status.

SUMMARY

Many options have been proposed for surgical correction of HFM as well as patients with TCS. The most popular autogenous bone grafts used for treatment of ipsilateral (HFM) or bilateral (TCS) mandibular/condylar hypoplasia or aplasia includes rib grafts and SCG. Distraction osteogenesis has also become popular for lengthening the hypoplastic mandible. In our extensive experience, autogenous bone grafts are not reliable in providing predictable treatment outcomes relative to stability of skeletal and occlusal relationships, because significant relapse can be expected related to graft flexibility, extended healing time, and biological effects of graft loading and response. In addition, there can be significant donor and recipient site complications. It is difficult to control the vectors in distraction techniques and it is difficult to achieve decent functional, occlusal, and esthetic results without additional surgery.

TMJ Concepts patient-fitted total joint prosthesis in conjunction with orthognathic surgery for TMJ and jaw reconstruction is a valid option for patients with HFM because (1) there is less morbidity because no bone grafting donor site is required, resulting in shorter operating time; (2) outcomes are highly predictable relative to stability and TMJ and occlusal function, as well as esthetics; (3) bony reconstruction of glenoid fossa is not required; and (4) TMJ Concepts total joint prostheses is a patient-fitted device that meets the patient's specific anatomic requirements for mandibular advancement, vertical lengthening, and TMJ reconstruction. Potential risks and concerns with the use of total joint prostheses include (1) the functional service life of TMJ total joint prostheses is unknown, but our recent study[47] evaluated 56 patients with 19 to 24 years follow-up, with improved function and quality of life compared to presurgery, all prostheses were still in place and none removed related to material wear or failure, (2) surgical risks associated with TMJ reconstruction, (3) infection, and (4) development of hypersensitivity to the materials in the prostheses.

It is our opinion that, whenever possible, delayed 1-stage reconstruction during the adolescent stages of the deformity, using an alloplastic device in conjunction with orthognathic surgery, provides the patient with a better, more predictable, and more functional result than multiple staged autogenous reconstructions done early. No other surgical technique is able to provide the amount of mandibular advancement, ramus lengthening, and stability necessary to correct the severe deformities in this patient population.

REFERENCES

1. Grabb WC. The first and second branchial arch syndrome. Plast Reconstr Surg 1965;36:485.
2. Gorlin RJ, Cohen MM Jr, Hemekam RC. Syndromes of the head and neck. 4th edition. New York: Oxford Universe Press; 2001. p. 790–7.
3. Pruzansky S. Not all dwarfed mandibles are alike. Birth Defects. Original Articles Series 1969;1(2):120.
4. Kaban LB, Moses MH, Mulliken JB. Surgical correction of hemifacial microsomia in the growing child. Plast Reconstr Surg 1988;82:9.
5. Ware WH, Brown SL. Growth centre transplantation to replace mandibular condyles. J Maxillofac Surg 1981;9:50.
6. Peltomaki T, Quevedo LA, Jeldes G, et al. Histology of surgically removed overgrown osteochondral rib grafts. J Craniomaxillofac Surg 2002;30:355.
7. Munro IR, Phillips JH, Griffin G. Growth after construction of the temporomandibular joint in children with hemifacial microsomia. Cleft Palate J 1989;26:303.
8. Mulliken JB, Ferraro NF, Vento RA. A retrospective analysis of growth of the constructed condyle-ramus in children with hemifacial microsomia. Cleft Palate J 1989;26:312.
9. Wolford LM, Cottrell DA, Henry CH. Sternoclavicular grafts for temporomandibular joint reconstruction. J Oral Maxillofac Surg 1994;52:119.
10. McCarty JG, Schreiber J, Karp N, et al. Lengthening of the human mandible by gradual distraction. Plast Reconstr Surg 1992;89:1.
11. Rachmiel A, Levy M, Laufer D. Lengthening of the mandible by distraction osteogenesis: report of cases. J Oral Maxillofac Surg 1995;53:838.
12. Riolo ML, Moyers RE, McNamara JA, et al. An atlas of craniofacial growth: cephalometric standards from the University School Growth Study, The University of Michigan. Ann Arbor (MI): University of Michigan; 1974. p. 105–6.
13. Wolford LM, Karras SC, Mehra P. Considerations for orthognathic surgery during growth, part 1: mandibular deformities. Am J Orthod Dentofacial Orthop 2001;119:95.
14. Wolford LM, Karras SC, Mehra P. Considerations for orthognathic surgery during growth, part 2: maxillary deformities. Am J Orthod Dentofacial Orthop 2001;119:102.
15. Wolford LM. Facial asymmetry: diagnosis and treatment considerations. In: Fonseca RJ, Marciani RD, Turvey TA, editors. Oral and maxillofacial surgery, vol. III, 2nd edition. Philadelphia: WB Saunders; 2008. p. 272–315.
16. Coleta KE, Wolford LM, Gonçalves JR, et al. Maxillomandibular counter-clockwise rotation and mandibular advancement with TMJ Concepts total joint prostheses, 2009 concepts total joint prostheses: part I–skeletal and dental stability. Int J Oral Maxillofac Surg 2009;38:126.
17. Coleta KE, Wolford LM, Gonçalves JR, et al. Maxillomandibular counter-clockwise rotation and mandibular advancement with TMJ Concepts total joint prostheses: part II–airway changes and stability. Int J Oral Maxillofac Surg 2009;38:228.
18. Pinto LP, Wolford LM, Buschang PH, et al. Maxillo-mandibular counter-clockwise rotation and mandibular advancement with TMJ Concepts total joint prostheses: part III–pain and dysfunction outcomes. Int J Oral Maxillofac Surg 2009;38:326.
19. Wolford LM, Pitta MC, Reiche-Fischel O, et al. TMJ Concepts/Techmedica custom-made TMJ total joint prosthesis: 5-year follow-up. Int J Oral Maxillofac Surg 2003;32:268.
20. Mercuri LG, Wolford LM, Sanders B, et al. Long-term follow-up of the CAD/CAM patient fitted total temporomandibular joint reconstruction system. J Oral Maxillofac Surg 2002;60:1440.
21. Mehra P, Wolford LM, Baran S, et al. Single-stage comprehensive surgical treatment of the rheumatoid arthritis temporomandibular joint patient. J Oral Maxillofac Surg 2009;67:1859.
22. Wolford LM, Cottrell DA, Henry CH. Temporomandibular joint reconstruction of the complex patient with the Techmedica custom-made total joint prosthesis. J Oral Maxillofac Surg 1994;52:2.
23. Wolford LM, Karras SC. Autologous fat transplantation around temporomandibular joint total joint prostheses: preliminary treatment outcomes. J Oral Maxillofac Surg 1997;55:245.
24. Wolford LM, Morales-Ryan CA, Garcia-Morales P, et al. Autologous fat grafts placed around temporomandibular joint total joint prostheses to prevent heterotopic bone formation. Proc (Bayl Univ Med Cent) 2008;21:248.

25. Wolford LM, Cassano DS. Autologous fat grafts around temporomandibular joint (TMJ) total joint prostheses to prevent heterotopic bone. In: Shiffman MA, editor. Autologous fat transfer. Berlin; Heidelberg (Germany): Springer-Verlag; 2010. p. 361–82.

26. Reiche-Fischel O, Wolford LM, Pitta M. Facial contour reconstruction using an autologous free fat graft: a case report with 18-year follow-up. J Ora Surg 2000;58:103.

27. Henry CH, Wolford LM. Treatment outcomes for temporomandibular joint reconstruction after Proplast-Teflon implant failure. J Oral Maxillofac Surg 1993;51(4):352–8.

28. Freitas RZ, Pitta MC, Wolford LM. The use of cranial bone grafts in jaw and craniofacial anomalies: results and outcomes. J Oral Maxillofac Surg 1998; 56(Suppl 1):97.

29. McPhillips A, Wolford LM, Rodrigues DB. SAPHO syndrome with TMJ involvement: review of the literature and case presentation. Int J Oral Maxillofac Surg 2010;39(12):1160–7.

30. Saeed NR, Kent JN. A retrospective study of the costochondral graft in TMJ reconstruction. Int J Oral Maxillofac Surg 2003;32(6):606–9.

31. Wolford LM, Fields RT. Diagnosis and treatment planning for orthognathic surgery. In: Fonseca RJ, Betts NJ, Turvey T, editors. Oral and maxillofacial surgery, vol. 2. Philadelphia: WB Saunders; 2000. p. 24–55.

32. Wolford LM. Surgical planning in orthognathic surgery (chapter 60). In: Booth PW, Schendel SA, Hausamen JE, editors. Maxillofacial surgery, vol. 2. St Louis (MO): Churchill Livingstone; 2007. p. 1155–210.

33. Wolford LM, Chemello PD, Hilliard FW. Occlusal plane alteration in orthognathic surgery. J Oral Maxillofac Surg 1993;51:730.

34. Wolford LM, Chemello PD, Hilliard FW. Occlusal plane alteration in orthognathic surgery-part I: effects on function and esthetics. Am J Orthod Dentofacial Orthop 1994;106:304.

35. Chemello PD, Wolford LM, Buschang MS. Occlusal plane alteration in orthognathic surgery-part II: long-term stability of results. Am J Orthod Dentofacial Orthop 1994;106:434.

36. Cottrell DA, Wolford LM. Altered orthognathic surgical sequencing and a modified approach to model surgery. J Oral Maxillofac Surg 1994;52:1010.

37. Wolford LM. Post surgical patient management. In: Fonseca RJ, editor. Oral and maxillofacial surgery. Philadelphia: WB Saunders; 2008. p. 396–418. ·

38. Movahed R, Teschke M, Wolford LM. Protocol for concomitant temporomandibular joint custom-fitted total joint reconstruction and orthognathic surgery utilizing computer-assisted surgical simulation. J Oral Maxillofac Surg 2013;71(12):2123–9.

39. Mehra P, Wolford LM. Surgical management of obstructive sleep apnea. Proc (Bayl Univ Med Cent) 2000;13:338.

40. Mehra P, Downie M, Pitta MC, et al. Pharyngeal airway space changes after counterclockwise rotation of the maxillo mandibular complex. Am J Orthod Dentofacial Orthop 2001;120:154.

41. Goncalves JR, Buschang PH, Goncalves DG, et al. Postsurgical stability of oropharyngeal airway changes following counter-clockwise maxillomandibular advancement surgery. J Oral Maxillofac Surg 2006;64:755.

42. Wolford LM, Cottrell DA, Karras SC. Mitek mini anchor in maxillofacial surgery. Proceedings of SMST-94, the First International Conference on Shape Memory and Superelastic Technologies. Monterey (CA): MIAS; 1995. p. 477–82.

43. Mehra P, Wolford LM. The Mitek mini anchor for TMJ disc repositioning: surgical technique and results. Int J Oral Maxillofac Surg 2001;30:497.

44. Wolford LM, Davis WM Jr. The mandibular inferior border split: a modification in the sagittal split osteotomy. J Oral Maxillofac Surg 1990;48:92.

45. Wolford LM. Clinical indications for simultaneous TMJ and orthognathic surgery. Cranio 2007;25:273.

46. Guymon M, Crosby DR, Wolford LM. The alar base cinch suture to control nasal width in maxillary osteotomies. Int J Adult Orthodon Orthognath Surg 1988;2:89.

47. Wolford LM, Bourland TC, Rodrigues D, et al. Successful reconstruction of nongrowing hemifacial microsomia patients with unilateral temporomandibular joint total joint prosthesis and orthognathic surgery. J Oral Maxillofac Surg 2012;70(12):2835–53.

48. Wolford LM, Mercuri LG, Schneiderman ED, et al. A cohort study on the Techmedica/TMJ Concepts patient-fitted temporomandibular joint prosthesis with a median follow-up of 21 years. J Oral Maxillofac Surg 2014. [Epub ahead of print].

Condylar Hyperplasia of the Temporomandibular Joint

Types, Treatment, and Surgical Implications

Daniel B. Rodrigues, DDS[a,b],*, Vanessa Castro, DDS[c]

KEYWORDS

- Condylar hyperplasia • Osteochondroma • Condylar tumor • Condylar hyperactivity
- Condylectomies

KEY POINTS

- Not all prognathic mandibles are caused by condylar hyperplasia (CH), only those showing accelerated, excessive mandibular growth continuing beyond the normal growth years.
- Diagnosis is made through serial radiographs, dental models, clinical evaluations, and bone scan techniques.
- The earlier the operation is done, the less pronounced the mandibular deformity.
- Identifying the specific CH pathology will provide insight into its progression if untreated and will guide the treatment plan.
- The more severe the pathology, the greater clinical asymmetry and the degree of morphologic alterations.
- The type of CH, and the presence or lack of activity will define whether condylectomies are necessary.

INTRODUCTION

Condylar hyperplasia (CH) is a progressive and pathologic overgrowth of either or both mandibular condyles. These condylar pathology can adversely affect the size and morphology of the mandible, alter the occlusion, and indirectly affect the maxilla, with the resultant development or worsening of dentofacial deformities, such as mandibular prognathism; unilateral enlargement of the condyle, neck, ramus, and body; facial asymmetry; malocclusion; and pain.[1] There are many suggested etiologies of CH, including neoplasia, trauma, infection, abnormal condylar loading,[2] hormonal influence, heredity, and aberrant growth factors.[2]

Some CH occurs more commonly within particular age ranges and genders. Identifying the specific CH pathology will provide insight to its progression if untreated and will guide the treatment plan. The type of CH, and the presence or lack of activity will determine if condylectomies are necessary. The diagnosis is usually made by clinical, radiologic examinations, and bone scintigraphy.[3] Since the first description of the treatment of CH with condylectomies by Adams in 1836 and Humphry in 1856, several therapeutic options have been proposed. The treatment objective is to eliminate the pathologic processes and provide optimal functional and esthetic outcomes.[1]

[a] Residency of Oral and Maxillofacial Surgery, Federal Bahia University, Salvador, Bahia, Brazil; [b] Private Practice, Avenida ACM, n 3244, sala 917, Caminho das Árvores, Salvador, Bahia CEP 41800-700, Brazil; [c] Private Practice, Avenida ACM, n585, sala 606, Itaigara, Salvador, Bahia CEP 41825-000, Brazil
* Corresponding author. Private Practice, Avenida ACM, n 3244, sala 917, Caminho das Árvores, Salvador, Bahia CEP 41800-700.
E-mail address: dbarrosr@yahoo.com.br

Oral Maxillofacial Surg Clin N Am 27 (2015) 155–167
http://dx.doi.org/10.1016/j.coms.2014.09.011
1042-3699/15/$ – see front matter © 2015 Elsevier Inc. All rights reserved.

CLASSIFICATION

CH is a generic term describing conditions that create excessive growth and that can cause alterations in the bony architecture of the mandible, malocclusion, and dentofacial deformity. Several classifications have been proposed for CH. Obewegeser and Makek[4] classified CH into 3 categories: hemimandibular hyperplasia, causing asymmetry in the vertical plane; hemimandibular elongation, resulting in asymmetry in the transverse plane; and a combination of the 2 entities. Nitzan and colleagues[5] described CH as a unilateral disorder in which the pathology occurs at the head of the condyle, creating facial asymmetry in the vertical or horizontal direction or a combination of both. In 2014, Wolford, Movahed, and Perez[1] proposed a classification encompassing the various CH pathologies.

Condylar Hyperplasia Type 1

The onset of this condition usually occurs during puberty; it is an accelerated and prolonged growth aberration of the normal condylar growth mechanism, and it can occur bilaterally (CH type 1A) or unilaterally (CH type 1B). The growth vector is usually in a horizontal direction creating mandibular prognathism and is self-limiting, with growth termination usually in the early to mid 20s.

Condylar Hyperplasia Type 2

This condylar pathology, osteochondroma, is the most commonly occurring mandibular condylar tumor; it can develop at any age (although more commonly during the teen years), with a unilateral vertical overgrowth deformity of the jaws. The growth process can continue indefinitely, with progressive worsening of the facial asymmetry. One growth vector causes predominantly vertical elongation and enlargement of the condylar head and neck (CH type 2A) and the other form also has a horizontal exophytic tumor growth off of the condyle (CH type 2 B).

Condylar Hyperplasia Type 3

These are other types of benign tumors that can cause condylar enlargement such as osteoma, neurofibroma, giant cell tumor, fibrous dysplasia, chondroma, chondroblastoma, and arteriovenous malformation.

Condylar Hyperplasia Type 4

These are malignant tumors arising from the mandibular condyle that cause condylar enlargement such as chondrosarcoma, multiple myeloma, osteosarcoma, Ewing sarcoma, and metastatic lesion.

This article will use the Wolford's classification,[1] and since types 1 and 2 are the most common CH pathologies,[1,6] the following sections will address those 2 types of CH.

CONDYLAR HYPERPLASIA TYPE 1
Clinical Diagnosis

Common clinical characteristics observed in bilateral, symmetrically growing CH type 1A patients usually include (**Table 1**)[1]

- Accelerated mandibular growth
- Mandibular growth continuing beyond the normal growth years into the early to middle 20s
- Worsening class 3 skeletal and occlusal relationship
- Obtuse gonial angles
- Facial shape more triangular and tapered

Additionally, unilateral cases of CH type 1 B may have (**Fig. 1**)[1,5]

- Worsening facial and occlusal asymmetry, with the mandible progressively shifting toward the contralateral side
- Unilateral posterior cross-bite on the contralateral side
- Transverse bowing of the mandibular body on the affected side
- Transverse flattening of the mandibular body on the contralateral side
- Worsening unilateral class 3 occlusion on the ipsilateral side

A horizontal mandibular growth vector extending beyond the normal growth years will likely be CH type 1, and the growth can continue into the middle 20s until cessation. Conditions that initiate excessive accelerated mandibular growth after the pubertal growth phase (15 years of age for girls, 17–18 years of age for boys) are most often unilateral and related to CH type 2 (osteochondroma) or other types of proliferative condylar pathology.[1]

Imaging Diagnosis

Radiographic analysis will show increased length of the condylar head and neck, without a significant volumetric increase in the size of the condylar head. MRI scans will show that the articular discs are commonly thin and may be difficult to identify. Occasionally, the articular discs can be posteriorly displaced (**Fig. 2**).[1]

Table 1
Condylar hyperplasia features (types 1 and 2)

CH	Age at Onset	Clinical Findings	Imaging	Histology
Type 1A	• Pubertal growth	• Bilateral accelerated symmetric growth • Self-limiting; can grow into mid-20s • Class III occlusion; • Prognathic mandible.	• Bilateral elongated condylar head, neck, body • Normal condylar head shape • MRI: thin discs; asymmetric cases may involve contralateral disc displacement	• Normally growing condyle • May show chondrocyte proliferation during initial and active phases, with normal bone after growth ceases
Type 1B	• Pubertal growth	• Unilateral accelerated asymmetric growth • Self-limiting, can grow into mid-20s • Deviated mandibular prognathism; • Ipsilateral class 3 occlusion; anterior and contralateral cross-bite	• Unilateral elongated condylar head, neck, body • Normal condylar head shape • Mandibular deviated prognathism; • MRI: thin disc; may have ipsilateral/contralateral disc displacement	• Normally growing condyle • May show chondrocyte proliferation during initial and active phases, with normal bone after growth ceases
Type 2	• Two-thirds of cases begin in second decade	• Unilateral vertical elongation of face and jaws • Not self-limiting; can grow indefinitely • Ipsilateral posterior open bite	• Unilateral vertical enlarged condylar head, neck, ramus, body • Type 2A: enlargement without horizontal exophytic growth off condyle • Type 2B: enlargement with exophytic growth off condyle • MRI: ipsilateral disc commonly in place contralateral TMJ arthritis, displaced disc, 75% of cases	• Bony mass • Cap of fibrocartilage, hyaline cartilage, fibrous tissue of perichondrium, endochondral ossification

Adapted from Wolford LM, Movahed R, Perez, DE. A classification system for conditions causing condylar hyperplasia. J Oral Maxillofac Surg 2014;72:568; with permission.

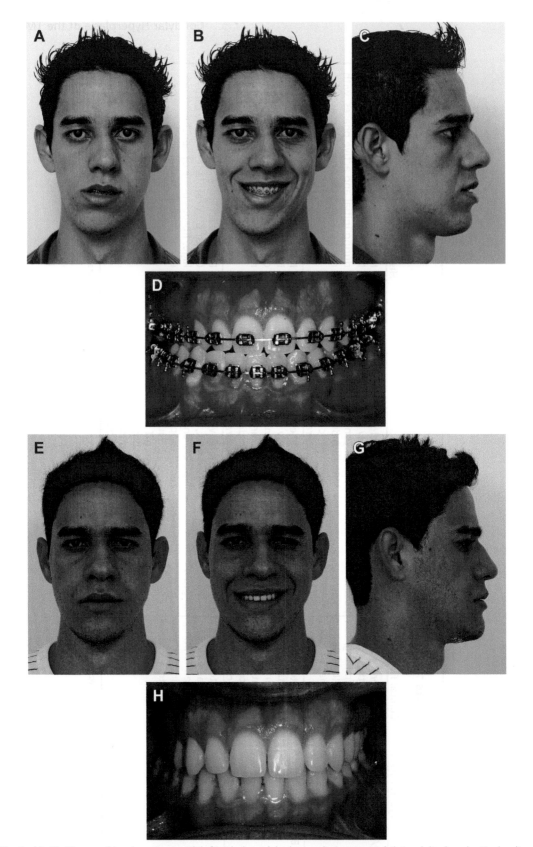

Fig. 1. (*A–D*), 19-year-old male patient with left-sided condylar hyperplasia type 1B, bilateral displaced articular discs, and mild temporomandibular joint pain. He was treated in a single surgical stage with (1) unilateral left high condylectomy; (2) bilateral disc repositioning; (3) bilateral ramus osteotomies; and (4) maxillary osteotomies. (*E–H*) At 3 years after surgery, the patient has good facial balance, stable skeletal and occlusal relations, and is pain free.

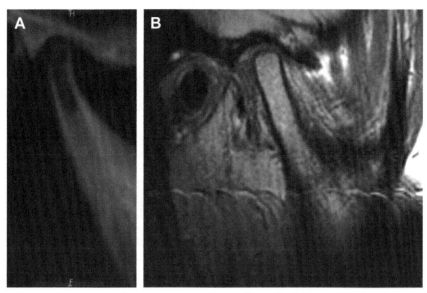

Fig. 2. (*A*) At CT scan, the CH type 1 shows an increased vertical length of the condylar head and neck. (*B*) At the MRI, the CH type 1 shows a thin disc that is difficult to identify, and can be posteriorly displaced.

Histologic Diagnosis

The histology of the affected condyle commonly resembles a normally growing condyle without any notable pathologic abnormalities. In some cases, the proliferative layer may exhibit greater thickness in some areas. The activity of the proliferative layer may regulate the rate at which the condyle and condylar neck (which is formed from the condyle by remodeling) will grow.[1,7,8]

Therapeutic Options

Not all prognathic mandibles are caused by CH, only those exhibiting accelerated, excessive mandibular growth that continues beyond the normal growth years. CH type 1 is self-limiting relative to growth; patients in their mid-20s or older will not have further jaw growth related to CH type 1, so routine orthognathic surgical procedures can usually be performed to correct the dentofacial deformity and malocclusion.[1] The treatment options for CH type 1B are similar to those for CH type 1A, in which patients with confirmed nongrowth can be treated with traditional orthognathic surgery. If active growth is confirmed, then there are 2 options for treatment (**Fig. 3**).[9]

Option 1

The surgical protocol for active CH type 1 consists of (**Fig. 4**)

- Bilateral or unilateral (depending if type 1A or 1B) high condylectomy (4–5 mm of the top of the condylar head), including the medial and lateral pole areas

- Disc repositioning, using a bone anchor
- Orthognathic surgical procedures, often requiring double jaw surgery to optimize the functional and esthetic outcomes
- Other ancillary procedures as indicated

This protocol predictably stops mandibular growth and provides highly predictable and stable outcomes, with normal jaw function and good esthetics.[7–9]

Option 2

Surgery is delayed until growth is complete, which could be in the early to mid-20s, and then only orthognathic surgery is performed. However, the longer the abnormal growth is allowed to precede, the worse the facial deformity, asymmetry, occlusion, and dental compensations will become, in addition to warping of the mandible and ipsilateral excessive soft tissue development. This will increase the difficulties in obtaining optimal functional and esthetic results, in addition to the adverse effects on occlusion, dental compensations, mastication, speech, and psychosocial development.[1,9,10]

Surgical correction of bilateral CH can predictably be performed from the ages of 14 in girls and 16 in boys. The vector of facial growth will change to a vertical direction, because the antero-posterior mandibular growth is stopped, but the maxillary vertical alveolar growth will continue until maturation. In unilateral cases (CH type 1B), it is recommend to delay surgery until the age of 15 for girls and 17 for boys, when most of the normal facial growth is complete. A

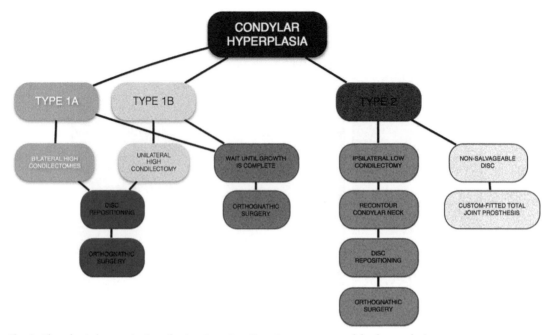

Fig. 3. Flowchart demonstrating the treatment options to manage condylar hyperplasia.

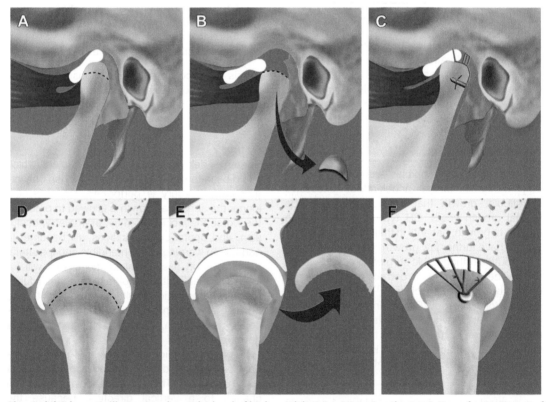

Fig. 4. (*A*) Schematic illustration shows the level of high condylectomy removing the top 4–5 mm for treatment of condylar hyperplasia type 1. (*B, C*) For CH type 1 in active growth, a high condylectomy will arrest any further anteroposterior mandibular growth. The articular disc is repositioned and stabilized on the condyle with a bone anchor. (*D, E*) Coronal view, the osteotomy must include the medial and lateral pole areas. (*F*) The anchor is placed into the posterior head 4 to 5 mm below the crown of the condyle just lateral to the midsagittal plane. The sutures are attached to the posterior aspect of the posterior band with 3 over-and-over sutures for each set of artificial ligaments (0-Ethibond) suture (Ehicon, Inc, Somerville, NJ); 1 set placed medial and 1 placed more lateral.

unilateral high condylectomy will arrest growth on the operated side, but normal growth can continue on the contralateral side and could cause development of facial and occlusal asymmetry later if the surgery is performed at a younger age.[8]

CONDYLAR HYPERPLASIA TYPE 2
Clinical Diagnosis

CH type 2 can develop at any age, but for most cases, in the second decade (68% of cases), it occurs predominantly in female patients (76% of cases). Specific characteristics of type 2 CH include (**Fig. 5**)[1,6,9]

- Increased unilateral mandibular vertical height
- Increased soft tissue volume on the ipsilateral side of the face
- Low mandibular plane angle facial-type morphology
- Chin asymmetry vertically and transversely, with shifting toward the contralateral side
- Compensatory downward growth of the ipsilateral maxillary dentoalveolus
- Lateral open bite on the ipsilateral side, particularly in more rapidly growing pathology
- Labial tipping of the mandibular ipsilateral posterior teeth and lingual tipping of the contralateral posterior teeth may occur
- Transverse cant in the occlusal plane

Imaging Diagnosis

Imaging features will include the following (**Fig. 6**)[9]

- Mandibular asymmetry particularly in a vertical plane
- Enlarged, elongated, deformed condyle
- Increased vertical height of the ipsilateral mandibular condyle, neck, ramus, body, symphysis, and dentoalveolus
- Increased thickness of the condylar neck compared with the contralateral side
- Loss of antegonial notching with downward bowing of the inferior border on the mandible
- MRI may show a displaced articular disc on the contralateral side (76% of the cases) and associated arthritic condylar changes; the disc is commonly in position on the ipsilateral side, although it also can be displaced (see **Fig. 6**E)

CH type 2A indicates an enlargement of the condylar head and neck with a predominant vertical growth vector of the osteochondroma without significant exophytic tumor development (see **Fig. 6**A, B). There can be unevenness or lumpiness on the condyle. CH type 2B indicates exophytic tumor extensions off the condyle, usually forward and medially, with the head becoming significantly enlarged and deformed (see **Fig. 6**C, D).[1]

Histologic Diagnosis

Histologically, osteochondroma has been described as a cartilage-capped lesion that undergoes endochondral ossification deep in the tumor. The cartilage is often hyaline, and of varying thickness and cellularity. Chondrocytes can form rows perpendicular to the surface and overlie a zone of endochondral ossification, producing cancellous bone that blends without distinction into that of the normal underlying bone.[11] The cartilaginous islands in the subcortical bone may have direct correlation with the scintigraphic activity. The cartilage islands are mini-growth centers producing bone, causing enlargement of the condyle. As the osteochondroma enlarges, the bone-producing islands of cartilage may become further separated from each other so that in the more mature tumors, the cartilaginous islands become more difficult to identify histologically.[1]

Therapeutic Options

Treatment considerations would include (see **Fig. 3** and **Fig. 7**)[12]

1. Low condylectomy to remove the tumor in its entirety
2. Reshape the condylar neck
3. Reposition the articular disc over the remaining condylar neck
4. An ipsilateral sagittal split osteotomy is then performed, and the disc/condylar stump complex is seated into the fossa
5. If indicated, perform orthognathic surgery to correct the maxillary and mandibular asymmetries
6. If needed, inferior border ostectomy on the involved side to reestablish vertical balance of the mandible; this may require dissection in preservation of the inferior alveolar nerve

The risk of recurrence of this benign lesion is low after surgical removal.[13]

This protocol will provide predictable and stable outcomes and optimize the functional and esthetic results. If the disc is not salvageable, a custom-fitted total joint prosthesis may be indicated to reconstruct the ipsilateral or contralateral TMJ.[9,12]

When CH type 2 is identified during the normal growth years, then surgery to resect the osteochondroma and correct the jaw's deformity (orthognathic surgery) should be deferred, if possible, until 15 years of age for girls and 17 to 18 years of age for boys, after normal jaw growth

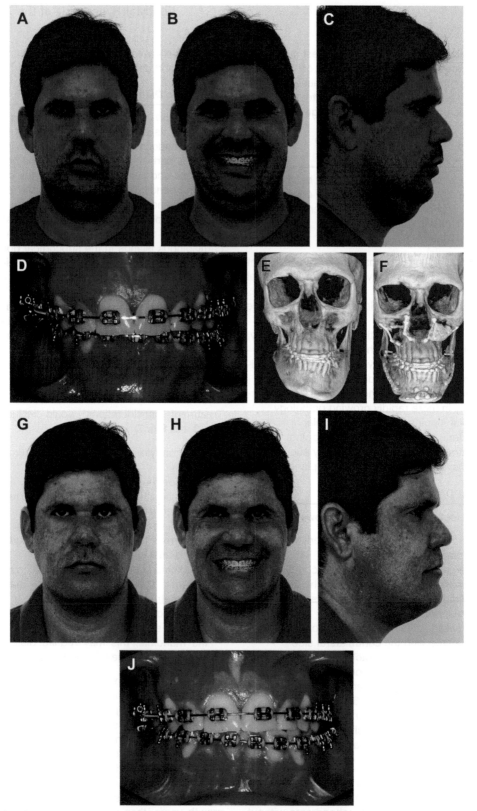

Fig. 5. (*A–D*) 34-year-old male patient presented with condylar hyperplasia type 2. He developed significant elongation of the left side of the face, retruded mandible, transverse cant in the occlusal plane. (*E, F*) 3-dimensional reconstruction before and after surgical treatment in a single stage included (1) left low condylectomy; (2) temporomandibular joint disc repositioning; (3) bilateral mandibular ramus osteotomies; (4) Le Fort I maxillary osteotomy; and (5) left inferior border ostectomy with preservation of the inferior alveolar nerve. (*G–J*) The patient 1.5 years after surgery shows good facial balance and a stable skeletal and occlusal result.

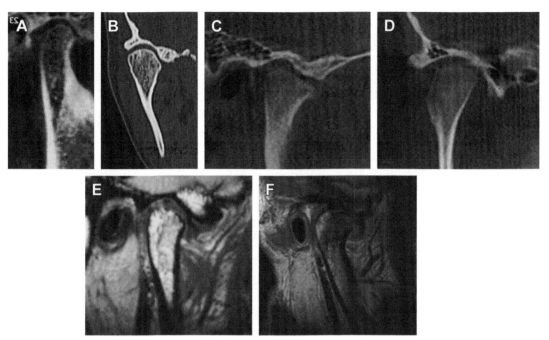

Fig. 6. At CT scan, (*A*) CH type 2A shows a larger condyle with increased vertical height of the condylar head and neck. (*B*) In the coronal view, the crown of the condyle may be more rounded than a normal condyle, (*C, D*) condylar hyperplasia type 2B have exophytic growths extending from the condylar head. At MRI, (*E*) the CH type 2A, and (*F*) CH type 2B, even with large exophytic growth development, the articular disc will commonly be in place.

is relatively complete. However, the severity of the deformity may warrant surgery at a younger age, and then an option would be to perform the unilateral condylectomy and plan for orthognathic surgery as a second stage after cessation of growth (**Fig. 8**). If the ipsilateral low condylectomy is performed in conjunction with orthognathic surgery when normal jaw growth is still occurring (<15 years of age in girls and <17–18 years of age in boys), then there is the risk of the contralateral condyle continuing with normal growth, shifting the mandible toward the ipsilateral side until growth cessation.[1,12]

COMPLEMENTARY TOOLS FOR DIAGNOSIS

Information regarding whether the abnormal growth is still active can be also provided by skeletal scintigraphy using technetium-99m methylene diphosphate.[13] Two frequently used scanning techniques are planar bone scanning and single-photon emission computed tomography (SPECT), both of which use the same basic technology. SPECT produces a tomographic bone scan image that may be more reliable than planar scanning.[14] Another scanning technique that can be used is positron emission tomography (PET) using a radiolabeled glucose

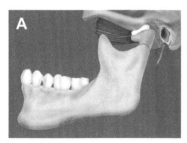
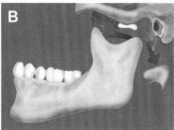
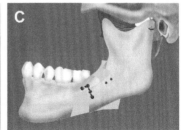

Fig. 7. (*A*) Schematic for the treatment of CH type 2 includes a low condylectomy, preserving the condylar neck as outlined to remove the osteochondroma. Commonly, but not always, osteochondromas have exophytic growths extending from the condylar head. (*B*) The condyle is removed; the condylar neck is recontoured. (*C*) The articular disc is repositioned with a bone anchor; sagittal split osteotomies are completed. Most of these cases also had an indication for maxillary osteotomies.

164

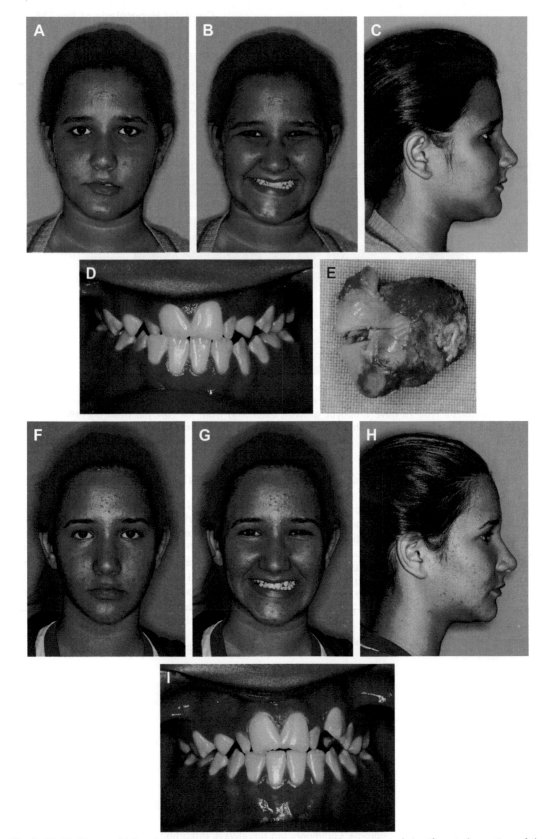

Fig. 8. (*A–D*) 11-year-old female patient presented with CH type 2. She developed significant elongation of the left side of the face, transverse cant in the occlusal plane. (*E*) Surgical treatment included left low condylectomy. The thickness of the cartilage on the condylar head can be seen. (*F–I*) The patient 1.5 years after surgery shows improvement on facial symmetry.

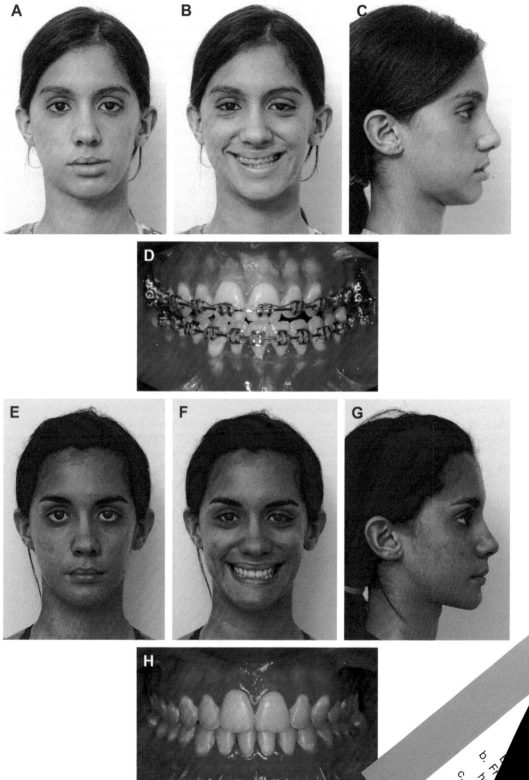

Fig. 9. (*A–D*) 18-year-old female patient with facial severe asymmetry. She was treat... osteotomies; (2) maxillary osteotomies; and (3) genioplasty. No TMJ surgery (condyle... since no evidence of growth/activity was found. (*E–H*) at 4 years after surgery, the patient... and stable skeletal and occlusal relations.

analog, 18F-2-fluoro-2-de- oxyglucose (FDG), as a tracer, alone or combined with CT (PET/CT). Dedicated (full ring) PET provides better spatial resolution than a conventional gamma camera and SPECT.[15] All methods might indicate increased cellular activity on the affected side.[13]

For asymmetric cases, the data indicate that an activity difference of more than 10% between the left and right condylar regions, found with bone scintigraphy, is suggestive of CH.[14]

Bone scintigraphy of the TMJs may detect active growth in the more rapidly growing CH type 1 conditions. However, in most cases, it will not be diagnostic in determining active CH type 1 growth. Healthy growing TMJs normally have some uptake at scintigraphy. The growth rate of CH type 1 is not growing at a tumorous rate, as seen in CH type 2, but only somewhat faster than the normal condylar growth rate; thus, it is usually difficult to differentiate CH type 1 from normal growth, particularly if both joints are involved.[1] In addition, the cellular growth activity is confined to a narrow band at the normal growth center resulting in low uptake, as compared to CH type 2 where there is diffuse cellular activity throughout the tumor in the condylar head. In unilateral cases, it can be more effective, especially if applied after the normal growing years, when condylar growth should have finished.[6] In CH type 2, unless the tumor is very slow growing, bone scintigraphy will usually show increased uptake, particularly in the more active tumors.

IDENTIFYING CONDYLAR HYPERPLASIA ACTIVITY

Active CH growth can usually be determined by worsening functional and esthetic changes with serial assessments (preferably at 6- to 12-month intervals) consisting of clinical evaluation (surgeon's, orthodontist's, patient's report), photograph records, dental model analysis with orthodontically trimmed models or models mounted in centric relation, and radiographic evaluation by superimposition. Radiographic evaluation includes

a. Lateral cephalometric radiographs; during pubertal growth, the normal yearly growth rate of the mandible measuring from condylion to point B is 1.6 mm for girls and 2.2 mm for boys[16]

   [fr]ontal cephalometric radiographs (particularly [use]ful in unilateral CH cases)

   [ ]al cephalometric tomograms that include [T]MJ, the mandibular ramus, the body, [po]sterior teeth to analyze the amount of [ ]growth over time for each side[1]

Bone scintigraphy or PET/CT scan are used to evaluate the metabolic activity of the bone. When all the information, photographs, study models, radiographs, and bone scans are correlated over time, some indication of the activity can be made.[17]

In evaluating the patient with suspected CH type 1, if no evidence of growth/activity is found, orthognathic surgery can be performed without condylectomy(ies) (**Fig. 9**). However, when evaluating CH type 2, if the records point to no evidence of growth/activity, a careful decision must be made whether to perform the condylectomy, since it is still a tumor. The data have not supported corrective orthognathic surgery of the maxillary and/or mandibular arches without accessing the tumor to confirm the histopathologic diagnosis.[13]

REFERENCES

1. Wolford LM, Movahed R, Perez DE. A classification system for conditions causing condylar hyperplasia. J Oral Maxillofac Surg 2014;72:567–95.
2. Hayward JD, Walker RV, Poulton G, et al. Asymmetric mandibular excess. In: Bell W, Proffit W, White R, editors. Surgical correction of dentofacial deformities. Philadelphia: WB Saunders; 1980. p. 947–53.
3. Kaban LB. Mandibular asymmetry and the fourth dimension. J Craniofac Surg 2009;20(Suppl 1):622–31.
4. Obwegeser HL, Makek MS. Hemimandibular hyperplasia—hemimandibular elongation. J Maxillofac Surg 1986;14(4):183–208.
5. Nitzan DW, Katsnelson A, Bermanis I, et al. The clinical characteristics of condylar hyperplasia: experience with 61 patients. J Oral Maxillofac Surg 2008;66:312–8.
6. Wolford LM, Movahed R, Dhameja A, et al. Surgical treatment of condylar hyperplasia type 2: retrospective study of 37 cases of osteochondroma. Abstract Presented at: Temporomandibular Joint Disorder, Bioengineering Conference. Pittsburgh, PA, September 20, 2012.
7. Wolford LM, Morales-Ryan CA, García-Morales P, et al. Surgical management of mandibular condylar hyperplasia type 1. Proc (Bayl Univ Med Cent) 2009;22(4):321–9.
8. Wolford LM, Mehra P, Reiche-Fischel O, et al. Efficacy of high condylectomy for management of condylar hyperplasia. Am J Orthod Dentofacial Orthop 2002;121:136–51.
9. Wolford LM. Mandibular asymmetry: temporomandibular joint degeneration. In: Bagheri SC, Bell RB, Khan HA, editors. Current therapy in oral and maxillofacial surgery. St. Louis (MO): 2012. p. 696–725. Chapter 82.
10. Wolford LM, Cassano DS, Goncalves JR. Common TMJ disorders: orthodontic and surgical

management. In: McNamara JA, Kapila SD, editors. Temporomandibular disorders and orofacial pain: separating controversy from consensus. Monograph 46, Craniofacial Growth Series, Department of Orthodontics and Pediatric Dentistry and Center for Human Growth and Development. Ann Arbor (MI): The University of Michigan; 2009. p. 159–98.

11. Vezeau PJ, Fridrich KL, Vincent SD. Osteochondroma of the mandibular condyle: literature review and report of two atypical cases. J Oral Maxillofac Surg 1995;53(8):954–63.

12. Wolford LM, Movahed R, Dhameja A, et al. Low condylectomy and orthognathic surgery to treat mandibular condylar osteochondroma: retrospective review of 37 cases. J Oral Maxillofac Surg 2014;72(9):1704–28.

13. Venturin JS, Shintaku WH, Shigeta Y, et al. Temporomandibular joint condylar abnormality: evaluation, treatment planning, and surgical approach. J Oral Maxillofac Surg 2010;68(5): 1189–96.

14. Saridin CP, Raijmakers PG, Tuinzing DB, et al. Bone scintigraphy as a diagnostic method in unilateral hyperactivity of the mandibular condyles: a review and meta- analysis of the literature. Int J Oral Maxillofac Surg 2011;40:11–7.

15. Laverick S, Bounds G, Wong WL. [18F]-fluoride positron emission tomography for imaging condylar hyperplasia. Br J Oral Maxillofac Surg 2009;47:196–9.

16. Riolo ML, Moyers RE, McNamara JA, et al. Growth: cephalometric standards from the University School Growth Study. Ann Arbor, MI: University of Michigan; 1974. p. 101.

17. Jones RH, Tier GA. Correction of facial asymmetry as a result of unilateral condylar hyperplasia. J Oral Maxillofac Surg 2012;70(6):1413–25.

Index

Note: Page numbers of article titles are in **boldface** type.

Oral Maxillofacial Surg Clin N Am 27 (2015) 169–173
http://dx.doi.org/10.1016/S1042-3699(14)00144-7
1042-3699/15/$ – see front matter © 2015 Elsevier Inc. All rights reserved.

Printed and bound by CPI Group (UK) Ltd, Croydon, CR0 4YY

03/10/2024

01040377-0015